HUMAN ANATOMY AND PHYSIOLOGY

TESTOSTERONE

BIOCHEMISTRY, THERAPEUTIC USES AND PHYSIOLOGICAL EFFECTS

Human Anatomy and Physiology

Additional books in this series can be found on Nova's website under the Series tab.

Additional E-books in this series can be found on Nova's website under the E-book tab.

HUMAN ANATOMY AND PHYSIOLOGY

TESTOSTERONE

BIOCHEMISTRY, THERAPEUTIC USES AND PHYSIOLOGICAL EFFECTS

KONSTANTIN CHICHINADZE
EDITOR

Nova Biomedical Books
New York

Library of Congress Cataloging-in-Publication Data

ISBN 978-1-62100-492-9

Library of Contress Control Number: 2011035504

Published by Nova Science Publishers, Inc. † New York

Contents

Preface

This book provides information on testosterone and its role in human anatomy, physiology, psychology and pathology. In particular, it proposes articles on testosterone biosynthesis and metabolism peculiarities; on the regulation of dominant behavior; on cognitive and emotional factors and the cardiovascular system involving testosterone and on androgen suppression mechanisms during stress. The book includes topics on the therapeutic effects of testosterone and effective methods of detecting androgens in the human body and presents a variety of clinical, experimental, theoretical and review articles. This collection gathers the latest research from around the world in this field and will be of value for researchers studying the effects of hormones, as well as for androgen deficiency therapists

Chapter I - Social power is one of the psychosocial aspects of human life that has been associated to dominance behavior and, in some circumstances, to testosterone concentration. Dominant individuals commonly describe themselves as more assertive, and self-confident. In addition, dominant personality is recognized by an observer because of the facial symmetry and emotion expressions commonly associated to it. For instance, symmetry is considered the result of a good ontogenetic development, so faces are an important source for inferences about an individual health, and the potential for being an adequate partner. On the other hand, some of the cues related to high social status are testosterone levels, which rely on the ability to grow different body structures like bones, skeletal muscle or other androgen-sensitive traits. These roles of testosterone enhance mate attraction and competitive ability with conspecifics for the access to potential mates. Overall, these revision will discuss some research mainly with humans suggesting that individuals higher in baseline testosterone are 1) more driven to gain and maintain status; 2) more responsive to information about their status in a situation. 3) To develop a more masculine and symmetrical facial traits. This could account for an accurate Resource Holding Power evaluation of an opponent in a competition.

Chapter II- Studies in monkey models of menopause have greatly advanced scientists' understanding of the effects of estrogens on women's cognitive health. Yet, parallel studies in male monkeys have been critically lacking and it remains unclear whether testosterone (T) replacement is a desirable intervention against age-related cognitive decline in men. In this chapter, the authors argue that male rhesus monkeys are excellent models to investigate this issue and describe the first studies using this species to test the effects of T on cognitive and emotional function. They present a series of studies from their laboratory, in which intact male macaques temporarily castrated with a gonadotropin-releasing hormone agonist were administered cognitive and emotional tests when treated with T vs. placebo. The cognitive tasks included tests of visual recognition memory, spatial memory and working memory. The emotional tasks consisted of an approach-avoidance task of objects, a video playback task of social stimuli, and a computerized test of attention to emotional stimuli. The results indicate that T manipulations in pharmacologically-castrated young male monkeys have only modest effects on cognitive function but significantly affect selective aspects of emotion. The authors' current studies in aged male monkeys should determine whether T benefits cognitive function and emotional reactivity later in life. The authors conclude that research in male nonhuman primates is essential to test the efficacy of T therapy as an intervention for maintaining cognitive and emotional health throughout the lifespan in men.

Chapter III- Testosterone has been described in scientific literature as one of the principal inducers of aggressive behavior. At the same time, aggressive behavior is mainly viewed in association with negative emotions, such as anger, rage, and fury. On the other hand, substantial amount of information has been collected on inhibition of androgen synthesis under the influence of negative emotions and stressful events. Taking into consideration the fact that aggressive encounter is stressful for both losers and winners, above-mentioned statements clearly contradict each other to a certain extent.

Chapter IV- Tissues in both sexes can be regulated by a balance of androgenic and estrogenic effects. The predominant secretion of androgens from the testes and estrogens from the ovaries sets the stage, and the dominant position of the liver in metabolism has a significant part to play. In addition, an important component in the response of the target tissues is the presence and concentration of specific hormone receptors. Less well recognized and studied is the role of local metabolism: enzymes in target tissues themselves constitute a final step in the delivery of the appropriate, or inappropriate, steroid product to the target cell. The complement of enzymes can lead to steroid inactivation, a weaker agent or even an enhanced activity. Examples of these are testosterone sulfate, androstenedione and 5α-dihydrotestosterone, respectively. However, another potential fate for an androgen in some target tissues is the formation of C_{18} products from the C_{19} androgens by action of an aromatase enzyme—just as occurs for estrogen biosynthesis in the ovaries, and in the testes to some extent. In the latter case, some species are remarkable for the large amounts of estrogens secreted from the testes. The importance of estrogens in the male is well documented, for the most part; the actions include those on bone, muscle and skin along with those more directly associated with reproduction (e.g. efferent ductules of the testes and libido itself). Lastly, aromatase activity in target tissues—and in the testes of some species—can result in the formation of C19-norandrogens that are recognized as endogenous anabolic agents. With the tremendous interest in 19-nortestosterone and efforts to replicate its properties with acceptable commercial products, the formation of 19-nortestosterone and its local metabolism is frequently underappreciated. This review will attempt to redress some aspects of testosterone metabolism that seem to deserve more consideration than usually given.

Chapter V- In mammals, chronic exposure to stressors of different nature, strength or quality has long been recognized as a profound disruptive factor in reproductive function. In males, stress suppresses testosterone secretion, spermatogenesis and sexual arousal. Severe suppression of reproduction appears to be caused by several hormones that are secreted when the hypothalamic-pituitary-adrenal (HPA) axis is activated during stress. Since Hans Selye suggested in 1946 that chronic stress increases activity in the HPA axis and at the same time suppresses activity in the hypothalamic-pituitary-gonadal (HGA) axis, there has been much work demonstrating this opposite relationship. Corticotropin releasing hormone (CRH), corticotrophin (ACTH), β-endorphins, and glucocorticoids can inhibit HGA axis function. The centrally mediated inhibition of Gonadotropin Releasing Hormone (GnRH) by the hormones of the HPA and the recently discovered Gonadotropin inhibitory hormone (GnIH), the decrease in pituitary responsiveness to GnRH, and the direct effects of stress-hormones on testis leading to the reduction in testosterone secretion are discussed. This chapter focuses on the suppression of testicular testosterone caused by stress, as well as its reproductive consequences in fertility and sexual behavior in males.

Chapter VI- Stead-state sex steroid concentrations in the circulations show significant inter-individual variations within and across populations. Such variations are also associated with predisposition to various diseases. Genetic polymorphisms in genes encoding enzymes in the biosynthesis and metabolism pathways of sex hormones are likely to account for such inter-individual variations. In this study of over 1400 Chinese men, single nucleotide polyporphisms (SNPs) of candidate genes involved in sex steroid metabolic pathway were investigated for their association with blood androgens concentrations. The authors found that blood androgen concentrations correlated with SNPs in *SRD5A1* and *AKR1C4* genes. The genotype of rs11738248 in *SRD5A1* was significantly associated with circulating dihydrotestosterone(DHT) to testosterone (T) ratio while the C-T-T haplotype on *SRD5A1* could be a predictor for low DHT level. As for AKR1C4, it was found that the genotype rs17134607 was associated with androsterone level in a linear regression model. In addition, it was also observed that the G-A haplotype could be a risk haplotype for high androsterone level. This chapter is the first to reveal the potential association between circulating androgen levels and the genetic variations in *SRD5A1* and *AKR1C4* in a large cohort of healthy general population. Future studies may examine their underlying functional genetic elements that affected the sex steroid level in blood and their potential association with diseases

Chapter VII- Testosterone, a potent androgen, is mainly synthesized in the testicular Leydig cells. It is well known that biosynthesis and the secretion of testosterone are stimulated by gonadotropin, especially the luteinizing hormone (LH) released from the anterior pituitary gland resulting from the activation of the hypothalamus-pituitary-testis (H-P-T) axis. A significant negative feedback regulation between testosterone and LH had been well established. In addition to gonadotropin, some factors may regulate testosterone production by acting, either directly or indirectly, on the Leydig cells. For example, thyroxine (T_4) and prolactin enhance testosterone production by acting directly at the testicular interstitial cells (TIC) or Leydig cells. However, some cardiac glycosides, e.g. digoxin and digitoxin, as well as the cardiotonic steroid isolated from Chausu, such as bufalin, may inhibit testosterone production *via* attenuation of the activities of adenylyl cyclase and cytochrome P450scc, and cause a decrease of testicular accumulation of adenosine 3', 5'-cyclic monophosphate (cAMP). Not only the cardiotonic steroids, some other Chinese herbs, such as evodiamine, *S*-petasin and the extracts of adlay hull can also decrease testosterone production *via* the inhibition of cAMP production, 17β-hydroxysteroid dehydrogenase (17β-HSD) enzyme activity in Leydig cells and gonadotropin-releasing hormone (GnRH)-induced LH secretion. Meanwhile, testosterone production can be altered by some abusive drug (e.g. amphetamine) and environmental pollutants (e.g. nonylphenol, polybrominated diphenol ethers). The authors have previously demonstrated that testosterone production can be increased by a gonadotropin-independent mechanism through a direct action of lactate on

Leydig cells. They have also found out that hypoxia increases cell proliferation and testosterone production in Leydig cells *via* an increase of the production of vascular endothelial growth factor (VEGF). These results indicate that many factors, including Chinese herb medicine, toxicants, environmental pollutants and lactate, as well as VEGF, may alter the biosynthesis of testosterone *via* a gonadotropin-independent mechanism, such as the changes of the activities of cAMP pathway, intracellular calcium and steroidogenic enzymes. The changes of testosterone production, either synthesis or secretion, might be associated with the alterations of metabolisms and carcinogenesis in the reproduction organs, e.g. prostate gland.

Chapter VIII- High performance liquid chromatography-tandem mass spectrometry (HPLC-MS/MS) is a powerful method for microanalysis of compounds in biological matrices. In this review, the authors introduce the recent development of HPLC-MS/MS analysis for the quantification of testosterone (T) and dihydrotestosterone (DHT). By adding an effective proton-affinitive tag to T and DHT, T and DHT were determined simultaneously with limits of quantification LOQs) of 1 pg/0.2 ml serum, and T and DHT with LOQs of 0.5 pg and 1 pg/3 mg prostate tissue, respectively. In addition, sufficient specificity of this method was achieved by selected reaction monitoring (SRM).

Chapter IX- Testosterone has classically been considered to exert an unfavourable effect upon the cardiovascular system. However, numerous recent clinical and epidemiological studies have reported a controversial relationship between testosterone and lipid profiles, inflammatory responses, hypertension, and altered vascular smooth muscle reactivity with regard to cardiovascular disease. Previous animal studies have demonstrated that testosterone exhibits a vasodilatory action in vasculature of experimental animals and more recently in isolated human pulmonary artery. Accordingly, the authors have recently shown that testosterone relaxes isolated human spermatic vein and corpus cavernosum as well as isolated human mesenteric, internal mammary and radial arteries. Because these effects occur in seconds to minutes, they and others have suggested that this action is likely to be mediated via the interactions with receptors on the membrane (nongenomic effect) rather than by interaction with the nucleus (genomic effect). Furthermore, several studies have shown the presence of the androgen receptor on the membrane of vascular smooth muscle cells, suggesting that the proposed mechanism is likely. While this effect frequently has been observed in large arteries at micromolar concentrations, more recent studies have reported vasorelaxation of smaller resistance arteries at nanomolar (physiological) concentrations. The data from in vitro studies suggest that vasodilatory effect of testosterone is mediated via inhibition of Ca^{2+} influx into the smooth muscle cell. On the basis of the data reported to date, the exact mechanisms underlying this physiological effect of testosterone remain unclear and might involve activation of K^{+} channels and antagonism of Ca^{2+} channels, are likely to be of nongenomic signaling, and might not require the endothelium. Taken as a whole, a considerable body of evidence suggests that testosterone causes relaxation of the vasculature and it could have useful therapeutic roles in hypertension, angina, erectile dysfunction, prostatic ischemia, or other vascular dysfunctions.

In: Testosterone
Editor: Konstantin Chichinadze
ISBN 978-1-62100-492-9

Chapter I

Testosterone: Physiological Effects, Dominance and Fluctuating Asymmetry

Ana Lilia Cerda Molina, Javier Iván Borráz León
Ethology Departament, Instituto Nacional de Psiquiatría Ramón de la Fuente Muñiz, Mexico City, Mexico

Abstract

Social power is one of the psychosocial aspects of human life that has been associated to dominance behavior and, in some circumstances, to testosterone concentration. Dominant individuals commonly describe themselves as more assertive, and self-confident. In addition, dominant personality is recognized by an observer because of the facial symmetry and emotion expressions commonly associated to it. For instance, symmetry is considered the result of a good ontogenetic development, so faces are an important source for inferences about an individual health, and the potential for being an adequate partner. On the other hand, some of the cues related to high social status are testosterone levels, which rely on the ability to grow different body structures like bones, skeletal muscle or other androgen-sensitive traits. These roles of testosterone enhance mate attraction and competitive ability with conspecifics for the access to potential mates. Overall, these revision will discuss some research mainly with humans suggesting that individuals higher in baseline testosterone are 1) more driven to gain and maintain status; 2) more responsive to information about their status in a situation. 3) To develop a more masculine and symmetrical facial traits. This could account for an accurate Resource Holding Power evaluation of an opponent in a competition.

Introduction

The phylogenetic history of competitiveness for rank and resources has become of growing interest to evolutionary psychiatrist since the 1960s. Three hundred million years ago our ancestors competed for resources (food, territory, mates), as many vertebrates continue to do this day. Then, as group living became established and territory began to be shared, individuals ceased competing directly for territory and instead started to compete for social status. So, rather than competing in energetically expensive interactions –e.g. contest– sexual selection could favor a strategy of assessment on the basis of which opponent is likely to represent a potential rival.

In this revision we would like to use the model of Stevens and Price (2000) of behavioral system for explaining some personality disorders and mental illness, based on the Parker's Resource Holding Power (RHP). In biology, RHP refers to the motivation to persevere in a fight, but not precisely the fighting ability to win a contest. Instead it is more important how many resources are at stake. For example, if many resources are at risk, the animal that has less to gain will lose the battle. In addition, animal aggression is favored when there are fewer resources than competitors; so an individual should gain the battle of resource guarding. Selection for aggression will be more intense the more discrete the resource, so most animal aggression relates to food fighting and especially to mating. In addition to aggression, dominance behavior could be favored depending on the social organization or the kind of resource individuals are competing for (Parker 1974).

Two advantageous strategies arise from RHP behavior. One is the ability and motivation to fight by means of the exhibition of physical cues indicating high probability of winning. The other is the ability to compare the own RHP with that of the opponent. These two strategies could withdraw the weaker RHP individual from the competition without being damage, and at the same time will reduce the cost of interaction escalation. But how an individual could recognize its own RHP and even to compare it to the opponent? Could the model be applied to humans?

Animals evaluate body size and sexual secondary characteristics meaning great ability to compete. They need visual and cognitive systems to "make" evaluations. In humans, Stevens and Price (2000) suggested that the human equivalent of RHP is self-esteem, and defeat can have similar effects on both, the behavior and self-esteem of human beings as it has on the behavior and RHP of reptiles, mammals and non-human primates. Probably, body size could have been more important in our ancestors, as a direct cue of the opponent's RHP. Nowadays, body size is not as important in humans for sexual competition; but other cues are being tested, for example dominance, fluctuating asymmetry and masculinity facial appearance, all of which are indirect signals of general health, including mental health. Recent evidence, points out that some of these parameters are related to testosterone (T) concentration.

Next, we will explore the most recent information about the relationship of T with some social behaviors and physical appearance in humans that could account for an accurate RHP as an evaluation of an opponent in a competition.

Testosterone Secretion and Function

From the group of the many biologically active androgens, testosterone is the most potent, followed by dihydrotestosterone, androstenediol, androstenedione and dehydroepiandrosterone.

Testosterone is one of the steroid hormones which is synthesized in the Leydig cells of the male testis. Most literature refers to the male's hormone because of its androgenic biological actions (Stoco, 1999). Nonetheless it is important to point out that estrogens are found in both males and females. In fact, the synthesis of estrogens in the brain of males by the aromatization of testosterone is responsible for masculinization of the male brain and plays major role in activating male sexual behavior during adulthood. The major production of testosterone, around 95%, comes from the testis of the adult man; the remainder arises from metabolic conversion of precursor steroids, predominantly secreted by the adrenal cortex (Roy, 2006). Testosterone is secreted in increased amount during three independent periods in the life of a human male. These are during intrauterine life, neonatal period, and during puberty. The initial secretory surge in intrauterine life is critical for genital sexual differentiation, whereas the neonatal surges may play an important role in gender-associated behavior and structural and functional gender differences in cognition. At the onset of puberty, the development of male secondary sexual characteristics is caused primarily by testosterone and other adrenal androgens. In the pilosebaceous unit of the skin, T and its active metabolite, dihydrotestosterone, increase sebum production and transform the thin vellous hair into darker, thicker terminal hair. In the skin, muscles, and bone, T has anabolic effects increasing protein production and the hypertrophy of the laryngeal mucosa causing deepening of the voice (Smikle 1999).

One of the most important functions of testosterone is on bone growth. The androgen participates in osteoblast/osteoclast activation and remodeling cycle for bone mineral density (Notelovitz, 2002; Vignozzi et al., 2010). Androgen nuclear receptors are found in all three bone cells: osteoblast, osteoclast and osteocytes; the greater degree of receptors is found in inactive osteoblast at the site of bone formation. The mechanism of action is the classical steroid nuclear receptor acting at genomic level to promote the synthesis of procollagen and growth factors; although a rapid non-genomic mechanism has been proposed (Peterziel et al., 1999). In addition, lots of clinical applications support the fact of the deep involvement of T on bone and muscle mass. For instance, a well-known effect of androgens is on growth of the prostate which affects both the non-cancerous and potentially cancerous cells in the organ. The best therapy to control prostate cancer is androgen deprivation; but under this condition, up to 20% of men will suffer osteoporosis and fractures within 5 years of treatment (Adler, 2011). Androgens can also affect red blood cell production and they appear to have an effect on blood fats and cholesterol.

Beyond their immediate physiological effects on reproductive and metabolic functions, gonadal steroid hormones are involved in activating cognitive functions throughout life, keeping men alert and during motivational processes related to dominance, sex drive and attachment. As serum T levels begin to decline as early as 30 years of age, T aging decline contribute to the progressive reduction in some cognitive functions, although ethnic differences has been described (Gray et al., 1991; Harman et al., 2001)

Fortunately, the new methods for measurements of salivary hormones have been useful to unravel many questions about function of steroid hormones. These techniques have allowed exploring normal individual variations in androgen concentration and to explore its influence on psychological and social parameters.

DOMINANCE

Aggression, competition and cooperation are common behaviors, taking place as a consequence of social lives in both human and animal societies. Because of the multiple interactions animals have to face during the conformation of complex social groups, constant conflicts arise. Hence individuals compete with each other for a wide range of resources that include such basics as food, space, mating opportunities and dominance.

Dominance could be seen as a mechanism to maintain order inside the social groups. In primate context, De Waal (1989) made a distinction between three kinds of dominance behaviors. Agonistic dominance is expressed by means of agonistic aggressive encounters, in order to limit the behavior of subordinates. Formal dominance, which takes place once the linear hierarchy is established, and submissive exhibitions by the subordinates are accepted by the dominants. This way agonistic encounters could be minimized or avoid. The third type, competitive ability, is more related to tolerance behavior because it happens when some individuals obtain privileges e.g. food access, without the need to engage in conflicts. This last alternative constitutes a way to resolve a conflict by deference of the loser without ending in escalation (Vervaecke et al., 2000). In any case, the main mechanism to establish rank order is competition, where the winners will be those better positioned and better able to fight and defend their rank.

Under customarily conditions in humans there is no need to spend energy in every day competition. According to Metha et al., (2008) dominance is referred to those behaviors intended to gain or maintain high status. In higher anthropoid primates dominance rank position and social success often depends predominantly on physical capacities, for example, physical strength, big fangs, aggressiveness or the ability to conform coalitions (Tatersall, 1998). Instead, in humans the acquisition of high status is mainly by using more cognitive abilities and personality: a more formal dominance.

On the other hand, dominance has been associated to testosterone concentration under some circumstances (Booth et al., 2006). It is important to make a distinction between those dominant behaviors only destined to maintain status without causing someone harms, and those aggressive behaviors. Evidence from animal studies in rodents shows that testosterone causes aggressive behavior towards conspecifics (Archer, 2006). In some non-human primates, T predicts how aggressive an individual could react to defend their valued resources. It is common that under social instability or sexual conflict, dominant males show higher rates of aggression associated to elevated circulating testosterone, whereas lower ranking males decrease androgen concentration. Wingfield et al., (1990) proposed an original integrating assumption "The challenge hypothesis" which suggests that testosterone levels and aggression in male adult animals are closely associated to the context of intense reproductive competition, particularly when males challenge one another for the access to receptive females or in the context of territory formation. So, sexual arousal and challenges would raise the androgen concentration to facilitate direct competitive behavior e.g. by increasing muscle mass and strength (Notelovitz, 2002) or by rapid actions involving neuronal excitability and sexual motivation (Remage-Healey and Bass, 2007). Although not always all aggressive behavior is associated to testosterone concentration, the most common observation is that aggressive winners corresponds to the most dominant individuals and T levels could predict this association when a challenge situation is imminent (Sapolsky, 1987; Wingfield, 1990). High ranking individuals enhance their condition displaying a variety of postural and gestural symbols of confidence. In humans, those displays –e.g. eye contact– are exhibited either during normal conversations or during face to face confrontations. Such behaviors could stress other individuals holding lower social status. Shultheiss et al., (2004) showed that there are men with high and low basal T concentration, but only men with high T levels increase even more the androgen levels after they watched a power-arousing movie compared to men with low basal T concentrations. It has been tested that females tend to prefer testosterone driven traits in males such as broad shoulders and prominent jaws. For females, all those traits are cues of fitness and self confidence proportioning security. For other males it could be a clear sign of a potential competitor during mating choice.

Although some authors have associated T to behaviors such as aggression and antisocial personality (Booth et al., 2006), others have suggested that those behaviors are predicted by the androgen, only when status is at stage. Under normal circumstances it seems no to be any relationship alone. Recently, Metha and Josephs (2010) adequate a new multiple regression analyses which evidenced that in humans facing a challenge, testosterone could predict dominance, but only in those men whose cortisol concentration is low. Recent investigation showed that if social status is not at risk, dominance is not related to testosterone concentration (Borraz-León et al., in preparation, figure 1).

The Handicap of Testosterone and Dominance

Many authors argue that dominance implicate some cost on the one hand, because those individuals easily get involved in social conflicts. On the other hand the association to T concentration represents a handicap because of the adverse immunosuppressive effects. Beyond anabolic function above described, the role of T also extends to the regulation of the immune system. This hypothesis has been probed specially in small mammals and birds, but little research has arisen in human and non-human primates.

The immune responses to any infection are complex; it implies activation of a variety of immune cells and the secretions of factors like cytokines. This system exhibit different energetic and nutritional needs which themselves can be subject to allocation mechanisms. According to Muehlenbein and Bribiescas (2005), a trade-off between two energetically expensive physiological processes occurs. During a dominance challenge episode, rises in testosterone may suppress certain kind of immune responses and instead augment anabolic processes regulating the relative amount of energy invested into either contest behavior or reproductive effort (i.e. muscle metabolism). This way, the cost of facing a stress situation is reduced. Those healthy individuals could face the handicap of high T concentration and face the immunosupression effect (Folstad and Karter, 1992).

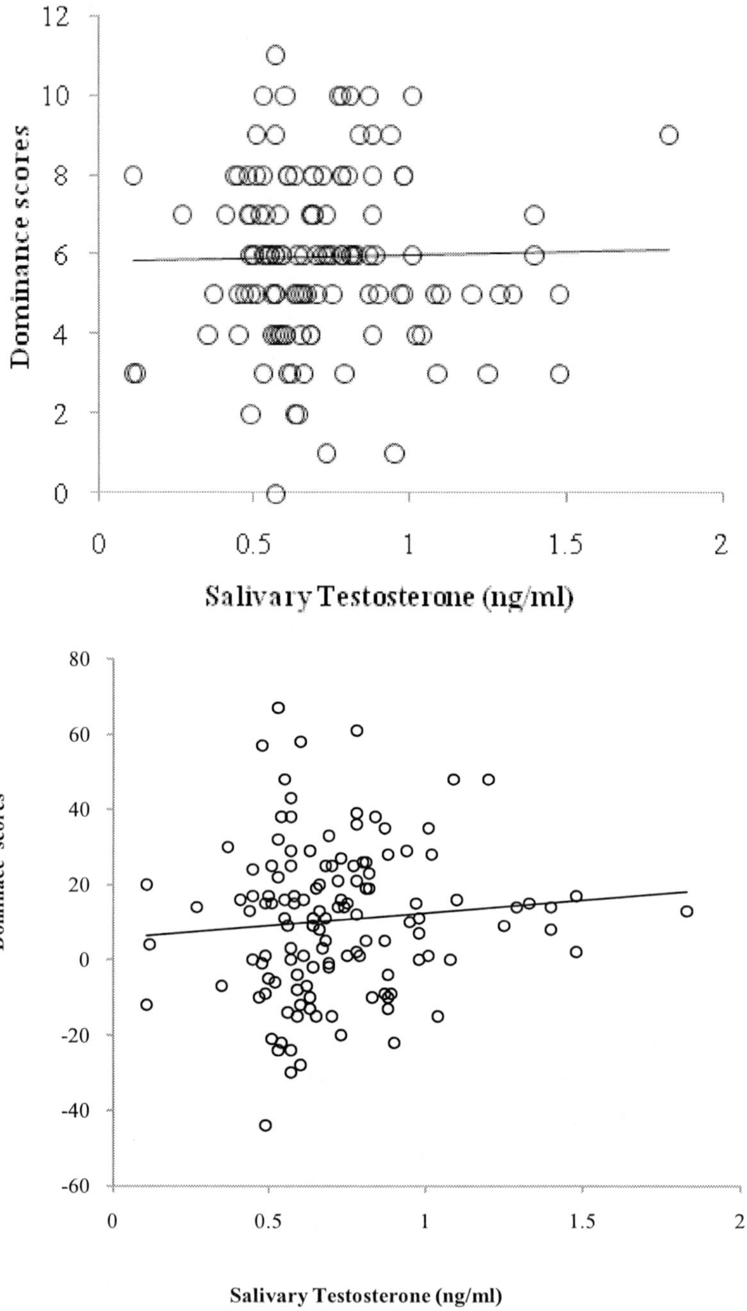

Figure 1. Dominance scores of 131 male volunteers around 21-28 years old as a function of testosterone. Left, direct verbal personality questions on 11 point scale. Right, written personality test on a -60-80 point scale) (Borraz-León et al., in preparation).

Testosterone normal metabolic actions and, individual's health in general, are mediated by other environmental factors such as stress response. Stress refers to a situation that causes a serious threaten of the homeostasis. The immediate response of the body to overcome an adverse stimulus is to secrete some hormones affecting physiological and behavioral reactions. Glucocorticoids, cortisol in most primates and corticosterone in the rest of the mammalian species, are the main adrenal gland hormones responsible for the stress reaction, along with catecholamines. Longer periods of stress, could compromise the immune system and alter the susceptibility of an illness by reducing the production of antibodies. Similar to the above mention trade-off model, stress reaction could suppress some systems as adaptive response, for example digestive, growth, and immune (Sapolsky et al., 2000). With this information we might suggest that under a challenge situation accompanied by a stress response, cortisol might contribute to the adaptive suppression of energetically systems when testosterone increases.

TESTOSTERONE AND COGNITION

Social cognition research as a branch of the evolutionary psychology has produce new interpretations on interpersonal attraction. Through the study of mental adaptations, it has been demonstrated the existence of behavioral gender differences in visuo-spatial task performance, and cognitive abilities, reflecting that males and females process spatial information in different ways (Kimura, 2002). Choi and Silverman (2002) provided evidence that supports these sexual differences in cognitive abilities, by administering spatial tasks to a group of males and females. The authors found that males make use of more landmarks and relative directions (left, right) than males, when they have to describe a particular route to get to a town. On the contrary males use more cardinal and distances directions; this last frequency was correlated to salivary testosterone concentration.

Androgens are capable of acting in the brain by shaping developing structures or by activating some areas after the hormonal rise during puberty. Newman et al., (2005) found that individuals holding a high status position and with high testosterone concentration performed better on spatial and verbal test than low status individuals, independently of the T levels. These findings agree with those of Metha and Joseph (2010) describing that high T concentration predicts dominance personality only when cortisol is low. Elevated concentration of cortisol is a sign of stress condition, so if some individuals have high T levels, then the adrenal hormone could be decreasing the role of the androgen to express a strong personality.

Although researchers agree with the hypothesis that testosterone in males improves spatial cognitive test, it has been probed that the androgen lessen the capacity for recognize some facial expressions. For instance, Van Honk and Schutter (2007) described that males administered with testosterone, experimented a reduced capacity in the conscious recognition of angry facial expressions.

This is important because, humans appear to have evolved to be more sensitive to social signals that indicate someone is angry with us or someone else. In evolutionary sense, being quick to identify when someone is angry with us will help us avoid being caught unawares and attacked. Here comes relevant the fact that testosterone during a challenge participates increasing and maintaining a cognitive vigilance behavior.

Facial expressions and the visual mechanism of perception became essential in human survival and reproductive strategies (Gallup, 2008). Facial expressions signal status which describes the power associated with the individuals's role and dominance. According to some authors, information get through a high status appearance is of someone with high power, assertive, self-assured and in general dealing with problems easily. On the contrary low dominance status expression, are related to sadness, shame, guilt and less ability to handle a stressful situation. At the same time, these same low dominant emotional states, affect the perceptions of other faces, and the sensitivity of feeling stress when dealing with a dominant personality.

In general, facial expression recognition represents and evolutionary advantage success because decoding faces allows the control of behavior of individuals and social groups. However, there is still the debate about whether testosterone has a direct role in neural mechanisms dedicated to facial recognition

Sexual differences in the perception of facial cues indicate that, for females, integrating those cues to estimate underlaying trait values such as health, intelligence, social status, symmetry, and masculinity could be more important to get reliable information about possible partners.

Fluctuating Asymmetry

The human body like most animals in nature possesses a similar pattern of bilateral symmetry, which most cultures agree with the coincidence of being aesthetic forms. Since early times the great philosophers Plato and Aristotle associated symmetry with beauty and thought that our brain and our sense of vision are really sensitive to perceive those symmetrical forms. But, it could be a matter of simplicity, because it is easier to appreciate and recognize a symmetrical –more organized– structure than an asymmetrical form.

We talk about symmetry when the position and size of objects on one side of an axis of a body are duplicated exactly on the other side of the axis (like a mirror image). In fact, the word symmetry comes from the Greek *sym* and *metria* which means "the same measure", or according to Livio (2005), a more mathematical sense: "immunity to a possible change". View this way, symmetry should be an indirect cue of stable development.

Literature largely in fishes, avian and reptiles species, suggest that bilateral symmetry indicates good health and resistance to environmental stressors; hence it could be an important cue to mate selection strategies. Actually the information reveals that high concentrations of glucocorticoids early in life in non-human animals are the consequence of environmental stressors e.g. nutritional deficits, low temperatures, pollutant exposure, etc. Those animals which were largely exposed to constant stress are adversely affected in their symmetrical development of bilateral characters. However, in humans, no empirical findings have been reported about a relationship of stress response and symmetry. Most information about the judgments of people exposed to manipulated faces indicates that symmetry correlates with beauty, attractiveness and health. But other research using natural faces show that symmetry not always predicts attractiveness ratings. In addition, judgments about attractiveness and masculinity are more pronounced in the case of females, consequently is an important aspect of mate selection.

Many studies have shown that, symmetry alone does not make people attractive, instead, symmetry plus masculinity or dominance act together to generate a preference for an attractive partner. Moller and Thornhill (1998) suggested that healthy individuals can maintain symmetric development under environmental and genetic stress, and therefore, symmetry can serve as an indicator of phenotypic and genotypic quality: the ability to resist diseases. Gangestad and Thornhill (2003) reveal that facial masculinity –using unmanipulated faces– was correlated with bilateral symmetry of the face and body, and described that men tended to have more masculine features, including wider jaws, prominent brows and longer chins. No direct evidence has arisen about a direct correlation between T and symmetry, but indirect cues relate both parameters as judgments of symmetry are linked to other traits like masculinity (large jaws and prominent brows), good health or dominance. Faces recognition has a neural substrate in the brain for the evaluation of fine deviations of symmetry, so probably T receptors might have a role in that ability.

Resource Holding Power Model and T

The overall preferences for symmetry are in line with what has been observed in all the studies: symmetry was generally preferred in both male and female faces. These preferences are coincident with judges of masculinity, large jaws and prominent brows, traits that depend on testosterone concentration. The influence of testosterone should be during the critical weeks of action: the first weeks of gestations, and few weeks of postnatal life, and under the resumption during adolescence with the pubertal surge. Most research on symmetry has evidenced that more symmetrical individuals could advertise quality in terms of immune function. In addition dominant individuals tend to have high concentrations of testosterone and are more competitive, but this capacity is possible only when cortisol is low (Metha and Joseph, 2010). According to the RHP model, dominant individuals could recognize themselves as a potent candidate for winning a competition wherever the resource. Taking into account that testosterone influence cognitive abilities, males might have evolved perceptual mechanism of facial recognition of a potential rival. Dominance not always is associated to aggressive behavior and masculine facial traits of dominants should be enough to transmit information about a possible victory. Resource holding power, as a model to evaluate its own ability or the others, could be applied in a situation of competition for social valuable resources. Recognizing others capacities would predict who's going to win a competition; as a result, one of the opponents should avoid the dispute. In humans the dispute could be in the context of mate selection strategies, or other social context implying communication, e.g. negotiation.

Conclusions

According to the bio-social model proposed by Booth and Mazur (2006) testosterone increases competitiveness and competitiveness increases T. Dominant individuals tends to have higher concentration of T and this encourage more predisposition to win a competition. On the contrary, losing a competition would depress the androgen, which would prevent further competition. Perhaps there is a pre-disposition to show dominance competitive behavior which account for the self-reinforcing effects of winning. Most studies in humans assumed that facial traits signal parameters such as symmetry, masculinity and social status.

Thus it is possible that brain has evolved visual and perceptual mechanism to recognize those traits in an opponent, in order to expend less energy in a contest. On the other hand recognizing a lower self RHP, would avoid a stressful situation, and the consequences of the stress physiological response. It would be useful to have future research on those cues to get information about the opponents T concentration and the opponents self evaluation.

REFERENCES

Adler R.A., *Maturitas*. 68, 143 (2011).

Archer J., *Neurosci. Biobehav. Rev*. 30, 319 (2006).

Booth A., Granger D. A., Mazur A., Kivlighan K. T., *Social Forces*. 85, 167 (2006).

Choi J. and Silverman I., *Brain and Cognition*. 50, 116 (2002).

de Waal F. B. M., *Comparative Socioecology*. Blackwell, Oxford, (1989).

Folstad I. and Karter A.J., *Am. Nat.* 139, 603 (1992).

Gallup G.G., *Evol. Psychol.* 6, 469 (2008).

Gangestad R. and Thornhill R., *Evolution and Human Behavior*. 24, 231 (2003).

Gray A., Feldman H.A., McKinlay J.B., Longcope C., *J. Clin. Endocrinol. Metab*. 73, 1016 (1991).

Harman S.M., Metter E.J., Tobin J.D., Pearson J., Blackman M.R., *J Clin Endocrinol Metab*. 86, 724 (2001).

Kimura D., *Neuro Endocrinol Lett.* 23, 67 (2002).

Livio M., *The Equation That Couldn't Be Solved*, Simon & Schuster, New York (2005).

Metha P. H., and Josephs R. A., *Horm. Behav*. 58, 898 (2010).

Metha P. H., Jones A.C., Josephs R. A., *J. Pers. Soc. Psychol.* 94, 1078 (2008).

Moller A. P. and Thornhill R., *Am. Nat.* 151, 174 (1998).

Muehlenbein M. and Bribiescas R., *Am J Hum Biol.* 17, 527 (2005).

Newman M., Sellers J.G., Josephs R.A., *Horm. Behav*. 47, 205 (2005).

Notelovitz M., *Fertil. Steril.* 77, S34 (2002).

Parker G.A., *J. Theor. Biol*. 47, 223 (1974).

Peterziel H., Mink S., Schonert M., Becker M., Klocker H., A.C. Cato, *Oncogene*. 18, 6322 (1999).

Remage-Healey L., Bass A.H., *J Neurosci*. 27, 1114 (2007).

Roy S.N., *Textbook of biochemistry and human biology*. Prentice-Hall, New Delhi (2006).

Sapolsky R.M., *Psychobiology and Reproductive Behavior*. Prentice-Hall, Englewood Cliffs, New Jersey (1987).

Sapolsky R.M., Romero L. M., Munck A.U., *Endocr. Rev*. 21, 55 (2000).

Schultheiss O.C., Wirth M.M., Stanton S.J., *Horm. Behav*. 46, 592 (2004).

Smikle C., *Encyclopedia of Reproduction*, 4. San Diego, California, Academic Press (1999).

Stevens A., and J. Price, *Evolutionary Psychiatry*. Routledge, London and Philadelphia. (2000).

Stocco D. M., *Encyclopedia of Reproduction*, 4. San Diego, California, Academic Press (1999).

Tatersall I., *Becoming Human*, Harcourt Brace & Company, Orlando Florida (1998).

Van Honk J. and Schutter D., *Psychol. Sci.* 18, 663 (2007).
Vervaecke H., de Vries H., and van Elsacker L., *Int. J. Primatol.* 21, 47 (2000).
Vignozzi L., Morelli A., Filippi S., Maggi M., Forti G., *J. Endocrinol. Invest.* 33, 27 (2010).
Wingfield J. C., Hegner R., Dufti A.M, Ball G., 1990. *Am. Nat.* 136, 830.

In: Testosterone
Editor: Konstantin Chichinadze

ISBN 978-1-62100-492-9

Chapter II

The Male Rhesus Monkey as a Model to Study the Effects of Testosterone on Cognitive and Emotional Function

Agnès Lacreuse [*] ***and Andrea Simoni***
Department of Psychology, University of Massachusetts,
Amherst, MA, US

Abstract

Studies in monkey models of menopause have greatly advanced our understanding of the effects of estrogens on women's cognitive health. Yet, parallel studies in male monkeys have been critically lacking and it remains unclear whether testosterone (T) replacement is a desirable intervention against age-related cognitive decline in men. In this chapter, we argue that male rhesus monkeys are excellent models to investigate this issue and describe the first studies using this species to test the effects of T on cognitive and emotional function. We present a series of studies from our laboratory, in which intact male macaques temporarily castrated with a gonadotropin-releasing hormone agonist were administered cognitive and emotional tests when treated with T vs. placebo. The cognitive tasks included tests of visual recognition memory, spatial memory and working memory. The emotional tasks consisted of an approach-avoidance task of objects, a video playback task of social stimuli, and a computerized test of attention to emotional stimuli. The results indicate that T manipulations in pharmacologically-castrated young male monkeys have only modest effects on cognitive function but significantly affect selective aspects of emotion. Our current studies in aged male monkeys should determine whether T benefits cognitive function and emotional reactivity later in life. We conclude that research in male nonhuman primates is essential to test the efficacy of T therapy as an intervention for maintaining cognitive and emotional health throughout the lifespan in men.

* Correspondence to: Agnès Lacreuse, Ph.D. Department of Psychology, Tobin Hall, 135 Hicks Way, University of Massachusetts, Amherst, MA 01003; Phone:413-545-2183; Fax:413-545-0996; Email: alacreuse@psych.umass.edu.

Introduction

The older population is growing at an unprecedented rate, and is expected to reach 14% of the World's population by 2040 [1]. As people live longer, alleviating the physical and cognitive burden of aging becomes a central issue. Currently at the forefront of possible interventions against age-related cognitive decline, diet and exercise show promising results and are extensively studied. In addition, hormonal replacement therapy, which enjoyed tremendous popularity before falling from grace shortly after the publication of the Women's Health Study in 2003, remains an intervention with great potential for women's cognitive health. Indeed, considerable evidence from animal studies suggest that estrogens protect against age-related cognitive decline in females (rodents: [2, 3]; nonhuman primates: [4, 5]) and trigger a cascade of neurobiological and functional changes in brain areas important for learning and memory, such as the prefrontal cortex [6, 7] and the hippocampus [8, 9]. While the results of clinical studies are more mixed [10], the main debate has slowly shifted from general safety concerns about estrogen use in women [11], to specific considerations regarding optimal regimens and timing of replacement [12, 13].

While great advances have been made in understanding the impact of estrogens on women's cognitive health, much less is known about the effects of androgens on male cognitive aging [14, 15]. Unlike women, in whom sex hormones decline abruptly after menopause at an average age of 52, men experience a progressive decline in testosterone (T) from the 30's onward [16, 17]. Despite a substantial loss of T with age, recognition that low T may have an impact beyond sexual and physical health has taken some time. Progress in this area has been slowed by health concerns related to androgen use in men [18] as well as by the paucity of animal studies. Not only have very few studies examined the effects of T on cognition in rodent models, but until recently no study had been conducted in nonhuman primates. Studies in nonhuman primates are particularly valuable for translating findings from basic studies into clinical applications [4, 5, 19, 20].

This chapter begins with a brief review of the consequences of T deficiency and T replacement for cognitive function and emotion in younger and older men. In the next section, we argue that the mixed results of the human literature can be clarified by studying nonhuman primates and describe some of the characteristics that make male rhesus monkeys particularly suitable for such investigations. We then present a series of crossover studies from our laboratory, in which intact male macaques temporarily castrated with a gonadotropin releasing hormone agonist (GnRH-a) were administered cognitive and emotional tests when treated with T and placebo. Throughout the chapter, we discuss the data in the context of the human literature and emphasize the unique contributions of nonhuman primate studies. We conclude that research in male macaques should help determine whether T therapy is a desirable intervention for maintaining cognitive and emotional health in aged men.

Testosterone, Cognition and Emotion: Studies in Men

The human brain contains androgen receptors in regions important for cognition and emotion, including the temporal cortex [21, 22] and the hippocampus [23]. In addition, T has been found to promote neuronal function and survival in these regions, through a range of neuroprotective and neurotrophic effects [24-26]. These findings suggest that androgens have the potential to modulate cognition and emotion dependent on these brain regions. Yet, while androgen deficiency in men has been associated with bone loss, muscle mass loss, increased fat mass, impairments in physical and sexual function as well as decreased quality of life [27-29], whether it also increases the risk of cognitive impairment and emotional dysfunction remains unclear to date. Below, we briefly review the literature on the relationships between T, cognition and emotion in younger and older men. More extensive reviews can be found in [14, 30-34].

T and Cognition in Younger Men

Many studies have investigated the relationships between endogenous T levels and cognitive function in healthy young men. Most studies have detected either a curvilinear [35-39] or a linear relationship between T levels and various tests of visuospatial ability [35, 39-44]. However, the findings are not entirely consistent, as some have reported a negative [45] or no relationship [46] between endogenous T and visuospatial ability. Only a few studies have explored the relationships between endogenous T and other cognitive domains (e.g, verbal fluency, episodic memory), and they have reported either small or nonexistent associations [35, 43, 44].

Due to health concerns, studies on exogenous T administration in healthy, eugonadal young men are rare. In one study, T was administered to young eugonadal and hypogonadal men for 8 weeks and men were tested on a battery of tests measuring spatial and verbal ability [47]. Supraphysiological T levels were found to decrease spatial ability and increase verbal fluency. Three other studies in young men used pharmacological suppression of T followed by T supplementation. Bhasin et al [48] treated men with a GnRH-a (Lupron) and several doses (25 mg to 600 mg, weekly injections) of T enanthate (TE) for 20 weeks and failed to find an effect of T on cognitive function at any dose. In contrast, Cherrier et al [49] found that T depletion induced by a synthetic progestin was associated with a decline in verbal memory that was restored by TE supplementation (weekly injections of 100 mg for 6 weeks). Finally, a recent study using Lupron and treatment with either placebo, Lupron alone, T (physiological levels) or T + anatrozole (aromatase inhibitor) for 6 weeks found no effect of T manipulations on tests of executive function, memory, and spatial cognition [50]. Thus, the effects of T on cognition in healthy young men are far from being clear-cut. As suggested by some authors [37, 47], there may be an optimal range for T to exert positive effects on cognitive function, with too low and too high levels of T being detrimental to cognition. Additionally, some cognitive domains may be more sensitive than others.

T and Cognition in Older Men

In older men, several studies have reported positive associations between endogenous T levels and measures of memory, including visual and verbal memory, visuospatial functioning, and global measures of memory [33, 51-55]. Reduced T levels have also been linked to a higher risk of developing Alzheimer's disease [56-58]. Yet, there are many inconsistencies. Negative correlations have been found between T and verbal fluency in older men [55] and a recent study reported that higher total and free T levels were associated with poorer verbal and executive function performance [59]. The effects of androgen deprivation therapy (ADT) on cognition in older men with prostate cancer are also inconsistent. A few studies found evidence for cognitive impairment in some aspects of memory following ADT [60, 61], while others studies have found no cognitive change [62]. ADT findings are difficult to interpret however, as the studies often have a small number of participants, lack appropriate controls and use various treatment regimens [63].

T therapy is recommended in men with symptomatic androgen deficiency to maintain secondary sex characteristics and improve sexual function, well-being, muscle mass, muscle strength, and bone mineral density [27]. Whether T therapy is effective in improving cognition and emotion in older men awaits more definitive data, however. While many studies have reported enhanced performance in several cognitive domains following T treatment, including visuospatial ability, verbal memory, verbal fluency and working memory [33, 47, 64-69], not all studies have found a positive effect [70-73]. In fact, in three recent studies, T treatment had either no effect [50, 74] or a negative effect [75] on cognition. The cognitive domains examined, the T regimen used, and health and demographic factors [34] are likely to mediate differences across studies. Well-controlled experiments in animal models could help clarify these inconsistencies.

T and Emotion in Younger Men

Evidence from animals and humans suggest that T influences a wide range of emotional behaviors. T is best known for its influence on aggressive behavior. Higher levels of T were positively correlated with aggressive behavior in several studies in boys, adolescent and adult men [76-83]. Increases in aggressive behavior have also been observed in adolescent men taking supraphysiological doses of anabolic steroids [84] and adult men tested in placebo-controlled studies with anabolic steroids [85, 86]. Several recent studies have emphasized the role of T in increasing risk-taking in tasks measuring decision-making [87-92]. Finally, T may also enhance attention to threatening facial expressions [93, 94], perhaps via increased activation of the amygdala. Indeed, recent neuroimaging studies have observed T-related increases in amygdala activation to threat-related cues in young men [95-97] and women [98, 99].

Paradoxically, there is also evidence for fear/anxiety-reducing properties of T in humans. T administration reduced fear-potentiated startle and non-conscious responses to anxiety-related stimuli in two studies in women [100, 101]. In another study, a 4-week hypogonadism induced by Lupron administration was sufficient for a small subset of young healthy men to develop a clinically significant depressive mood [102], suggesting that T may play a role in emotional regulation. Consistent with this idea, O'Connor [103], found that supraphysiological T levels significantly reduced negative mood (tension, fatigue and anger) in hypogonadal men.

T and Emotion in Older Men

A number of studies have documented positive correlations between low T levels and negative mood states, as reviewed by Margolese [104]. In particular, low levels of T have been associated with depressive symptoms, anxiety, and irritability in several studies in older men [105-109]. Significant improvements in mood following T treatment were also noted in middle-aged hypogonadal men [110, 111] and middle-aged depressed men [105, 112]. Yet, other studies found that T supplementation had no effect on mood scores or quality of life in older hypogonadal men [71] or in older men temporarily suppressed by a GnRH agonist [68].

Thus, the effects of T on emotion in men are particularly inconsistent. The discrepancies of the human literature may be related to the widely different methodologies and treatment regimens used across studies, as well as differences in the population studied (such as age, physical health, and psychological status). In addition, many studies use self-reports as measures of emotion. These measures should be supplemented with experimental measures for a more objective assessment of emotion. Studies in animal models, and in nonhuman primates in particular, may help resolve these discrepancies. In the next section, we propose that male rhesus monkeys are particularly well-suited for studying the effects of T on cognition and emotion throughout the lifespan.

The Male Macaque as a Model for Understanding the Effects of T on Cognition and Emotion

Rhesus monkeys (*Macaca mulatta*) are found ubiquitously throughout Asia. In adulthood, they typically weigh between 5 to 20 kg. They reach puberty around 3 (females) or 4 years old (males) and can live until 40 years, with very few individuals surviving past 30 years [113]. On this basis, 15-19 year old monkeys are generally considered as "middle-aged", 20-25 monkeys as "early-aged" and monkeys over 25 as "oldest old".

The rhesus monkey is a particularly relevant model for studying the effects of gonadal hormones on cognition and emotion because of its close genetic proximity to humans (97.5 % genetic homology [114]) and similarities with humans in many neural, cognitive, behavioral and physiological characteristics. First, the rhesus monkey shares with humans a complex neural organization characterized by a highly developed cerebral cortex, a large prefrontal cortex and many functionally homologous cortical regions. For these reasons, the rhesus monkey is the most widely used primate for neuroscience research [115]. Yet, the macaque brain is by no means a scaled version of the human brain: important differences between the two brains have been emphasized in several recent papers [116, 117]. Despite these differences, rhesus monkeys are capable of performing complex tasks which assess various aspects of cognition such as working memory, visuospatial ability, attention, executive function, categorization, and abstract concept learning, that are relevant to human cognitive abilities. These tasks can be administered in settings similar to those in use with humans, using manual systems such as the Wisconsin General Testing Apparatus [118], or automated systems relying on joysticks [119] or touchscreen methodologies [120]. Secondly, there are also many similarities between rhesus monkeys and humans in social and emotional behavior, with rhesus monkeys expressing psychopathology resembling that observed in humans [121, 122]. Finally, due to close similarities between the reproductive endocrinology of female macaques and women [123], female macaques have been particularly useful for research on women's health issues [19], in particular as models for understanding the effects of ovarian hormones on cognitive aging [4, 5]. Surprisingly, it is only very recently that male rhesus monkeys have been used in similar studies to study the effects of testicular hormones on cognition.

As previously described in several extensive reviews [28, 124, 125], men's reproductive aging is characterized by a dysregulation at all levels of the Hypothalamic-Pituitary-Testicular axis. Men experience a progressive decrease in total T levels with age, of about a 1-2% decline per year from the 30s onward [16, 17]. Importantly, total circulating T in the blood includes only 1-2% of free T. The remaining 98% is bound to proteins, with about 40% bound to sex hormone binding globulin (SHBG) and about 60% to albumin. Only the non-SHBG bound fraction is biologically active (bioavailable T), and therefore is considered by many as the clinically relevant marker [29, 33, 53, 126]. As SHBG increases significantly with age [16, 29], steeper age-related declines are typically observed in free T and bioavailable T compared to total T. In addition to age-related changes in circulating T levels, reduced sensitivity of the hypothalamus/pituitary to T feedback, alterations in pulsatile GnRH secretion and LH secretion (lower amplitude, more frequent pulses), and reduced sensitivity of the testes to LH stimulation [124] are also observed. Furthermore, the normal circadian rhythm of T secretion, characterized by lower T levels during the day compared to during the night, is reduced in older men [127-129].

The endocrine control of testicular function is, in many respects, similar in men and male macaques [130, 131]. Therefore, aged male rhesus monkeys could be excellent models for men's reproductive senescence. Yet, important differences have also been noted between the two species. For example, Schlatt et al (2008) [132] recently reported that aged male monkeys (16-19 years old) showed a more pronounced (instead of blunted) T circadian rhythm compared to younger male monkeys (6-9 years old). This finding should be confirmed in monkeys of older ages, however, since the older monkeys used in this study were only middle-aged. Conflicting results have also been reported concerning age-related decline in T levels. Early studies found no evidence for age-related declines in T levels in rhesus monkeys [133-137]. In contrast, more recent data detailing 24-hour hormone profiles with remote sampling indicate significantly reduced T levels in aged compared to younger rhesus monkeys [138]. Obviously, additional studies are needed to confirm that aged male monkeys show an age-related decline in T levels similar to that of men.

T Studies in the Intact, GnRH-a Suppressed, Adult Male Rhesus Monkey

In male macaques, androgen receptors are found in many brain regions involved in cognition and emotion, including limbic structures and cortical regions [139-143]. Evidence in male rodents has shown that T increases synaptic density in the CA1 region of the hippocampus [144, 145]. Although comparable studies have not been conducted in primates, indirect evidence in male vervet monkeys suggests that circulating androgens are essential for maintaining synaptic density in CA1, with castrated monkeys exhibiting reduced synaptic density in this region relative to intact monkeys [146]. These findings suggest that androgens have the potential to modulate cognitive and emotional processes involving these brain regions. Two studies in rhesus monkeys have shown that pre- or perinatal exposure to androgens indeed modulates cognitive abilities. Early in infancy, T accelerates the development of frontal regions and slows the development of inferotemporal areas, leading to transient cognitive sex differences in rhesus monkeys younger than 6 months [147-150]. Prenatal T treatment also modulates spatial abilities later in adulthood [151]. However, it is only recently, that the activational effects of T on cognition have been investigated in male nonhuman primates.

Effects of T Manipulations on Cognition in Young Male Rhesus Monkeys

To study the activational effects of T on cognitive function in male rhesus monkeys, we used a paradigm in which intact males were treated with the GnRH-a Depot Lupron and replaced with TE or placebo in a cross-over, double-blind design. In our first study [152], 6 young adult males (5-6 years old) were tested in 3 memory tasks. The Delayed Non-Matching-to-Sample (DNMS), that assessed visual recognition memory, required the monkeys to recognize a novel from a familiar object after various delays (10, 60, 120, 300 and 600 s). In the Delayed Response task (DR), that assessed working memory, monkeys had to remember the location of a reward after various delays (5, 10, 15, 30 and 60 s). In the spatial version of the Delayed Recognition Span Test (spatial-DRST), monkeys were presented with a series of identical disks added one at a time on a 18-location board. The task was to select the disk placed in a new location at each trial. Both random locations sequences and a unique, repeated sequence were used, allowing to measure spatial working memory and reference memory, respectively. The tasks were administered in a miniature version of the WGTA that could be attached to the home cage. Monkeys learned each task in succession for several months before the initiation of treatment. Following a 4-week baseline period, monkeys were treated with Depot Lupron (200 μg/kg) before being randomly assigned, 4 weeks later, to one of 2 treatment groups: Lupron + TE (20 mg/kg) or Lupron + oil vehicle. In each treatment group, monkeys received Lupron + TE (or Lupron + oil) for 4 weeks before crossing over to the alternate treatment for an additional 4 weeks.

Monkeys were tested on the cognitive tasks during 3 experimental conditions: the Baseline, Lupron + TE and Lupron + oil conditions. No testing occurred during the Lupron alone condition, as T levels were progressively declining during this phase. Testing took place 4 days a week on each successive task, one task per week. On day 5 of each week, monkeys were anesthetized for blood collection. As predicted, suppressed T levels were observed about 4 weeks after Lupron injection and TE injection induced supraphysiological T levels decreasing progressively over 4 weeks, as found in a prior study in male macaques [153]. Contrary to our hypotheses, however, DR and spatial-DRST measures were not affected by T. In addition, DNMS performance was significantly impaired when the longest delay (600 s) was imposed between the encoding of the sample object and the recognition phase. Since DNMS performance is largely dependent on medial temporal function, we suggested that supraphysiological T levels may compromise medial temporal lobe function when memory is heavily taxed. These results are consistent with those obtained by Maki et al. (2007) [75] in a crossover study in older men treated with supraphysiological doses of TE. Relative to oil vehicle, T treatment was found to be associated with significant declines in verbal memory and altered patterns of frontal and temporal cerebral metabolic rates for glucose, as measured by Positron Emission Tomography [75]. Altogether, these data suggest that supraphysiological T levels may adversely affect medial temporal lobe function.

Effects of T Manipulations on Emotional Reactivity in Young Male Rhesus Monkeys

Many studies focusing on the effects of T on cognition have failed to examine whether T may induce cognitive changes through its influence on emotion. Our second report [154] specifically addressed the effects of T on emotion in male rhesus monkeys. Previous studies in this species had shown positive correlations between T levels and social dominance [155, 156], sexual competition [157], and low-intensity aggressive behaviors, such as stares, threats and displacements [155, 158, 159]. Based on these results and the human literature reviewed above, we hypothesized that exogenous T would increase aggressive behaviors and/or facilitate approach or attention towards threatening stimuli.

To test these hypotheses, monkeys were tested in two emotional tasks: the Approach-Avoidance task assessed behavioral responses of the monkeys when exposed for 5 min to familiar, novel, or threatening objects baited with a banana. Objects from the neutral category consisted of familiar enrichment toys, objects from the novel category included enrichment toys that the monkeys had never seen before, and objects from the threatening category included items such as large capture gloves, costume masks and plastic snakes. The second task, the Social Playback task, assessed the monkeys' behavioral responses during exposure to 3 min-long videos of neutral (sleeping), positive (grooming), and negative (fighting) scenes displaying unfamiliar conspecifics. Monkeys were tested at baseline and during the Lupron + TE and Lupron + oil treatments, as described above. For each task, the monkeys' behavior was videotaped and the frequency and/or duration of specific behaviors were analyzed to identify differences between the treatment and placebo conditions. In the

Approach-Avoidance task, we had predicted that T would facilitate approach towards threatening objects and/or increase the duration spent at proximity of a threatening object. We found no support for this prediction, despite evidence that the monkeys perceived the different objects as familiar, novel and threatening, based on increasing latencies to approach each object type, respectively.

For the Social Playback task, we had predicted that monkeys would be more likely to watch negative videos when treated with T compared to oil, based on reports that exogenous T increases attention to negative social stimuli in humans [93, 94]. Indeed, we found that T treatment significantly increased the amount of time the monkeys spent watching the negative videos, without affecting watching time for the other types of videos. This result suggested that T may increase attention to social threatening stimuli.

We specifically tested this assumption in a subsequent study (King et al, unpublished data), in which monkeys were presented with a modified Dot-Probe task, a task traditionally used to test attentional biases to emotional stimuli in humans (e.g, [160]). Monkeys were first required to touch a fixation cross in the middle of a touchscreen. Immediately after, two side-by-side images were briefly flashed for 1 s after which a small yellow dot appeared in place of one of the images. The monkey was rewarded for touching the dot and response times were recorded. Faster response times to touch the dot indicated greater attention allocation to the image preceding it. One of the images was always a neutral stimulus while the other image was always an emotional stimulus, either positive or negative. Both social and nonsocial images were presented. Social images consisted of photographs of unfamiliar rhesus monkeys with neutral, positive (i.e, lipsmack) and negative (i.e, threat) facial expressions. Nonsocial images consisted of photographs such as cage parts (neutral), food items (positive) or syringes (negative). Our predictions were that monkeys would pay more attention to negative stimuli, as generally found in humans [161, 162], and that T treatment would increase this attentional bias, as suggested by the findings of [94] and [93] in humans. Monkeys were tested 4 days a week during each of 4-week long experimental conditions, the Baseline, Lupron alone, Lupron +TE and Lupron + oil conditions, and were treated with TE 5mg/kg (biweekly injections) or oil vehicle. Three important results were obtained. First, we confirmed that monkeys, like humans, show an attentional bias for threatening stimuli at baseline, but only when social stimuli (faces) are displayed. Second, contrary to our predictions, T did not enhance this bias, perhaps due to repeated exposure to the stimuli across several months of testing. In contrast, the majority of human studies have examined changes in emotion within *a few hours* of administering acute doses of T [98, 163-166]. We are currently examining whether selective attention to threat is enhanced by T shortly after initial exposure to emotional stimuli. Third, we found that monkeys treated with T had faster response times compared to when treated with oil, independently of stimulus exposure. These results suggest that T may increase generalized arousal, defined as "increased sensory alertness, motor activity and emotional reactivity" [167].

Finally, we also examined potential effects of T on anxiety [168], using a test based on the Human Intruder Paradigm, that measures defensive responses to a potential threatening human intruder in primates [169]. In this task, each monkey was placed in a plexiglas cage. After a 2 min period acclimatation, an unfamiliar intruder entered the room and stood 2.5 meters from the cage while staring directly into the monkey's eyes for a period of 2 min. Each monkey was tested every two weeks during the Baseline, Lupron+oil, and Lupron+TE treatment conditions for a total of six sessions per monkey. The videos were analyzed for the frequency and duration of aggressive, anxious and submissive behaviors using a standard ethogram. We found no evidence that T reduced anxiety. In contrast, anxious behaviors tended to increase (non significant trend) during T treatment. These results are consistent with the idea that T increases arousal in nonhuman primates. They also suggest that T, at least as administered in this study, is not effective in reducing anxiety. T has been found to reduce anxiety in many other animal models including rats [170-174], mice [175], cattle [176] and ewes [177]. In rhesus monkeys, Richards et al [178] found that castrated adolescents, compared to intact peers, were less likely to spend time in proximity of an unfamiliar monkey, a finding that they interpreted as indicative of increased anxiety.Another interpretation of these findings would suggest that the lack of T may decrease arousal and reduce motivation to approach an unfamiliar (negative) conspecific. Additional studies are critically needed to understand the effects of T on anxiety in nonhuman primates and reconcile the findings with those of the nonprimate literature.

T Studies in the Intact, GnRH-a Suppressed, Aged Male Rhesus Monkey

Ongoing studies in our laboratory examine the effects of T on cognition and emotional reactivity in aged male rhesus monkeys, using the same methodology used in our two previous reports in young adult males [152, 154]. Based on the consistent finding that exogenous estrogens benefit cognition in *aged* female macaques, but do not affect cognition in younger females [4, 179], we expect that T administration will significantly improve cognition in older males. As far as emotion is concerned, there is currently no data on emotional aging in nonhuman primates. As described above, we found evidence that young male macaques allocate more attention towards negative (social) stimuli, a finding consistent with the negativity bias exhibited by young people for a variety of stimuli. Interestingly, there is a well documented switch from a negativity bias to a positivity bias in human aging, in that older adults exhibit preferences away from negative information as compared to younger adults [180-182]. The Socioemotional Selectivity Theory (SST) has been proposed to account for these findings. The SST suggests that older and younger persons process emotional information differently due to differences in life goals [183]. This psychological interpretation fails to consider that specific biological differences between younger and older adults, such as age-related changes in T, may drive changes in emotional processing with age. Thus, it will be of particular interest to examine whether greater emotion regulation occurs in aged nonhuman primates and whether these changes might be driven by changes in T levels.

Conclusion

Our studies are the first to examine the effects of exogenous T on cognition and emotion in adult male monkeys. We selected a paradigm in which intact male rhesus monkeys are temporarily castrated with a GnRH-a (Lupron), treated with TE and crossover oil vehicle for 4 weeks and tested at baseline and during each treatment condition on a battery of cognitive and emotional tasks. So far, data collected in young males suggest that supraphysiological T has only modest effects on cognition and may impair medial temporal lobe function when memory is heavily taxed. The emotional assessments further indicate that monkeys have an attentional bias towards negative social stimuli and that T may enhance this bias, at least under high arousing conditions, i.e, when monkeys are watching videos of fights between conspecifics. Our failure to find an enhancing effect of T on attention to static stimuli (threats of conspecifics) in the Dot-Probe task, suggests caution with an interpretation relying exclusively on attentional processes. Rather than modulating attention *per se,* T may increase generalized arousal, as suggested by faster response times following T treatment in the Dot-Probe task. Finally, we found no evidence for anxiolytic properties of T, which contradicts a vast literature in other animal models. Further investigations are needed to reconcile these findings.

We have just begun to probe the effects of T on cognition and emotion in male nonhuman primates and it is clear that much remains to be understood. For example, the conversion of T to estradiol may very well underlie some of the effects that we have observed. Conversely, the lack of effect on some cognitive and emotional tasks may be directly related to the particular dose, duration or timing of administration of T selected for our studies. The role of these factors ought to be clarified in animal models, from rodents to nonhuman primates, before translation to clinical settings. Our ongoing studies will address whether T benefits cognition and modulates emotional reactivity in aged male monkeys tested in the same paradigm as the one used in young monkeys. The findings from these studies will be a first step in assessing the potential of T as a therapeutic agent to alleviate age-related cognitive deficits and emotional dysfunction in men.

Acknowledgments

These studies were supported by a Collaborative Biomedical Research grant between UMass and Baystate Medical Center, a Healey Endowment/Faculty Research grant, and a grant from the American Federation for Aging Research to Agnès Lacreuse and an Honors Research Grant from the Commonwealth Honors College to Andrea Simoni. We thank the UMass shop staff, veterinary staff and animal care staff for their support and the many students who assisted with the research. The monkeys were humanely treated in accordance with the standards of the PHS Policy on Humane Care and Use of Laboratory Animals.

References

[1] K. Kinsella and H. Wan, *US Census Bureau, International Population Reports, An Aging World,* US Government Printing Office Washington, DC (2009).
[2] J. M. Daniel, *J Neuroendocrinol,* 18, 787 (2006).
[3] K. M. Frick, *Horm Behav,* 55, 2 (2009).
[4] A. Lacreuse, *Neuroscience,* 138, 859 (2006).
[5] M. L. Voytko, *et al., Am J Primatol,* 71, 794 (2009).
[6] J. Hao, *et al., J Neurosci.,* 26, 2571 (2006).

[7] R. D. Brinton, *Trends Pharmacol Sci,* 30, 212 (2009).
[8] J. Hao, *et al.*, *J Comp Neurol,* 465, 540 (2003).
[9] C. S. Woolley, *Horm Behav,* 34, 140 (1998).
[10] P. M. Maki and E. Sundermann, *Hum Reprod Update* (2009).
[11] S. R. Rapp, *et al.*, *JAMA,* 289, 2663 May 28, 2003 (2003).
[12] B. B. Sherwin and J. F. Henry, *Front Neuroendocrinol,* 29, 88 (2008).
[13] B. B. Sherwin, *Nat Rev Endocrinol,* 5, 620 (2009).
[14] M. M. Cherrier, *Front Horm Res,* 37, 150 (2009).
[15] J. S. Janowsky, *Trends Cogn Sci,* 10, 77 (2006).
[16] H. A. Feldman, *et al.*, *J Clin Endocrinol Metab,* 87, 589 (2002).
[17] S. M. Harman, *et al.*, *J Clin Endocrinol Metab,* 86, 724 (2001).
[18] C. T. Liverman and D. G. Blazer, *Testosterone and aging: clinical research directions,* National Academies Press Washington DC (2004).
[19] C. A. Shively and T. B. Clarkson, *Am J Primatol,* 71, 715 (2009).
[20] J. H. Morrison, *et al.*, *J Neurosci.,* 26, 10332 (2006).
[21] L. Puy, *et al.*, *J Steroid Biochem & Mol Biol,* 55, 197 (1995).
[22] A. Sarrieau, *et al.*, *Neuroendocrinology,* 51, 713 (1990).
[23] S. Beyenburg, *et al.*, *Neurosci Lett,* 294, 25 (2000).
[24] C. J. Pike, *et al.*, *Front Neuroendocrinol,* 30, 239 (2009).
[25] T. V. Nguyen, *et al.*, *J Neuroendocrinol,* 22, 1013 (2010).
[26] K. N. Fargo, *et al.*, "Molecular Biology of Androgen Action: Perspectives on Neuroprotective and Neurotherapeutic Effects," in *Hormones, Brain and Behavior*, W. P. Donald, San Diego: Academic Press, 2009, pp. 1219.
[27] S. Bhasin, *J Clin Endocrinol Metab,* 95, 2536 (2010).
[28] S. Bhasin and K. L. Herbst, "Age-related changes in the male reproductive axis," in *Endocrinology of male reproduction*, R. McLachlan, Endotext.com, http://www.endotext.org/male/index.htm (2003).
[29] J. M. Kaufman and A. Vermeulen, *Endocr Rev,* 26, 833 (2005).
[30] I. Driscoll and S. M. Resnick, *Curr Alzheimer Res,* 4, 33 (2007).
[31] M. Zitzmann, *Aging Male,* 9, 195 (2006).
[32] J. S. Janowsky, *Neuroscience,* 138, 1015 (2006).
[33] S. D. Moffat, *Ann N Y Acad Sci,* 1055, 80 (2005).
[34] O. Beauchet, *Eur J Endocrinol,* 155, 773 (2006).
[35] K. Christiansen and R. Knussmann, *Neuropsychobiology,* 18, 27 (1987).
[36] C. Gouchie and D. Kimura, *Psychoneuroendocrinology,* 16, 323 (1991).
[37] S. D. Moffat and E. Hampson, *Psychoneuroendocrinology,* 21, 323 (1996).
[38] N. Neave, *et al.*, *Brain Cogn.,* 41, 245 (1999).
[39] I. Silverman, *et al.*, *Psychoneuroendocrinology,* 24, 813 (1999).
[40] J. Choi and I. Silverman, *Brain Cogn,* 50, 116 (2002).
[41] C. K. Hooven, *et al.*, *Neuropsychologia,* 42, 782 (2004).
[42] I. Driscoll, *et al.*, *Horm Behav,* 47, 326 (2005).
[43] P. P. Thilers, *et al.*, *Psychoneuroendocrinology,* 31, 565 (2006).
[44] H. W. Gordon, *et al.*, *Cortex,* 22, 399 (1986).
[45] J. E. Yonker, *et al.*, *Cortex,* 42, 376 (2006).
[46] D. A. Puts, *et al.*, *Horm Behav,* 58, 282 (2010).

[47] D. B. O'Connor, *et al.*, *Neuropsychologia,* 39, 1385 (2001).
[48] S. Bhasin, *et al.*, *Am J Physiol Endocrinol & Metab,* 281, E1172 (2001).
[49] M. M. Cherrier, *et al.*, *J Clin Endocrinol Metab,* 87, 3090, (2002).
[50] L. A. Young, *et al.*, *J Clin Endocrinol Metab,* 95, 280 (2010).
[51] E. Barrett-Connor, *et al.*, *J Clin Endocrinol Metab,* 84, 3681 (1999).
[52] K. Yaffe, *et al.*, *J Am Geriatr Soc,* 50, 707 (2002).
[53] S. D. Moffat, *et al.*, *J Clin Endocrinol Metab,* 87, 5001 (2002).
[54] M. Muller, *et al.*, *Neurology,* 64, 866 (2005).
[55] O. T. Wolf and C. Kirschbaum, *Horm Behav,* 41, 259 (2002).
[56] E. Hogervorst, *et al.*, *Neuroendocrinol Lett,* 22, 163 (2001).
[57] S. D. Moffat, *et al.*, *Neurology,* 62, 188 (2004).
[58] E. R. Rosario, *et al.*, *J Am Med Assoc,* 292, 1431 (2004).
[59] D. M. Martin, *et al.*, *Maturitas,* 57, 182 (2007).
[60] J. R. Bussiere, *et al.*, *Behav Neurosci,* 119, 1429 (2005).
[61] T. M. Beer, *et al.*, *J Urol,* 175, 130 (2006).
[62] E. Salminen, *et al.*, *Br J Cancer,* 89, 971 (2003).
[63] S. M. H. Alibhai, *et al.*, *Critical Rev Oncol/Hematol,* 60, 201 (2006).
[64] J. S. Janowsky, *et al.*, *Behav Neurosci.,* 108, 325 (1994).
[65] J. S. Janowsky, *et al.*, *J Cogn Neurosci,* 12, 407 (2000).
[66] M. M. Cherrier, *et al.*, *Neurology,* 57, 80 (2001).
[67] M. M. Cherrier, *et al.*, *Psychoneuroendocrinology,* 29, 65 (2004).
[68] P. B. Gray, *et al.*, *J Clin Endocrinol Metab,* 90, 3838 (2005).
[69] A. M. Kenny, *et al.*, *J Gerontol Biol Sci & Med Sci,* 57, M321 (2002).
[70] O. T. Wolf, *et al.*, *Biol Psychiatr,* 650 (2000).
[71] M. T. Haren, *et al.*, *Maturitas,* 50, 124 (2005).
[72] R. Sih, *et al.*, *J Clin Endocrinol Metab,* 82, 1661 (1997).
[73] P. H. Lu, *et al.*, *Arch Neurol,* 63, 177 (2005).
[74] M. H. Emmelot-Vonk, *et al.*, *J Am Med Assoc,* 299, 39 (2008).
[75] P. M. Maki, *et al.*, *J Clin Endocrinol Metab,* 92, 4107, 2007 (2007).
[76] D. Olweus, *et al.*, *Psychosom Med,* 42, 253 (1980).
[77] D. Olweus, *et al.*, *Psychosom Med,* 50, 261 (1988).
[78] R. Rowe, *et al.*, *BiolPsychiatry,* 55, 546 (2004).
[79] J. Archer, *Neurosci & Biobehavioral Rev,* 30, 319 (2006).
[80] A. Popma, *et al.*, *Biological Psychiatry,* 61, 405 (2007).
[81] J. M. Dabbs, Jr., *et al.*, *Psychosom Med,* 49, 174 (1987).
[82] D. R. Rubinow and P. J. Schmidt, *Am J Psychiatr,* 153, 974 (1996).
[83] A. Mazur and A. Booth, *Behav Brain Sci,* 21, 353 (1998).
[84] K. M. Beaver, *et al.*, *Am J Public Health,* 98, 2185 (2008).
[85] H. G. Pope, Jr., *et al.*, *Arch Gen Psychiatry,* 57, 133 (2000).
[86] T. P. Su, *et al.*, *J Am Med Assoc,* 269, 2760 (1993).
[87] R. Reavis and W. H. Overman, *Behav Neurosci,* 115, 196 (2001).
[88] J. van Honk, *et al.*, *Psychoneuroendocrinology,* 29, 937 (2004).
[89] J. M. Coates and J. Herbert, *Proc Natl Acad Sci,* 105, 6167 (2008).
[90] C. L. Apicella, *et al.*, *Evol Hum Behav,* 29, 384 (2008).
[91] A. E. Goudriaan, *et al.*, *Psychoneuroendocrinology,* 35, 1416 (2010).

[92] S. J. Stanton, *et al.*, *Horm Behav,* 59, 252 (2011).
[93] J. van Honk, *et al.*, *Horm Behav,* 36, 17 (1999).
[94] M. M. Wirth and O. C. Schultheiss, *Physiol Behav,* 90, 496 (2007).
[95] B. Derntl, *et al.*, *Psychoneuroendocrinology,* 34, 687 (2009).
[96] S. J. Stanton, *et al.*, *Biol Psychol,* 81, 118 (2009).
[97] S. B. Manuck, *et al.*, *Psychoneuroendocrinology,* 35, 94 (2010).
[98] E. J. Hermans, *et al.*, *Biol Psychiatry,* 63, 263 (2008).
[99] G. A. van Wingen, *et al.*, *Neuropsychopharmacology,* 34, 539 (2009).
[100] E. J. Hermans, *et al.*, *Biol Psychiatry,* 59, 872 (2006).
[101] J. van Honk, *et al.*, *Biol Psychiatry,* 58, 218 (2005).
[102] P. J. Schmidt, *et al.*, *Arch Gen Psychiatry,* 61, 997 (2004).
[103] D. B. O'Connor, *et al.*, *Physiol Behav,* 75, 557 (2002).
[104] H. C. Margolese, *J Geriatr Psychiatry Neurol,* 13, 93 (2000).
[105] S. N. Seidman and B. T. Walsh, *Am J Geriatr Psychiatry,* 7, 18 (1999).
[106] E. Barrett-Connor, *et al.*, *J Clin Endocrinol Metab,* 84, 573 (1999).
[107] O. P. Almeida, *et al.*, *Arch Gen Psychiatry,* 65, 283 (2008).
[108] A. Vermeulen, *Ann Med.,* 25, 531 (1993).
[109] J. L. Tenover, *J Androl,* 18, 103 (1997).
[110] C. Wang, *et al.*, *J Clin Endocrinol Metab,* 89, 2085 (2004).
[111] C. Wang, *et al.*, *J Clin Endocrinol Metab,* 85, 2839 (2000).
[112] H. G. Pope, Jr., *et al.*, *Am J Psychiatry,* 160, 105 (2003).
[113] J. Tigges, *et al.*, *Am J Primatol,* 15, 263 (1988).
[114] R. A. Gibbs, *et al.*, *Science,* 316, 222 (2007).
[115] J. P. Capitanio and M. E. Emborg, *The Lancet,* 371, (2008).
[116] J. K. Rilling, *Evol Anthropol,* 65 (2006).
[117] R. Passingham, *Curr Opinion Neurobiol,* 19, 6 (2009).
[118] H. Harlow and J. A. Bromer, *Psychol Rev,* 19, 434 (1938).
[119] D. A. Washburn and D. M. Rumbaugh, *Int J Primatol,* 12, 377 (1991).
[120] M. R. Weed, *et al.*, *Brain Res Cogn.Brain Res,* 8, 185 (1999).
[121] N. H. Kalin and S. E. Shelton, *Ann N Y Acad Sci,* 1008, (2003).
[122] V. P. Bakshi, *et al.*, *Prog Brain Res,* 122, 105 (2000).
[123] E. Knobil, *Rec Prog Horm Res,* 30, 1 (1974).
[124] J. D. Veldhuis, *et al.*, *Mol Cell Endocrinol,* 299, 14 (2009).
[125] N. Sampson, *et al.*, *J Pathol,* 211, 206 (2007).
[126] R. H. Matousek and B. B. Sherwin, *Horm Behav,* 57, 352 (2010).
[127] J. S. Tenover, *et al.*, *J Gerontol,* 43, M163 (1988).
[128] W. J. Bremner, *et al.*, *J Clin Endocrinol Metab,* 56, 1278 (1983).
[129] D. J. Brambilla, *et al.*, *J Clin Endocrinol Metab,* 94, 907 (2009).
[130] G. F. Weinbauer and R. Korte, *Reproduction in nonhuman primates: a model system for human reproductive physiology and toxicology.* Waxmann Publishers, Muenster, NY (1999).
[131] T. M. Plant, *Endocr Rev,* 7, 75 (1986).
[132] S. Schlatt, *et al.*, *Biol Reprod,* 79, 93 (2008).
[133] L. W. Kaler, *et al.*, *Endocrinology,* 119, 566 (1986).
[134] S. M. Schwartz and J. W. Kemnitz, *Am J Phys Anthropol,* 89, 109 (1992).
[135] C. H. Phoenix and K. C. Chambers, *Proc Soc Exp Biol Med,* 183, 151 (1986).

[136] K. C. Chambers, *et al.*, *Physiol Behav,* 27, 615 (1981).
[137] J. A. Robinson, *et al.*, *Biol Reprod,* 13, 203 (1975).
[138] H. F. Urbanski, "Neuroendocrine rhythms in the aged macaque," 37th Annual Meeting of the American Aging Association, Boulder, CO, 2008.
[139] S. E. Abdelgadir, *et al.*, *Biol Reprod,* 60, 1251 (1999).
[140] J. A. Resko, *et al.*, *J Clin Endocrinol Metab,* 76, 1588 (1993).
[141] R. P. Michael, *et al.*, *J Neuroendocrinol,* 7, 713 (1995).
[142] J. V. Choate, *et al.*, *Endocrine,* 8, 51 (1998).
[143] A. N. Clancy, *et al.*, *Life Sci,* 50, 409 (1992).
[144] C. Leranth, *et al.*, *J Neurosci,* 23, 1588 (2003).
[145] N. J. MacLusky, *et al.*, *Neuroscience,* 138, 957 (2006).
[146] C. Leranth, *et al.*, *Cereb Cortex,* 14, 503, 2004 (2004).
[147] J. Bachevalier, *et al.*, *Dev Psychobiol.,* 22, 585 (1989).
[148] P. S. Goldman, *et al.*, *Science,* 186, 540 (1974).
[149] A. S. Clark and P. S. Goldman-Rakic, *Behav Neurosci,* 103, 1287 (1989).
[150] C. Hagger and J. Bachevalier, *Behav Brain Res,* 45, 57 (1991).
[151] R. A. Herman and K. Wallen, *Horm Behav,* 51, 496 (2007).
[152] A. Lacreuse, *et al.*, *Physiol Behav,* 98, 524 (2009).
[153] A. Tyagi, *et al.*, *Int J Androl,* 22, 139 (1999).
[154] A. Lacreuse, *et al.*, *Horm Behav,* 58, 854 (2010).
[155] R. M. Rose, *et al.*, *Nature,* 231, 366 (1971).
[156] R. M. Rose, *et al.*, *Science,* 178, 643 (1972).
[157] J. K. Rilling, *et al.*, *Biol Psychiatry,* 56, 364 (2004).
[158] J. D. Higley, *et al.*, *Biol Psychiatry,* 40, 1067 (1996).
[159] N. H. Kalin, *J Clin Psychiatry,* 60, 29 (1999).
[160] M. Mather and L. L. Carstensen, *Psychol Sci,* 14, 409 (2003).
[161] T. A. Ito, *et al.*, *J Pers Soc Psychol,* 75, 887 (1998).
[162] L. Carretié, *et al.*, *Int J Psychophysiol,* 71, 57 (2009).
[163] E. J. Hermans, *et al.*, *Biol Psychiatry,* 59, 872 (2006).
[164] E. J. Hermans, *et al.*, *Psychoneuroendocrinology,* 32, 1052 (2007).
[165] J. van Honk, *et al.*, *Behav Neurosci,* 115, 238 (2001).
[166] J. van Honk and D. J. Schutter, *Psychol Sci,* 18, 663 (2007).
[167] D. Pfaff, *et al.*, *Trends Neurosci,* 25, 45 (2002).
[168] H. M. King, *et al.* (2010). *Effects of testosterone on anxiety in male rhesus monkeys.* 14th annual meeting of the Society for Behavioral Neuroendocrinology, Toronto, CA.
[169] N. H. Kalin and S. E. Shelton, *Science,* 243, 1718 (1989).
[170] D. Bitran, *et al.*, *Horm Behav,* 27, 568 (1993).
[171] C. A. Frye and A. M. Seliga, *Cogn Affect Behav Neurosci,* 1, 371 (2001).
[172] D. Toufexis, *et al.*, *J Neurosci,* 25, 9010 (2005).
[173] A. Fernandez-Guasti and L. Martinez-Mota, *Psychoneuroendocrinology,* 30, 762 (2005).
[174] V. Viau, *J Neuroendocrinol,* 14, 506 (2002).
[175] J. L. Aikey, *et al.*, *Horm Behav,* 42, 448 (2002).
[176] A. Boissy and M. F. Bouissou, *Horm Behav,* 28, 66 (1994).
[177] M. F. Bouissou and M. Vandenheede, *Horm Behav,* 30, 93 (1996).
[178] A. B. Richards, *et al.*, *Horm Behav,* 56, 140 (2009).

[179] J. Hao, *et al.*, *Proc Natl Acad Sci,* 104, 11465 (2007).
[180] S. T. Charles, *et al.*, *J Exp Psychol Gen,* 132, 310 (2003).
[181] M. L. Keightley, *et al.*, *Psychol Aging,* 21, 558 (2006).
[182] D. M. Isaacowitz, *et al.*, *Emotion,* 6, 511 (2006).
[183] L. L. Carstensen, *Science,* 312, 1913 (2006).

In: Testosterone
Editor: Konstantin Chichinadze

ISBN 978-1-62100-492-9

Chapter III

Testosterone – Inducer of Aggression or Pleasure-related Hormone?

Konstantin Chichinadze[a,b,*]***, Nodar Chichinadze***[c]***,***
Ledi Gachechiladze[c]***, Ann Lazarashvili***[c]
[a]Life Science Research Center, Tbilisi, Georgia
[b]I. Javakhishvili Tbilisi State University, Georgia
[c]A. Natishvili Institute of Morphology, Tbilisi, Georgia

Abstract

Testosterone has been described in scientific literature as one of the principal inducers of aggressive behavior. At the same time, aggressive behavior is mainly viewed in association with negative emotions, such as anger, rage, and fury. On the other hand, substantial amount of information has been collected on inhibition of androgen synthesis under the influence of negative emotions and stressful events. Taking into consideration the fact that aggressive encounter is stressful for both losers and winners, above-mentioned statements clearly contradict each other to a certain extent.

The present article represents an effort to explain pre-encounter and post-encounter increase in testosterone level, as well as different dynamics of androgen levels in dominant and subordinate males in the frames of one concept.

The concept states:

1) Post-encounter increase of testosterone level is related to the pleasure received as a result of victory and sharp decrease of emotional tension. Besides, increased secretion of testosterone plays a role of positive reward for the type of behavior that has led to the victory.
2) Pre-encounter increase of testosterone is a result of excitement caused by anticipated victory. Individuals, who do not experience this kind of emotion before encounter, usually do not demonstrate increase of secretion and release of androgens.

* Corresponding author: k.chichinadze@lifescience.org.ge; ss_433@yahoo.com.

3) High basal level of testosterone in dominant males is present only in those instances, when dominating not only results in profit related to possession of resources, but is associated with low emotional tension, as well.

1. Introduction

It is widely accepted that among all hormones, testosterone (T) is most consistently linked to aggressive behavior (Baron & Richardson, 1994; Giammanco *et al.*, 2005; Simon & Lu 2006). Individuals with higher endogenous levels of T can be more aggressive and may be dominant over conspecifics with lower circulating T levels (Beehner et al. 2006; Cavigelli & Pereira 2000). This relationship between aggression and T is not exclusive to mammals and is observed in a variety of vertebrate taxa (Francis 1992). It is also known that territorial aggression associated with reproductive maturity appears to be mediated with few exceptions, by androgens resulting from gonadal maturation in all vertebrate classes (Wingfield *et al.* 2006). Despite these data there can be few hormone-behavior mechanisms that have been more controversial than the interaction of testosterone and aggression (Chichinadze et al., 2009, 2010, 2011; Mazur 2006; Wingfield et al., 2006). The fact is that, according to some researchers, T levels are positively related to aggression only in individuals with low cortisole (Mehta & Josephs 2010). Other scientists, contrary to the popular impressions, think that heightened T does not contribute directly to male violence (Mazur 2006) and T is importantly involved only in dominance behavior (Mazur 2009; Scotti et al. 2008). The cause of this contradiction is the undeniable fact that the administration of testosterone in the organism of animals increases, as a rule, their aggressiveness, also that the level of testosterone in aggressive/dominant individuals is higher than in other individuals, on the one hand. However, on the other hand, an agonistic encounter, during which an individual gains the dominant status, represents a stressful event, being very frequently such for both winners and losers (Summers & Windberg, 2006). According to Collins (2008), violent confrontation is fraught with tension and fear, while negative emotions lead to a suppression of testosterone synthesis (Davies et al. 1992).

So how do matters stand in fact? Is the gaining by organism of a higher hierarchic status caused by stimulation of aggression through testosterone, or is it associated with other processes?

This article is an attempt to demonstrate that a difference in T dynamics in dominants/winners and subordinates/losers is very largely associated with psychological/mental mechanisms, and that the gaining by the organism of a higher status upon stimulation with testosterone is not directly linked to an increase in aggressiveness but is rather a consequence of a formation in animals of the human-assertiveness analog. We would like to note that the psychological mechanism of differences in the T dynamics in dominants/winners and subordinates/losers had been discussed in greater detail earlier (Chichinadze & Chichinadze 2008). In the same article, we had analyzed a psychological component of this event as well, although not so thoroughly.

It is known that androgens influence or regulate the development or expression of suites of many morphological, physiological and behavioral traits that are closely related to male fitness (Adkins-Regan 2005). For example, in birds, it has been reported that plasma T levels correlate with testes size (Denk & Kempenaers 2005; Garamszegi et al. 2005), ornament size or color (Buchanan et al. 2001; Redpath et al. 2006), territorial and aggressive behavior, including mate guarding (Soma 2006), singing behavior (De Ridder et al. 2000; Foerster et al. 2002), courtship behavior (Fusani et al. 2007), mating success, etc. (Kempenaers et al. 2008; Raouf et al. 1997; Redpath et al. 2006). The same holds true in respect of mammals.

Analysis of literature concerning the linkage of T to aggressive/dominant behavior has revealed several main types of data in humans and animals: 1) pre-encounter/competition T growth in winners, 2) post-encounter/competition T growth in winners, 3) a higher basal level of T in dominants against subordinates, 4) increase in aggressive/dominant behavior under exogenously administered T, 5) increase in aggressive/dominant behavior during maximum rise in the endogenous T level (for example, during the reproduction period/mating).

In this article, we shall try to propose a new concept explaining these events within the framework of one paradigm.

There are several main hypotheses to explain the relationship between T level and aggressive/dominant behavior. Van der Meij *et al.* (2010) pointed out two of them: biosocial theory of status (Mazur & Booth, 1998) and the challenge hypothesis (Archer, 2006). Gleason *et al.* (2009) suggested three hypothesis: 1. Hypothesis about reinforce effect of T; 2. "Winner-Challenge Hypothesis"; 3. Hypothesis that elevated T following a competitive dispute might affect behaviors associated with winning and territoriality, without necessarily influencing aggressive behavior directly, *per se*. Wobber *et al.* (2010) wrote that two main psychological factors have been implicated in governing the endocrine changes surrounding competition within and between species: implicit power motive and coping style.

According to the biosocial theory of status, the relationship between status and T is reciprocal. The model predicts that in physical or non-physical competition, winning and thereby gaining status causes an increase in T, while losing decreases T levels. It has been proposed that winning or losing is not in itself enough to cause T levels to shift, but that T responses in reaction to competition are moderated by psychological processes (Salvador & Costa, 2009). In support of this it has been shown that a high motivation to win is positively related to T changes during competition (Suay et al., 1999) and a high power motivation predicts T increases among winners and decreases among losers (Schultheiss et al., 2005; Van der Meij et al. 2010). The challenge hypothesis predicts that T increases throughout a competitive interaction and may in the long-term cause a further rise of T in the winner of the competition. The outcome of such an interaction can be relevant for reproductive success, since it could affect the status, and thus the mating success of the winner. Therefore, according to the challenge hypothesis, in reaction to a challenging and evolving competition, T should first rise throughout the competition for both winners and losers and, only when considering a long-time interval, further increase among the winners (Van der Meij et al. 2010). These hypotheses have had notable success in explaining both inter- and intraspecific patterns of testosterone production across more than 60 species (Muller & Wrangham 2004; Wingfield et al. 2000). According to hypothesis about reinforce effect of T, this hormone reinforces learning associated with an aggressive encounter (Gleason et al. 2009).

Our concept, while not contradicting many provisions of the above concepts in the least, provides a better explanation of some facts. Let us first formulate our hypothesis and then attempt to analyze the available data on T dynamics with its help.

2. Hypothesis

The pivot of our concept consists of the following theses: (1) the strengthening of T synthesis is a result of not only the existence of challenges but also of a positive mood before an encounter associated with the "anticipation with pleasure" of a victory; (2) an increased T release to blood while decreasing anxiety, elevates mood of the body, increasing thus assertiveness and, consequently, aggressiveness of the organism.

When analyzing articles dealing with T level rise in humans and animals, we noted one peculiarity – the elevated T in the winners of agonistic contests is frequently observed both before and after an encounter. In losers such growth is not observed before encounters and is very seldom observed after encounters (see discussion of the issue in paragraphs 3.1 and 3.2). If in connection with the "after" situation all is clear, then how do organisms manage to "find out" whether they will win or lose before an encounter?

We assumed that in dominants and/or animals with experience of permanent victories in agonistic encounters any such challenge provokes the "anticipation" of a victory (probabilistic forecasting of a victory because of confidence thereof, and therefore the individual as if forecasting his/its victory – gets positive emotions. Probably, this process underlies positive dynamics of T before an encounter. In its turn, such discharge of T further improves mood. And the improvement of mood before an encounter tends to improve chances of the organism for winning. Of course, the unsuccessful party (loser) might also have the "anticipation" of a victory before an encounter. Perhaps this circumstance explains a high level of pre-encounter T in the blood of losers that had been fixed only in several studies (e.g., Oliveira et al. 2009). But one thing is to plan and anticipate and other is to realize what is anticipated. Nevertheless, most losers (especially permanent losers) most often can themselves forecast a loss with high probability, and such a forecast, like strong negative emotions in general, cannot stimulate synthesis and discharge of T.

The post-encounter T dynamics does not require a special explanation, since the victory-related positive emotions stimulate the production of T, while the loss-related negative emotions lead to its suppression.

According to our concept, a rise of T in an individual in the beginning of an agonistic encounter is observed only when it is associated with the anticipation of winning and increases after the encounter only if the individual wins in the given encounter or predicts winning in future encounters. It is obvious that in all these cases the body experiences positive emotions. T is found to function as a certain "pleasure" hormone being released in the situations (including upon occurrence of definite challenges) when the individual obtains or anticipates the obtaining of satisfaction. Being a product of comfort, T, in its turn, by reducing anxiety, enhances the sensation of comfort and (self-) confidence in the body/organism.

Animals, after several losses, rarely show an increase in T level before a new agonistic encounter, although at that the animal's level of aggressiveness might be rather high. This fact evidences that androgens are related but rather indirectly to the induction of an aggressive behavior. Very likely, the anticipation of a win upon occurrence of a challenge rather that existence of such challenge is the hormone growth booster.

As regards the biological sense/meaning of a post-encounter increase in synthesis and discharge of androgens, many researchers associate it with the positive reinforcing effects of androgens (Schultheiss & Rohde, 2002). Although, many authors consider that the biological function of the post-encounter T growth is associated with an increase of the mass bulk in animals (Newman et al. 2005). These observations will be analyzed below, yet we must note that such approach to the problems fails to explain why the level of T drops in losers. Do not they require an increase in the mass bulk?

3. Winners vs. Losers and Dominants vs. Subordinates: T Dynamics

3.1. Pre-encounter Increase of T Level

It is known that athletes' T rises shortly before their matches, as if in anticipation of the competition (Campbell et al. 1988; Booth, et al. 1989; Mazur et al., 1997). The anticipatory T response is described in several other studies (Mazur et al., 1992; Suay et al., 1999). Plasma T levels were higher in chess tournament winners, as well (Mazur et al. 1992). It is established that the athletes with higher anticipatory T growth before competition demonstrated greater motivation to win (Salvador et al. 2003). Other authors also note that men with a high power motive are more likely to show increases in testosterone before competition (Wobber et al. 2010). The same regularity is observed in animal species showing a high drive to achieve dominance rank, or power motive. In particular, in chimpanzees (Pan troglodytes), which, as compared with bonobos (Pan paniscus), have a higher power motive (Vervaecke et al., 2000; Wrangham & Pilbeam, 2001) and, unlike bonobos, their T level was observed to rise before competition (Wobber et al. 2010).

The results of the several studies convincingly proved that T is positively associated with a positive mood before competition (Salvador et al. 1991). Players with the highest pre-match testosterone had the most positive improvement in mood before their matches (Booth et al., 1989). If the mood elevation is absent or subjects do not regard the win as important, then the rise in T does not occur (Mazur & Lamb 1980) and in both winners and losers, T elevation is correlated to positive mood change (Mazur & Booth, 1998; McCaul, et al. 1992). In another study the authors did not find a statistically significant correlation between the level of T and positive mood of judo wrestlers; however, those wrestlers showing such a correlation had better results (Salvador et al. 2003).

Of course, the number of studies of T level in blood before competition significantly lags behind similar studies concerning plasma T levels after competition. At that, individual measurements of the given hormone concentration in dominants/winners and subordinates/losers were not carried out in all these studies. And, most important, rare studies have differentiated permanent winners from the first-time or accidental winners (Newman et al. 2005); notwithstanding the fact that it is primarily the frequency of victories that gives the winner an anticipatory feeling of a win before competition. We believe that this very factor is leading in T dynamics.

In spite of a wide recognition of the challenge theory, it seems strange how such directly inconsistent processes as challenges caused by different threats and the joy associated with a victory in an encounter (competition) can equally change the testosterone synthesis. In our opinion, challenges may stimulate the development and release of T only when they are associated with the prediction by animals or humans of their victory in a combat. Therefore, an anticipatory increase in T level is more frequently observed in winners.

3.2. Post-encounter Increase of T Level

The relevant literature contains many data on testosterone dynamics after an encounter and competition. Human studies have found that T level in winners of a sports contest increased after the winning even where the basal levels of the hormone in winners and losers did not differ. T levels in winners increase relative to losers in such physical contests as wrestling, martial arts, tennis, and in more cerebral contests, such as chess and coin flips (cited by Bernhardt et al. 1998). Plasma T levels were higher among sport supporters, even though they were not taking part in the competitions. It was reported that in 1994, after the victory of Brazil against Italy during the football World Cup, T significantly increased in those Brazilians who were watching the match on television, while it decreased in Italian supporters (Fielden et al. 1994; Giammanco et al. 2005).

Similar data have been also obtained in animal studies. Individuals that won the encounter had significantly higher T levels than those of controls, as found in several mammals: non-human primates (Cavigelli & Pereira, 2000), rodents (Buck & Barnes 2003; Oyegbile & Marler 2005). The same regularity is observed in many other vertebrates (Hirschenhauser & Oliveira 2006). At that, most pronouncedly such regularity occurred in territorial and highly aggressive animal species (Fuxjager & Marler 2010). These authors claim that post-encounter T increases only after a fight in home cage and it is possible that the residency-dependent nature of the winner effect is related to territoriality.

We think that the fact of T rise in the process of just watching an agonistic encounter, without participation therein ("audience effect") (Gleason et al. 2009) makes it clear that such an increase is linked to emotions experienced by an individual while watching the encounter; at that, the emotions are positive. After all, should the emotions be negative, no spike in androgens would have occurred, which fact was well demonstrated, for example, in supporters of losing teams in World Cup Soccer tournament (Bernhardt et al. 1998).

Animals (a) under stress and (b) with the permanent winning experience demonstrate negative emotions before an encounter and, especially, after losing, their T level being frequently dropped (see review by Chichinadze & Chichinadze 2008).

Obviously, if "anticipation" of winning is one of the factors enhancing T secretion in males (dominants), then it can be predicted that the presentation to the male of an a priori weak rival will cause the production of androgens in the former. An impression is created that this idea follows directly from our concept. However, this is not the case. Our concept states that only positive mood associated with the anticipation of a win is conducive to a rise in testosterone, rather than the anticipation of a victory as such. Where the anticipation of victory is present but the positive mood is lacking – no rise in T level will occur. This is indirectly confirmed by the results of several studies. In particular, as has been demonstrated in the already cited study, the lack in the winner of high motivation to win, or a victory won by luck rather than through own efforts does not lead to a rise in T level in winners (Booth et al. 1989; Giammanco et al. 2005; Mazur & Lamb 1980). Consequently, positive mood is the main factor conducive to a rise in the secretion of androgens before and after an encounter/game.

As we see, most available literary data correlate well with our concept. Schultheiss et al. (2005) have, however, advanced a concept on the relationship of T dynamics with the level of personal motive. They found that implicit power motivation enhanced implicit learning and T increases 15 min after the contest in winners and impaired implicit learning and T decreases 15 min after the contest in losers. We think these data are also consistent with our concept. The point is that under the term "anticipation of victory" we imply the presence of a strong power motive to win. Otherwise it would be simply expectation rather than anticipation of a victory. And expectation, unlike anticipation, may be emotionally neutral if the individual's motivation to win is low. Therefore, the individual's motivation in T level dynamics noted by Schultheiss et al. (2005) is part of our concept as well. Especially, as it is known that the fact of winning against the background of high motivation dramatically improves positive emotions, while a loss against the background of high motivation dramatically worsens mood and is associated with negative emotions. Conformation of the above is the work of the same team of researchers, which demonstrates that the increased cortisol post-contest was associated with high levels of power motivation among losers, suggesting that a social defeat is stressful for high-power individuals (Wirth et al. 2006).

But if the matter only concerned the power motive, then several defeats in an agonistic conflict for food would only reinforce in an individual the motive to win food because of the sense of hunger. We doubt that under such conditions (reinforcement of motive because of the sense of hunger, together with a rise in the level of stress because of the defeat) T level would tend to elevate. On the contrary, it is known that even a single defeat in an encounter might inhibit the plasma androgen level.

Mazur (2009) wrote that researchers "could in principle collect saliva samples before, during, and after fighting... Initially, cortisol would be high in most combatants. At the "tipping point" of a battle, as losers perceive their abysmal fate, their cortisol ought to measurably increase. Among winners, who now see the triumphant "light at the end of the tunnel," cortisol should decrease". Since expectation of a near victory sharply reduces the level of cortisole in winners, it can be assumed that if winners were sure of their victory, then the cortisol level would be low already at the beginning of fighting. And given the reciprocal relationship between cortisol and T, it is clear that the level of T in winners in such a situation can be high already at the beginning of fighting. All is in compliance with our concept.

3.3. High-ranking Individuals vs. Low-ranking Individuals: T Dynamics

Since positive emotions associated with a win in an agonistic encounter lead to an enhanced T synthesis, one might assume that the level of this hormone among the dominant in social hierarchy individuals will be higher than that of subordinates. Different studies carried out both under laboratory and field conditions confirm this assumption.

Across a variety of species, T levels regulate social dominance – a behavior intended to gain or maintain high status (Mazur & Booth, 1998). Higher T in humans is related to greater aggression and dominance motivation (Archer, 2006; Hermans et al., 2008; Josephs et al., 2003, 2006; Mehta & Josephs, 2006; Mehta et al., 2008, 2009; van Honk et al., 2001; Wirth & Schultheiss, 2007), especially when social status is up for grabs (Josephs et al., 2003, 2006; Mehta et al., 2008). Although most research on T and behavior has been conducted in men, a growing literature indicates that T also influences social dominance in women (Bateup et al., 2002; Hermans et al., 2008; Josephs et al., 2003, 2006; Mehta et al., 2008; van Honk et al., 1999, 2001). Overall, the evidence suggests that high T individuals are more motivated to gain status than low T individuals (Mehta et al. 2009). Nonhuman animal studies extend these observations (Kraus et al. 1999; Simon & Lu 2006). However, according to a number of studies this kind of patterns does not occur in all cases. In his research in wild baboons, Sapolsky (1991) demonstrated that T predicted status-related behaviors when the status hierarchy was unstable (after the α-male was crippled in fighting and social competition broke out). When the hierarchy was stable, however, T and behavior were unrelated (Mehta et al. 2008). A key to the explanation of the given phenomenon can become studies on stress and dominance interrelationship. Sapolsky's studies on stress and dominance status in Anubis baboons (Papio hamadryas anubis) revealed higher glucocorticoid levels in low-ranking compared to high-ranking individuals under stable conditions (Wingfield & Sapolsky, 2003). Data on a lesser stress level and correspondingly on glucocorticoids (GCs) among dominants and winners in agonistic encounters under stable conditions have been proved true in numerous studies (Abbott et al. 2003; Blanchard et al. 1993; Drews 1993; Hardy et al. 2002; Isovich et al. 2000; Kollack-Walker et al. 1997; Ostner et al. 2008; Stefanski 2001), whereas the idea that social stress might fall heavily on dominants has received much less attention (Creel, 2001; Creel & Sands, 2003). An exception to this regularity is the reproduction period among animals (for details see Chichinadze & Chichinadze 2008). But, on the other hand, as we have already mentioned, a difference between dominants and subordinates by the T blood level is generally observed under unstable conditions – the T concentration among dominants being raised against the basal level as well (Kraus et al. 1999; Sapolsky 1991). Consequently, under unstable conditions when the level of GCs among dominants is maximum, T level also attains peak values/tops out. It turns out that if GCs stimulate T synthesis in dominants. But contrary, it is known that GCs play an important role in the *inhibition* of T secretion (Consten et al. 2001; Dong et al. 2004; Gao et al 2002; Hardy et al. 2005; Sidibe et al. 1992). Experiments also confirm that a high level of GCs is combined with a low level of T (Castro and Matt 1997; Consten et al. 2001; Fenske 1997). The decrease of the blood level of testicular androgens during stress is probably the direct consequence of reduced synthesis of testicular androgens in the testicles, caused by GCs and adrenocorticotropic hormones. Besides the direct suppression of steroidogenesis, GCs enhance apoptosis of Leydig cells (Gao et al. 2002; Hardy et al. 2005) and increased apoptosis in the gonads is associated with decrease in the level of T in the blood (Jara et al. 2004). Based on all these data, a possible cause of a higher level of T in blood of dominants unstable conditions in population might be the fact that in such situation the number of agonistic encounters increases. It is logical to assume that dominants come into collision more frequently than other animals in expectation and in anticipation of a win. Hence the higher T level in their organism. Surely, the cause of different dynamics of T among dominants and subordinates can be of purely *physiological* origin (see for details Chichinadze & Chichinadze 2008). We, shall, however, content ourselves with the discussion in our paper of the psychological mechanisms of hormonal regulation only.

The fact that dominance exerts positive influence on T synthesis is noted by many researchers. In particular, Mazur (2009) wrote that "reciprocally, changes in dominance behavior can cause changes in testosterone level… Hypothetically, this provides a feedback loop in which success in competition heightens testosterone, which in turn facilitates future competitive success, and so on." The same opinion was suggested by Wingfield et al. (2006): "testosterone levels, even a single baseline measurement, correlate well with dominance behavior, that is, testosterone not only affects dominance behavior but also responds to it".

In the end of this section we would like to note that the difference between T levels among dominants/winners and subordinates/losers might be caused by both an enhanced T synthesis in the challenge situation among the former as well as by a reduced synthesis of the hormone under stressful events among the latter.

T increases vigilance toward dominance cues, such as angry, threatening faces (van Honk et al., 1999; Wirth & Schultheiss, 2007), and decreases vigilance toward submissive cues, such as fearful faces (van Honk et al., 2005). These effects of T on attention seem to be strongest when dominance-submission cues are presented outside conscious awareness (e.g., van Honk et al., 2005; Wirth & Schultheiss, 2007), suggesting that the relationship between T and dominant behaviors may be mediated, at least in part, by subconscious motivational and attentional processes (Mehta et al. 2008).

Without confidence of winning and/or the win itself in an encounter, angry emotion may generally stress the organism and consequently reduce rather than increase the production of T. It turns out that only upon availability of the "intrinsic" confidence of winning T can lead towards it, this being confirmed by the experimental data of Ruiz-de-la-Torre and Manteca (1991). In the study male lambs injected with T increased in dominant behaviors only after they were placed in a group of unfamiliar lambs and not when they were placed back in their original social group (Mehta et al. 2008). If T directly stimulated aggressiveness, then all the lambs injected with T would improve their status. But this did not happen. Apparently, T improves the status through reinforcing some other component, for example the animal assertiveness. It is clear that the growth of assertiveness will better improve the animal's status in the group where the hierarchic relations have not been yet established (in a group of unfamiliar lambs). Thus, androgens possesses dual-sided, aggression-increasing and fear-reducing, motivational properties (van Honk et al. 2005), for while increasing self-confidence of an individual, they reduce thereby the level of fear in him and increase aggressiveness.

4. "Home Advantage", Territoriality, Aggression and T

A rise in T levels during an agonistic encounter is known to be most frequently observed among territorial species (Fuxjager & Marler 2010; Wingfield et al. 2006). Moreover, post-encounter T pulses occur only after fights in the home cage (Fuxjager et al. 2009; Fuxjager & Marler 2010). Why does territoriality so affect the level of androgens during agonistic encounters? We think that the phenomenon lacks any logical explanations within the bounds of "classical" concepts. If we recall that most victories in the "resident-intruder" models are won by residents, it will become clear that our approach explains well this phenomenon. The point is that being in "own" territory significantly increases the confidence of winning among the residents of territorial species (it is quite natural – the "home advantage" effect is especially pronounced among territorial animal species), whereas the anticipation of winning is closely linked to the confidence of wining. According to our hypothesis, it is the anticipation of winning proper that participates in the enhancement of T synthesis. This can serve as an explanation of an intensive rise in the level of androgens among territorial animal species. Besides, males in the process of establishing a territory have higher plasma androgens than males that have already acquired a territory. Moreover, by simulating territorial intrusions the researchers revealed that the increase in plasma T and 11-ketotestosterone was due to male–male aggressive disputes, which occur more frequently during territory settlement (Gleason et al. 2009). The "home advantage" effect is also observed among men, representing a sporting phenomenon when a team wins oftener in home matches than in away matches (Neave & Wolfson, 2003). The analysis of the T level showed that soccer and hokey players' testosterone increases prior to a competition only when the match occurs at the home venue (Carre et al. 2006; Carre 2009; Gleason et al. 2009; Neave & Wolfson 2003). This is another corroboration of our idea concerning the role of anticipation of winning in the enhancement of T synthesis.

Sexual arousal in males is frequently associated with high plasma androgen levels and/or release of androgens in blood (Richardson et al. 2004). The fact that T is a leading factor during absolutely inconsistent processes, such as sexual arousal and dominant/aggressive behavior was noted by many other authors as well. Gleason et al. (2009) wrote that "we discuss how a steroid hormone such as testosterone can respond similarly to dissimilar social contexts and how this response can have different functional consequences for behavior". We believe that in fact a rise in T level in the challenge situation and upon sexual arousal is caused by the circumstance that both these processes are associated with positive emotions.

5. Behavioral/psychological Changes in the Organism under the Influence of T

In the previous sections we considered the influence of emotions on T synthesis. Now we shall analyze the influence of T on the behavioral/psychological parameters that determine the participation of the organism in agonistic encounters.

5.1. Reinforcing Effects of Androgens

In a natural environment, T secretion is intimately related to reinforcing social behaviors, including mating and aggression (Wood 2004). In laboratory environment this has been tested using two well established animal models for reward and reinforcement: conditioned place preference (CPP) and self-administration (Sato et al. 2008). Evidence from animal studies suggests T can have positive hedonic effects (Frye et al. 2002). Male hamsters preferentially self-administer testosterone orally (Johnson & Wood, 2001; Wood, 2002). In many studies of CPP, which is used to examine hedonic effects of drugs, a CPP was established by pairing systemic T (Alexander *et al.*, 1994; Packard *et al.*, 1997, 1998; Schroeder & Packard, 2000) or T applied centrally to the nucleus accumbens (Packard et al., 1997) or to the medial preoptic area (King et al., 1999), with a distinctive chamber (Frye 2007). As well, animals can be made to be physically dependent on anabolic-androgenic steroids (synthetic variants of the T) (Bonson *et al.*, 1994). Besides, reward and reinforcement with systemic T injections is not secondary to testosterone's systemic anabolic and androgenic actions (Sato *et al.* 2008). Packard et al. proved (1997) proved that injections of testosterone directly into the brain can produce a place preference. Likewise, Wood et al. (2004) has demonstrated intracerebroventricular (icv) T self-administration in male hamsters. Intracerebral CPP and icv self-administration with testosterone argue for central androgen reinforcement (Wood 2008). Reinforcement action of anabolic-androgenic steroids is also observed in humans (Frye 2007).

A. Mazur has speculated that post-victory testosterone surges, which can be observed within minutes and up to some hours after a dominance success, may serve to reinforce behavior that was instrumental for achieving the victory. This hypothesis has gained plausibility by recent findings that document rewarding (e.g., Packard *et al.* 1998) and mood-enhancing (e.g., Rabkin *et al.* 1996) effects of testosterone administration (Schultheiss & Rohde, 2002).

5.2. Androgens and Mood

5.2.1. Correlation between T Level and Mood

According to data from many studies, the enhancement of T synthesis positively correlates with improvement of mood after a win in the competition (Bernhardt et al. 1998), as well as with positive mood before the competition (Salvador et al. 1991). Although an interesting study by Gonzalez-Bono et al. (1999) did not detect a reliable growth of T in the winners before the match, it nevertheless demonstrated that tensions were significantly higher in the losers than in the winners before the match.

Furthermore, a correlation between mood and the level of different hormones participating in the regulation of T levels has been found, Fox example, it is known that participants having higher optimism scores exhibited less cortisol secretion in the awakening period (Lai et al. 2005).

Contrariwise, mood disturbances may be associated with decreased T level in men (Shores et al. 2009) and women (Rivera-Woll et al. 2004). Some studies came to the conclusion that testosterone levels are low in cases of dysthymic disorder and depression (Almeida et al., 2004; Barrett-Connor et al., 1999; Christiansen 2001; Ebinger et al. 2009; Heuser 2002; Seidman et al. 2002).

Surely, the available relevant literature contains many data evidencing the lack of a relationship between mood and T, between the fact of wining in an encounter and T., between dominance and T. The existence of any phenomenon or effect is to be proved by correct experiments/observations where it was observed, rather than by less correct experiments/observations where the given phenomenon could not be detected. The fact than someone failed to observe any phenomenon may not serve as the cause for refuting its existence

Since enhancement of the synthesis and excretion of T we have linked to positive emotions, then, taking into account the reinforcing action of androgens, it would be logical to expect that following the extraction T will contribute to mood elevation. This supposition is corroborated by the data on the action of exogenous T on mood, which will be discussed in the following section.

5.2.2. Improvement of Mood and Anxiolysis under the Influence of Exogenous T

One of the most replicated findings in research on the relationship between steroid hormones and emotional behavior involves reductions in fear after treatment with the T. This phenomenon has been demonstrated in a large variety of species using an excessive range of behavioral assessment paradigms (e.g., Aikey et al. 2002; Boissy & Bouissou 1994; Bouissou & Vandenheede 1996; Frye & Seliga 2001; Van Honk et al. 2005). Androgen administration can increase analgesia and anxiolysis in male and female rats (cited by Frye & Seliga 2001). T may also indirectly support sexual behavior via the ability of its androgenic metabolites to reduce anxiety (Gleason et al. 2009). The adrenal steroid hormone dehydroepiandrosterone (DHEA), which is a precursor to testosterone and estrogen, is able to prevent development of anxiety in a stressful environment (Ovsyukova et al. 2003).

In a randomized placebo-controlled cross-over trial of healthy premenopausal women complaining of loss of libido, testosterone cream resulted in not only an improvement in libido, but also in mood and general well being (Goldstat et al., 2003; Rivera-Woll et al. 2004).

T has the same effect during depression. A recent placebo-controlled study found that testosterone replacement was effective in older hypogonadal men with dysthymia or minor depression (Shores et al., 2009). DHEA also has an important role in mood regulation and may have significant antidepressant effects (Schmidt et al., 2005; Wolkowitz et al., 1999). Although, according to some researchers, it is possible that the positive effects of testosterone are restricted to dysthymic symptoms of androgen deficiency rather than major depressive episodes (Ebinger et al. 2009). This circumstance still more underlines the relationship between T and mood.

Given the data on i) the existence of a correlation between T level and mood, ii) the reinforcing action of androgens, as well as iii) the improvement of mood under influence of exogenously administered T, we can assume that similar mechanisms are responsible for pre-encounter and post-encounter increase of synthesis of T.

Conclusion

Analysis of literary and own data has demonstrated that T correlates with aggressiveness because its reinforced production/excretion is, at least partially, the result of self-assertion and positive mood. T acts as a pleasure hormone, being released in the situations when the organism gets pleasure and affords/increases the sense of pleasure. This is one of the most important conclusions from the submitted article/paper. By lessening anxiety and rendering the reinforcing action, T thus enhances the opportunity of aggressive response in both a short-term and long-term perspective. All the data denote T as modulator rather than inducer of aggressive/dominant behavior.

REFERENCES

Abbott, D.H., Keverne, E.B., Bercovitch, F.B., Shively, C.A., Mendoza, S.P., Saltzman, W., Snowdon, C.T., Ziegler, T.E., Banjevic, M., Garland, T.Jr., Sapolsky, R.M., 2003. Are subordinates always stressed? A comparative analysis of rank differences in cortisol levels among primates. *Horm Behav.* 43(1):67-82.

Adkins-Regan, E. 2005. Hormones and animal social behaviour. Princeton, NJ: Princeton University Press.

Aikey J.L., Nyby J.G., Anmuth D.M., James P.J. 2002. Testosterone rapidly reduces anxiety in male house mice (*Mus musculus*). *Horm Behav.* 42: 448-460.

Alexander G., Packard M., Hines M. Testosterone has rewarding affective properties in male rats: implications for the biological basis of sexual motivation. *Behav Neurosci.* 1994; 108:424-428.

Almeida, OP, Waterreus, A, Spry, N, Flicker, L, Martins, RN (2004). One year follow-up study of the association between chemical castration, sex hormones, beta-amyloid, memory and depression in men. *Psychoneuroendocrinology.* 29: 1071-1081.

Archer J. (2006). Testosterone and human aggression: an evaluation of the challenge hypothesis. *Neuroscience and Biobehavioral Reviews. 30(3)*:319-45.

Baron, R., & Richardson, D.R. (1994). *Human aggression.* New York: Plenum Press.

Barrett-Connor, E, Goodman-Gruen, D, Patay, B (1999). Endogenous sex hormones and cognitive function in older men. *J Clin Endocrinol Metab.* 84: 3681-3685.

Bateup, H.S., Booth, A., Shirtcliff, E.A., Granger, D.A., 2002. Testosterone, cortisol, and women's competition. *Evol Hum Behav.* 23:181-192.

Beehner JC, Bergman TJ, Cheney DL, Seyfarth RM, Whitten PL. Testosterone predicts future dominance rank and mating activity among male chacma baboons. *Behav Ecol Sociobiol* 2006; 59:469–79.

Bernhardt P.C., Dabbs Jr. J.M., Fielden J.A., Lutter C.D. 1998. Testosterone changes during vicarious experiences of winning and losing among fans at sporting events. *Physiol. Behav.* 65: 59-62.

Blanchard, D.C., Sakai, R.R., McEwen, B., Weiss, S.M., Blanchard, R.J., 1993. Subordination stress: behavioral, brain and neuroendocrine correlates. *Behav Brain Res.* 58(1-2):113-121.

Boissy A., Bouissou M.F. (1994). Effects of androgen treatment on behavioral and physiological responses of heifers to fear-eliciting situations. *Horm Behav.* 28:66-83.

Bonson K.R., Garrick N.A., Murphy D.L. Evidence for a withdrawal syndrome following chronic administration of an anabolic steroid to rats. *Soc Neurosci.* Abstr 1994. 20:1527.

Booth, A., Shelley, G., Mazur, A., Tharp, G. & Kittok, R. (1989) Testosterone, and winning and losing in human competition. *Hormones and Behavior.* 23:556–71.

Bouissou M.F., Vandenheede M. (1996). Long-term effects of androgen treatment on fear reactions in ewes. *Horm Behav.* 30:93-99.

Buchanan, K.L., Evans, M.R., Goldsmith, A.R., Bryant, D.M. & Rowe, L.V. 2001. Testosterone influences basal metabolic rate in male house sparrows: a new cost of dominance signalling? *Proc. R. Soc. B.* 268, 1337-1344.

Buck, C.L. and Barnes, B.M., 2003. Androgen in free-living arctic ground squirrels: seasonal changes and influence of staged male–male aggressive encounters. *Horm. Behav.* 43:318–326.

Campbell B., O'Rourke M., Rabow M. Pulsatile response of salivary testosterone and cortisol to aggressive competition in young males. Annual Meeting of the American Association of Physical Anthropologists, Kansas City, Missouri; 1988.

Carre J.M. 2009. No place like home: testosterone responses to victory depend on game location. *Am J Hum Biol.* 21:392–394.

Carre J., Muir C., Belanger J., Putnam S.K. 2006. Pre-competition hormonal and psychological levels of elite hockey players: relationship to the 'home advantage'. *Physiol. Behav.* 89: 392-398.

Castro, W.L. and Matt, K.S., 1997. Neuroendocrine correlates of separation stress in the Siberian dwarf hamster (*Phodopus sungorus*). *Physiol. Behav.* 61(4):477-484.

Cavigelli S.A., Pereira M.E. Mating season aggression and fecal testosterone levels in male ring-tailed lemurs (*Lemur catta*). *Horm Behav* 2000; 37:246-55.

Chichinadze K. & Chichinadze N. Stress-induced increase of testosterone: Contributions of social status and sympathetic reactivity. *Physiology & Behavior*. 2008. 94(4): 595-603.

Chichinadze K., Chichinadze N., Lazarashvili A. New Classification and Neurobiology of Aggressive Behavior. *Handbook of Aggressive Behavior Research*. Caitriona Quin and Scott Tawse (Editors). Nova Publishers. New York. 2009. pp. 183-213.

Chichinadze K., Chichinadze N., Lazarashili A. Hormonal and neurochemical mechanisms of aggression and a new classification of aggressive behavior. *Aggression and Violent Behavior*. 2011. DOI: 10.1016/j.avb.2011.03.002 (In press).

Chichinadze K.N., Domianidze T.R., Matitaishvili T.Ts., Chichinadze N.K. and Lazarashvili A.G. Possible Relation of Plasma Testosterone Level to Aggressive Behavior of Male Prisoners. *Bulletin of Experimental Biology and Medicine*. 2010. 149(1): 7-9

Christiansen, K (2001). Behavioural effects of androgen in men and women. *J Endocrinol.* 170: 39-48.

Collins, R. (2008) *Violence: A Micro-sociological Theory of Violence*. Princeton: Princeton University Press.

Consten, D., Lambert, J.G., Goos, H.J., 2001. Cortisol affects testicular development in male common carp, Cyprinus carpio L., but not via an effect on LH secretion. *Comp Biochem Physiol B Biochem Mol Biol.* 129(2-3):671-677.

Creel, S., 2001. Social dominance and stress hormones. *Trends Ecol. Evol.* 16: 491-497.

Creel, S. & Sands, J. L. 2003. Is social stress a consequence of subordination or a cost of dominance? In: Animal Social Complexity (Ed. by F. de Waal & P. Tyack), pp. 153-179. Cambridge, Massachusetts: Harvard University Press.

Davies R.H., Harris B., Thomas D.R., Cook N., Read G. & Riad-Fahmy D. 1992. Salivary testosterone levels and major depressive illness in men. *British Journal of Psychiatry*. 161: 629-632.

Denk, A.G. & Kempenaers, B. 2005 Testosterone and testes size in mallards (*Anas platyrhynchos*). *J Ornithol.* 147, 436-440.

De Ridder, E., Pinxten, R. & Eens, M. 2000. Experimental evidence of a testosterone-induced shift from paternal to mating behaviour in a facultatively polygynous songbird. *Behav. Ecol. Sociobiol.* 49:24-30.

Dong, Q., Salva, A., Sottas, C.M., Niu, E., Holmes, M., Hardy, M.P., 2004. Rapid glucocorticoid mediation of suppressed testosterone biosynthesis in male mice subjected to immobilization stress. *J Androl.* 25(6):973-981.

Drews, C., 1993. The concept and definition of dominance in animal behaviour. *Behaviour.* 125:283-313.

Ebinger M., Sievers C., Ivan D., Schneider H.J., Stalla G.K. Is there a neuroendocrinological rationale for testosterone as a therapeutic option in depression? *J Psychopharmacol.* 2009 Sep; 23(7): 841-53.

Fenske, M., 1997. Role of cortisol in the ACTH-induced suppression of testicular steroidogenesis in guinea pigs. *J Endocrinology.* 154:407-414.

Fielden J., Lutter C., Dabbs J. Basking in glory: Testosterone changes in World Cup soccer fans, Psychology Department, Georgia State University, 1994.

Foerster, K., Poesel, A., Kunc, H. & Kempenaers, B. 2002. The natural plasma testosterone profile of male blue tits during the breeding season and its relation to song output. *J. Avian Biol.* 33, 269-275.

Francis R.C., Jacobson B., Wingfield J.C., Fernald R.D. Castration lowers aggression but not social dominance in male *Haplochormis burtoni* (*Cichlidae*). *Ethology.* 1992. 90: 247-55.

Frye, C., 2007. Some rewarding effects of androgens may be mediated by actions of its 5α-reduced metabolite 3α-Androstanediol. *Pharmacol Biochem Behav.* 86: 354–367.

Frye, C.A., Rhodes, M.E., Rosellini, R., Svare, B., 2002. The nucleus accumbens as a site of action for rewarding properties of testosterone and its 5a-reduced metabolites. *Pharmacology, Biochemistry and Behavior.* 74:119-127.

Frye C.A., Seliga A.M. (2001). Testosterone increases analgesia, anxiolysis, and cognitive performance of male rats. *Cogn Affect Behav Neurosci.* 1:371-381.

Fusani, L., Day, L.B., Canoine, V., Reinemann, D., Hernandez, E. & Schlinger, B.A. 2007. Androgen and the elaborate courtship behavior of a tropical lekking bird. *Horm Behav.* 51: 62-68.

Fuxjager M., Marler C. (2010). How and why the winner effect forms: Influences of contest environment and species differences. *Behav Ecol.* 21:37-45.

Fuxjager MJ, Mast G, Becker EA, Marler CA. 2009. The 'home advantage' is necessary for a full winner effect and changes in postencounter testosterone. *Horm Behav.* 56:214-219.

Gao, H.B., Tong, M.H., Hu, Y.Q., Guo, Q.S., Ge, R., Hardy, M.P., 2002. Glucocorticoid induces apoptosis in rat leydig cells. *Endocrinology.* 143(1):130-138.

Garamszegi, L.Z., Eens, M., Hurtrez-Bousses, S. & Møller, A. P. 2005. Testosterone, testes size, and mating success in birds: a comparative study. *Horm. Behav.* 47, 389-409.

Giammanco, M., Tabacchi, G., Giammano, S., Di Majo, D., & La Guardia, M. (2005) Testosterone and aggressiveness. *Medical Science Monitor.* 11(4), RA 136-145.

Gleason E.D., Fuxjager M.J., Oyegbile T.O., Marler C.A. Testosterone release and social context: When it occurs and why. *Front Neuroendocrinol.* 2009. 30(4): 460-469.

Goldstat R., Briganti E., Tran J., Wolfe R. and Davis S. (2003). Transdermal testosterone improves mood, well being and sexual function in premenopausal women. *Menopause.* 10: 390-398.

Gonzalez-Bono E, Salvador A, Serrano MA, Ricarte J. Testosterone, cortisol, and mood in a sports team competition. *Horm Behav*. 1999. 35:55-62.

Hardy, M.P., Gao, H.B., Dong, Q., Ge, R., Wang, Q., Chai, W.R., Feng, X., Sottas, C., 2005. Stress hormone and male reproductive function. *Cell Tissue Res*. 322(1):147-53.

Hardy, M.P., Sottas, C.M., Ge, R., McKittrick, C.R., Tamashiro, K.L., McEwen, B.S., Haider, S.G., Markham, C.M., Blanchard, R.J., Blanchard, D.C., Sakai, R.R., 2002. Trends of reproductive hormones in male rats during psychosocial stress: role of glucocorticoid metabolism in behavioral dominance. *Biol Reprod*. 67(6):1750-1755.

Hermans, E., Ramsey, N., van Honk, J., 2008. Exogenous testosterone enhances responsiveness to social threat in the neural circuitry of social aggression in humans. *Biological Psychiatry*. 63(3): 263-270.

Heuser, I. (2002). Depression, endocrinologically a syndrome of premature aging. *Maturitas*. 41 (Suppl. 1): S19-S23.

Hirschenhauser, K. & Oliveira, R.F. 2006. Social modulation of androgens in male vertebrates: meta-analyses of the challenge hypothesis. *Animal Behaviour*. 71: 265-277.

Isovich, E., Mijnster, M.J., Flugge, G., Fuchs, E., 2000. Chronic psychosocial stress reduces the density of dopamine transporters. *Eur J Neurosci*. 12(3):1071-1078.

Jara, M., Carballada, R., Esponda, P., 2004. Age-induced apoptosis in the male genital tract of the mouse. *Reproduction*. 127(3):359-366.

Johnson L.R., Wood R.I. Oral testosterone self-administration in male hamsters. *Neuroendocrinology*. 2001. 73: 285-292.

Josephs, R.A., Newman, M.L., Brown, R.P., Beer, J.M., 2003. Status, testosterone, and human intellectual performance: stereotype threat as status concern. *Psychol Sci*. 14(2): 158-163.

Josephs, R.A., Sellers, J.G., Newman, M.L., Mehta, P.H., 2006. The mismatch effect: when testosterone and status are at odds. *J Pers Soc Psychol*. 90(6): 999-1013.

Kempenaers B, Peters A, Foerster K. 2008. Sources of individual variation in plasma testosterone levels. *Philos Trans R Soc Lond B Biol Sci*. 363(1497):1711-23.

King B.E., Packard M.G., Alexander G.M. Affective properties of intra-medial preoptic area injections of testosterone in male rats. *Neurosci Lett*. 1999. 269:149-152.

Kollack-Walker, S., Watson, S.J., Akil, H., 1997. Social Stress in Hamsters: Defeat Activates Specific Neurocircuits within the Brain. *The Journal of Neuroscience*. 17(22):8842–8855.

Kraus, C., Heistermann, M., & Kappeler, P.M. (1999). Physiological suppression of sexual function of subordinate males: A subtle form of intrasexual competition among male sifakas *(Propithesuc verreauxi)*. *Physiology and Behavior*, 66:855-861.

Lai JC, Evans PD, Ng SH, Chong AM, Siu OT, Chan CL, Ho SM, Ho RT, Chan P, Chan CC. Optimism, positive affectivity, and salivary cortisol. *Br J Health Psychol*. 2005. 10(Pt 4): 467-84

Mazur A. (2009). A Hormonal Interpretation of Collins's Micro-sociological Theory of Violence. *Journal for the Theory of Social Behaviour*, 39(4): 434-447.

Mazur A. (2006). The role of testosterone in male dominance contests that turn violent. *Biodemography and Social Biology*. 53(1-2): 24-29.

Mazur, A., Booth, A., 1998. Testosterone and dominance in men. *Behavioral and Brain Sciences*. 21 (3): 353-397.

Mazur A., Booth A., Dabbs J.M. Jr. Testosterone and chess competition. *Soc Psychol Q*, 1992; 55: 70–77.

Mazur, A. & Lamb, T. (1980) Testosterone, status, and mood in human males. *Hormones and Behavior*. 14: 236-246.

Mazur A., Susman E.J., Edelbrock S. (1997). Sex Difference in Testosterone Response to a Video Game Contest. *Evolution and Human Behavior*. 18: 317-326.

McCaul K., Gladue B. & Joppa M. (1992). Winning, losing, mood, and testosterone. *Hormones and Behavior*. 26: 486-506.

Mehta, P.H., Jones, A.C., Josephs, R.A., 2008. The social endocrinology of dominance: basal testosterone predicts cortisol changes and behavior following victory and defeat. *J. Pers. Soc. Psychol*. 94 (6), 1078–1093.

Mehta P.H. & Josephs R.A. (2010). Testosterone and cortisol jointly regulate dominance: Evidence for a dual-hormone hypothesis. *Hormones and Behavior*. 58: 898-906.

Mehta P.H., Wuehrmann E.V., Josephs R.A. (2009). When are low testosterone levels advantageous? The moderating role of individual versus intergroup competition. *Hormones and Behavior*. 56: 158-162.

Muller, M.N., & Wrangham, R.W. (2004). Dominance, aggression, and testosterone in wild chimpanzees: A test of the 'challenge hypothesis.' *Animal Behaviour,* 67, 113-123.

Neave N. & Wolfson S. 2003. Testosterone, territoriality, and the 'home advantage'. *Physiol. Behav*. 78: 269-275.

Newman M.L., Sellers J.G., & Josephs R.A. (2005). Testosterone, cognition, and social status. *Hormones and Behavior*. 47: 205-211.

Oliveira, T., Gouveia, M. J., & Oliveira, R. F. (2009). Testosterone responsiveness to winning and losing experiences in female soccer players. *Psychoneuroendocrinology*, 34, 1056-1064.

Ostner, J., Kappeler, P., Heistermann, M., 2008. Androgen and glucocorticoid levels re"ect seasonally occurring social challenges in male redfronted lemurs (*Eulemur fulvus rufus*). *Behav Ecol Sociobiol*. 62: 627-638.

Ovsiukova MV, Amikishieva AV, Kudriavtseva NN, Obut TA. Anxiolytic effect of dehydroepiandrosterone sulfate in male mice with high anxiety level. *Zh Vyssh Nerv Deiat Im I P Pavlova*. 2003. 53(6):789-93. Russian.

Oyegbile, T.O., Marler, C.A., (2005). Winning fights elevates testosterone levels in alifornia mice and enhances future ability to win fights. *Hormones and Behavior*. *48(3)*:259-267.

Rabkin, J.G., Wagner, G., and Rabkin, R. (1996). Treatment of depression in HIV+ men: Literature review and report of an ongoing study of testosterone replacement therapy. *Ann Behav Med*. 18: 24-29.

Packard M., Cornell A., Alexander G. Rewarding affective properties of intra-nucleus accumbens injections of testosterone. *Behav Neurosci*. 1997. 111:219-224.

Packard M., Schroeder J., Alexander G. Expression of testosterone conditioned place preference is blocked by peripheral or intra-accumbens injection of α-flupenthixol. *Horm Behav*. 1998. 34:39-47.

Raouf, S.A., Parker, P.G., Ketterson, E.D., Nolan, V. & Ziegenfus, C. 1997. Testosterone affects reproductive success by influencing extra-pair fertilizations in male dark-eyed juncos (Aves: *Junco hyemalis*). *Proc. R. Soc. B*. 264, 1599-1603.

Redpath, S.M., Mougeot, F., Leckie, F.M. & Evans, S.A. 2006. The effects of autumn testosterone on survival and productivity in red grouse, Lagopus lagopus scoticus. *Anim. Behav*. 71, 1297-1305.

Richardson H.N., Nelson A.L., Ahmed E.I., Parfitt D.B., Romeo R.D., Sisk C.L. 2004. Female pheromones stimulate release of luteinizing hormone and testosterone without altering GnRH mRNA in adult male Syrian hamsters (*Mesocricetus auratus*). *Gen. Comp. Endocrinol.* 138:211-217.

Rivera-Woll LM, Papalia M, Davis SR, Burger HG. Androgen insufficiency in women: Diagnostic and therapeutic implications. *Human Reproduction Update*. 2004. 10(5): 421-432.

Ruiz-de-la-Torre, J.L., & Manteca, X. (1999). Effects of testosterone on aggressive behaviour after social mixing in male lambs. *Physiology andBehavior*. 68: 109-113.

Salvador, A., & Costa, R. (2009). Coping with competition: Neuroendocrine responses and cognitive variables. *Neuroscience and Biobehavioral Reviews*, 33:160-170.

Salvador A, Martinez S, Suay F, Borras JJ, Perez M, Montoro JB. Relationship between testosterone and psychological mood states. II Congre s Mundial del COI de Cie`ncies de l'Esport, Barcelona; 1991.

Salvador, A., Suay, F., Gonzalez-Bono, E., Serrano, M.A., 2003. Anticipatory cortisol, testosterone and psychological responses to judo competition in young men. *Psychoneuroendocrinology*. 28:364–375.

Sapolsky, R.M. (1991). Testicular function, social rank, and personality among wild baboons. *Psychoneuroendocrinology*, 16, 281-293.

Sato S.M., Schulz K.M., Sisk C.L., and Wood R.I. (2008). Adolescents and androgens, receptors and rewards. *Hormones and Behavior*. 53: 647-658.

Schmidt P.J, Daly R.E., Bloch M., Smith MJ, Danaceau MA, Simpson St. Clair L, Murphy JH, Haq N, Rubinow DR. (2005). Dehydroepiandrosterone monotherapy in midlife-onset major and minor depression. *Archive of General Psychiatry*. 62: 154-162.

Shores M.M., Kivlahan D.R., Sadak T.I., Li E.J., Matsumoto A.M. A randomized, double-blind, placebo-controlled study of testosterone treatment in hypogonadal older men with subthreshold depression (dysthymia or minor depression). *J Clin Psychiatry*. 2009. 70(7):1009-1016.

Schultheiss, O.C., & Rohde, W. (2002). Implicit power motivation predicts men's testosterone changes and implicit learning in a contest situation. *Hormones & Behavior*. 41: 195–202.

Schultheiss O.C., Wirth M.M., Torges C.M., Pang J.S., Villacorta M.A., Welsh K.M. (2005). Effects of implicit power motivation on men's and women's implicit learning and testosterone changes after social victory or defeat. *J Pers Soc Psychol*. 88(1):174-188.

Schroeder J.P., Packard M.G. Role of dopamine receptor subtypes in the acquisition of a testosterone conditioned place preference in rats. *Neurosci Lett*. 2000. 282:17-20.

Scotti MA, Belén J, Jackson JE, Demas GE. The role of androgens in the mediation of seasonal territorial aggression in male Siberian hamsters (*Phodopus sungorus*). *Physiol Behav*. 2008. 95(5): 633-40.

Seidman, S.N., Araujo, A.B., Roose, S.P., Devanand, D.P., Xie, S., Cooper, T.B., et al. (2002). Low testosterone levels in elderly men with dysthymic disorder. *Am J Psychiatry*. 159: 456-459.

Sidibe, M., Franco, L.A., Fredriksson, G., Madej, A., Malmgren, L., 1992. Effects on testosterone, LH and cortisol concentrations, and on testicular ultrasonographic appearance of induced testicular degeneration in bulls. *Acta Vet Scand*. 33(3):191-196.

Simon N.G. & Lu S-F. 2006. Androgens and Aggression. In Randy J. Nelson (Eds.), *Biology of Aggression*. (pp. 211-230). New York, Oxford University Press.

Stefanski, V., 2001. Social stress in laboratory rats: behavior, immune function, and tumor metastasis. *Physiol. Behav*. 73(3):385-391.

Suay F, Salvador A, Gonzalez-Bono E, Sanchis C, Martinez M, Martinez-Sanchis S, Simon VM, Montoro JB. Effects of competition and its outcome on serum testosterone, cortisol and prolactin. *Psychoneuroendocrinology*. 1999 Jul; 24(5):551-566.

Soma, K.K. 2006. Testosterone and aggression: berthold, birds and beyond. *J. Neuroendocrinol*. 18, 543-551.

Summers, C.H., & Winberg, S. (2006). Interactions between the neural regulation of stress and aggression. *The Journal of Experimental Biology, 209*, 4581-4589.

Van der Meij L, Buunk AP, Almela M, Salvador A. Testosterone responses to competition: The opponent's psychological state makes it challenging. *Biol Psychol*. 2010 May; 84(2):330-335.

van Honk, J., Peper, J., & Schutter, D. (2005). Testosterone reduces unconscious fear but not consciously experienced anxiety: Implications for the disorders of fear and anxiety. *Biological Psychiatry, 58*: 218-225.

van Honk, J., Tuiten, A., Hermans, E., Putnam, P., Koppeschaar, H., Thijssen, J., et al., 2001. A single administration of testosterone induces cardiac accelerative responses to angry faces in healthy young women. *Behav Neurosci*. 115(1): 238-242.

van Honk, J., Tuiten, A., Verbaten, R., van den Hout, M., Koppeschaar, H., Thijssen, J., et al. (1999). Correlations among salivary testosterone, mood, and selective attention to threat in humans. *Hormones and Behavior*. 36: 17-24.

Vervaecke H., de Vries H., van Elsacker L. (2000). Dominance and its behavioral measures in a captive group of bonobos (*Pan paniscus*). *Int J Primatol*. 21:47–68.

Wingfield, J. C., Jacobs, J. D., Tramontin, A. D., Perfito, N., Meddle, S., Maney, D. L. & Soma, K. 2000. Toward an ecological basis of hormone-behavior interactions in reproduction of birds. In *Reproduction in Context: Social and Environmental Influences on Reproduction* (Ed. by K. Wallen & J. E. Schneider), pp. 85-128. Cambridge, Massachusetts: MIT Press.

Wingfield, J.C., Moore, I.T., Goymann, W., Wacker, D.W. & Sperry, T. (2006). Contexts and Ethology of Vertebrate Aggression: Implications for the Evolution of Hormone-Behavior Interactions. In Randy J. Nelson (Eds.), *Biology of Aggression*. (pp. 179-210). New York, Oxford University Press.

Wingfield, J.C., & Sapolsky R.M., (2003). Reproduction and resistance to stress: when and how. *Journal of Neuroendocrionology*. 15: 711-724.

Wirth, M.M., & Schultheiss, O.C. (2007). Basal testosterone moderates responses to anger faces in humans. *Physiology & Behavior*. 90: 496–505.

Wirth M.M., Welsh K.M., Schultheiss O.C. (2006). Salivary cortisol changes in humans after winning or losing a dominance contest depend on implicit power motivation. *Hormones and Behavior*. 49: 346-352.

Wobber V, Hare B, Maboto J, Lipson S, Wrangham R, Ellison PT. Differential changes in steroid hormones before competition in bonobos and chimpanzees. *Proc Natl Acad Sci U S A*. 2010 Jul 13; 107(28):12457-62.

Wolkowitz O.M., Reus V.I., Keebler A., Nelson N., Friedland M., Brizendine L., Roberts E. Double-blind treatment of major depression with dehydroepiandrosterone. *Am J Psychiatry*. 1999. 156:646-649.

Wood, R.I. Anabolic–androgenic steroid dependence? Insights from animals and humans. *Frontiers in Neuroendocrinology*. 2008. 29: 490-506

Wood, R.I. Reinforcing aspects of androgens. *Physiol Behav*. 2004. 83: 279-289.

Wood, R.I. Oral testosterone self-administration in male hamsters: dose-response, voluntary exercise, and individual differences. *Horm Behav*. 2002. 41(3):247-258.

Wood R.I., Johnson L.R., Chu L., Schad C.A., Self D.W. Testosterone reward: intravenous and intracerebroventricular self-administration. *Psychopharmacology*. 171 (2004) 298–305.

Wrangham R., Pilbeam D. (2001). *African apes as time machines*. All Apes Great and Small, eds Galdikas B, Briggs N, Sheeran L, Shapiro G, Goodall J (Kluwer Academic) Plenum Publishers, New York), pp 5-18.

In: Testosterone
Editor: Konstantin Chichinadze

ISBN 978-1-62100-492-9

Chapter IV

Testosterone Metabolism: The Significance of Aromatase Activity

James I. Raeside
Department of Biomedical Sciences, Ontario Veterinary College, University of Guelph, Guelph, Ontario, Canada

Abstract

Tissues in both sexes can be regulated by a balance of androgenic and estrogenic effects. The predominant secretion of androgens from the testes and estrogens from the ovaries sets the stage, and the dominant position of the liver in metabolism has a significant part to play. In addition, an important component in the response of the target tissues is the presence and concentration of specific hormone receptors. Less well recognized and studied is the role of local metabolism: enzymes in target tissues themselves constitute a final step in the delivery of the appropriate, or inappropriate, steroid product to the target cell. The complement of enzymes can lead to steroid inactivation, a weaker agent or even an enhanced activity. Examples of these are testosterone sulfate, androstenedione and 5α-dihydrotestosterone, respectively. However, another potential fate for an androgen in some target tissues is the formation of C_{18} products from the C_{19} androgens by action of an aromatase enzyme—just as occurs for estrogen biosynthesis in the ovaries, and in the testes to some extent. In the latter case, some species are remarkable for the large amounts of estrogens secreted from the testes. The importance of estrogens in the male is well documented, for the most part; the actions include those on bone, muscle and skin along with those more directly associated with reproduction (e.g. efferent ductules of the testes and libido itself). Lastly, aromatase activity in target tissues—and in the testes of some species—can result in the formation of C19-norandrogens that are recognized as endogenous anabolic agents. With the tremendous interest in 19-nortestosterone and efforts to replicate its properties with acceptable commercial products, the formation of 19-nortestosterone and its local metabolism is frequently underappreciated. This review will attempt to redress some aspects of testosterone metabolism that seem to deserve more consideration than usually given.

INTRODUCTION

It bears repeating that testosterone and other androgens are not the preserve of the male; likewise, estrogens are not restricted in their biosynthesis and biological actions to females of the species. In both sexes tissues can be regulated by a balance of androgenic and estrogenic actions. The stage is set initially by the secretion of androgens predominantly from the testes and estrogens from the ovaries—interesting exceptions to the 'rule' can be cited which present challenges for later consideration in this chapter. Meanwhile, the dominant position of the liver in steroid metabolism is acknowledged as having a major role in determining the amounts of the so-called 'sex hormones' that prevail at the level of the target tissues. The resulting response may then depend largely on the presence and concentrations of specific hormone receptors that are seen as a characteristic of the tissues involved. However, before the steroid hormones reach the receptors they may be subjected to 'local metabolism' by enzymes within the target tissues themselves [1]. This aspect of the biological action of steroid hormones has received less attention but has been gaining recognition over the past few decades since the classical demonstration of testosterone as a pro-hormone by its conversation to 5α-dihydrotestosterone (5α-DHT) in the prostate gland [2]. In addition to creating a more active product from testosterone, such as 5α-DHT, the presence of enzymes locally can lead to formation of a weaker androgen (androstenedione) or even inactivation by conjugation (testosterone sulfate or testosterone glucuronidate). Thus, local metabolism by enzymes in the target tissues constitutes a final step in the delivery of the appropriate, or inappropriate, steroid product to the target cell in a paracrine, or autocrine, rather than an endocrine manner.

There remains one further form of local metabolism that has been less well recognized and studied. A potential fate for an androgen in some target tissues is the formation of C_{18} products from the C_{19} androgens by the action of an aromatase enzyme—as occurs for estrogen biosynthesis in the ovaries, and in the testes to a lesser extent. Indeed, the high level of aromatase activity in the testes of the stallion results in the surprising situation in which the secretion of estrogens surpasses that of androgens by a factor of about one-hundred fold [3]. The importance of estrogens in the male from whatever source, testes or peripheral formation, is well documented; the actions include those on bone, muscle, brain and skin [4] as well as those more directly related to reproduction (e.g. prostate [5], efferent ductules of the testes [6], and libido itself [7,8]).

Besides the formation of estrogens, the activity of aromatase can result in the formation of C_{18} steroids that lose the methyl group at C19 but fail to undergo the remaining steps to complete the fully unsaturated ring A as seen in natural estrogens. This gives rise to the C19-norandrogens that are recognized as endogenous anabolic agents. Their formation is noted by relatively high amounts of 19-nortestosterone in the testes in some species [9, 10] and the presence of 19-norandrostenedione in ovarian follicular fluid [11, 12]. In fact, Short's finding 50 years ago [11] was the first time that a non-aromatic 19-nor steroid had been found as a natural product. Whether norandrogens can be metabolized further to estrogens in particular, and to other products, seems to depend on various factors—organ, species, and age. In view of the immense interest in 19-nortestosterone and efforts to replicate its biological properties with acceptable commercial products, the biosynthesis of 19-nortestosterone and its local metabolism is largely underappreciated. The aim of this review is to present the role of the aromatase enzyme(s) as a significant component of the total scheme of testosterone metabolism. Evidence is derived largely from studies on mammalian species; it is not restricted by sex or age, but has emphasis on the male. This bias seems justified insofar as recognition of a natural position for aromatase activity in the male gained full acceptance only after the discovery of human patients deficient in aromatase [13, 14].

OVERALL METABOLISM OF TESTOSTERONE

The position and importance of aromatase in the metabolism of testosterone can best be appreciated by starting with a brief overview of its metabolism, to be followed by a focus on aromatase itself. A scheme is presented that is a composite of the activities of a large number of enzymes distributed in many organs and tissues throughout the body (Figure 1). It is derived mainly from studies of mammalian species but makes no attempt to reflect the more limited range of steroid metabolizing enzymes found in any one species. With the exception of the liver, which plays a major role in testosterone metabolism, the complement of enzymes involved is very much limited in other tissues. The degree of restriction also applies, appropriately, to the testes and ovaries that are the principal source of testosterone in the male and estrogens through aromatase action on androgens in the female. In the gonads the 17β-hydroxysteroid dehydrogenases (17β-HSD) are especially prominent in ensuring that the most active form of the sex hormones is secreted by the testes and ovaries, respectively.

The two most important biologically active products of testosterone metabolism are 5α-dihydrotestosterone (5α-DHT) and 17β-estradiol (17β-E2). In both cases testosterone serves as a pro-hormone, mainly in target tissues in the male where the enzyme steroid 5α-reductase acts to reduce the double bond in the A ring of the steroid molecule. Two isozymes of 5α-reductase are recognized and their distribution is apparently tissue- and species-specific [15]. Beyond this, 5α-DHT can be converted by further reduction to 3α- and 3β-androstanediol (3α-Adiol and 3β-Adiol) by the enzymes 3α-hydroxysteroid dehydrogenase (3α-HSD) and 3β-hydroxysteroid dehydrogenase (3β-HSD), respectively. This takes place mainly in the liver but also in other peripheral tissues [16]. Moreover, an interconversion is possible between the active 5α-DHT and the inactive 3α-Adiol that defines the response to androgens in many tissues. In contrast the back conversion of 3β-Adiol → 5α-DHT does not occur and it should be noted that 3β-Adiol shows an affinity for the estrogen receptor β (ER-β, ER2) and thus may be considered a weak estrogen with a degree of specificity in its action [17].

The second major biological product of testosterone metabolism is estradiol which results from the aromatase activity of a cytochrome P450 enzyme (P450arom). Although this microsomal enzyme is present in Leydig cells the amounts of estrogens formed in the testes of adult males are decidedly modest—with the remarkable exception of members of the equine and porcine families where the male greatly surpasses the non-pregnant female in their respective species [3, 18]. The activity of P450arom in the ovaries and the placenta would otherwise account for the much higher estrogen levels in females. Several tissues in the body have the capability of converting testosterone to estradiol with important consequences (e.g. adipose tissue, brain) in a local ('intracrine') manner. These and other aspects of the aromatase enzyme will be considered in greater detail later in this chapter.

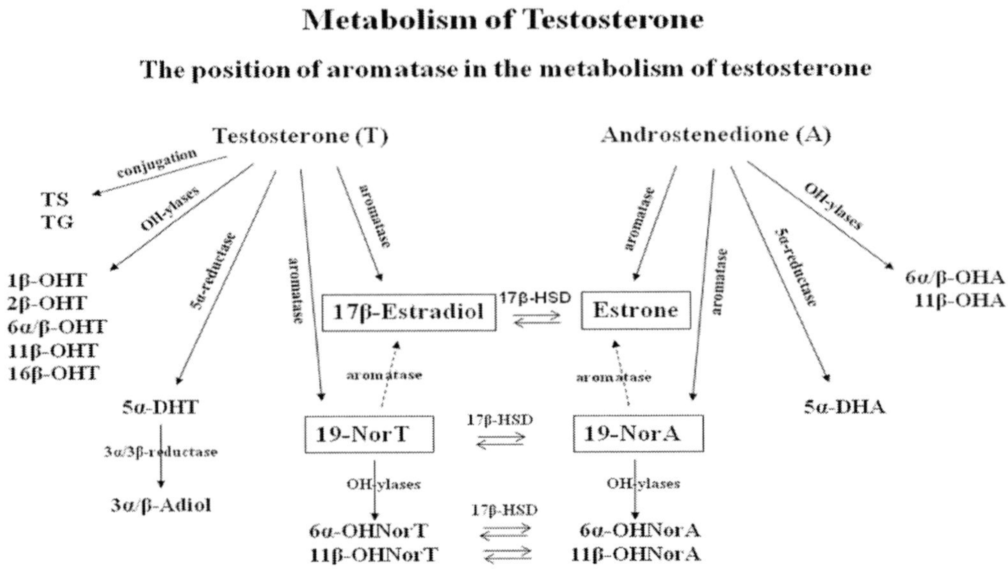

Figure 1. Abbreviations: 19-NorT, 19-nortestosterone; 19-NorA, 19-norandrostenedione; TS, testosterone sulfate; TG, testosterone glucuronoside; -OH, -hydroxy; 5α-DHT, 5α-dihydrotestosterone; 5α-DHA, 5α-dihydroandrostanedione; 3α/β-Adiol, 3α or 3β, 17β-androstanediol; 17β-HSD, 17β-hydroxysteroid dehydrogenase; OH-ylases, hydroxylases; conjugation – sulfotransferase, glucuronyltransferase.

Still on the subject of reductive activity there is a critical role played by 17β-HSDs in the testes and ovaries, as alluded to earlier, but not restricted to the gonads (Figure 2). The reductive action is dominant in the biosynthesis of the key sex hormones in the gonads whereas the preferential direction in the interconversion (oxidation/ reduction) largely determines the response in the peripheral tissues. For example, an isozyme that is a dehydrogenase would cause formation of the weaker 17-ketosteroid, androstenedione, to 'protect' the female from overexposure to testosterone.

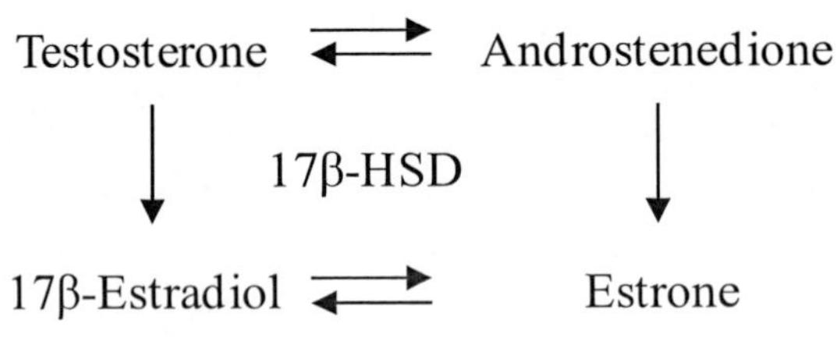

Figure 2. Role of 17β-hydroxysteroid dehydrogenase in steroidogenesis.

Another group of enzymes, found principally in the liver, is responsible for metabolism of testosterone to monohydroxylated products that serve in removal of the hormone in the urine and bile (see Dorfman and Ungar's monograph [19] for a comprehensive review of the earlier literature). Hydroxylation has been noted at carbons 2, 6, 7, 11 and 16 that results in hydrophilic compounds that are more readily excreted—especially when hydroxylation occurs at more than one site such as in androgen triol and tetrol metabolites. Few species other than primates show hydroxylation at C16. The situation with hydroxylation at C11 is particularly interesting in that the testes rather than the adrenal glands may be involved in some instances. In fact, the principal androgen in salmonid fish is not testosterone but 11-keto-testosterone from the testes [20]. Furthermore, in at least one mammalian species, the pig, 11β-OH-testosterone and 11β-OH-androstenedione have been shown to be secreted by the testes [21]; no biological function for these testicular products has been demonstrated, as yet, in the boar. Although the activity of the hydroxylases is less pronounced in tissues other than the liver, it is likely that local metabolism of testosterone has an influence on the action of the hormone in some target tissues, at least in reducing the exposure to testosterone itself. Moreover, there remains the possibility that a specific biological function for some of the hydroxylated derivatives of testosterone may exist— though not yet demonstrated.

The last group of enzymes to consider in a general review of testosterone metabolism is instrumental in the conjugation of testosterone and its hydroxylated products formed in the liver and other tissues. The role of conjugation is mainly to promote the elimination of testosterone from the body. Sulfotransferases and glucuronyltransferases are the principal ones in the liver giving water-soluble conjugates that are readily removed by the kidneys. Only minor amounts of testosterone (2%) are excreted unchanged in human subjects but much greater quantities of the more hydrophilic products of its further hydroxylation are found in urine. The bulk of the metabolites in urine nonetheless occur in some form of conjugation with sulfuric or glucuronic acid. Not all of the sulfate conjugation takes place in the liver (or kidneys), however. The male reproductive tracts of the stallion and boar show significant sulfotransferase activity with testosterone although much lower than with estrogens [22, 23]. An early report on the finding of sulfoconjugated neutral steroids in human testis tissues [24] is pertinent to later discussion in this chapter.

Aromatase Metabolism of Testosterone and Androstenedione

Part 1

Estrogen Action in Males

As preface to a discussion on the formation of estrogens from androgens it is apposite to briefly consider the actions of estrogens in the male—this would be redundant for the female. Earlier studies on the biological actions of estrogens were reviewed extensively by H. Burrows in 1949, comprising several chapters in his book on the "Biological Actions of Sex Hormones" [25]. They extend from embryonic gonads and the reproductive tract to effects on the adult gonads, external genitalia and accessory genital organs, and to a further broad array of actions on skin, bone, muscle, pituitary, brain, liver, pancreas, thymus, and the excretion of electrolytes and water. The scientific value of such studies naturally attained more acceptable levels after the first isolation of a crystalline estrogen was achieved in 1929; before that time an estrogen was a hypothetical substance which could be recognized only by its biological effects. Nevertheless, the broad range of responses was impressive especially when applied to the male. It became an interesting challenge when estrogen-like effects were observed after the administration of testosterone—which had not been obtained in crystalline form until 1935 [26]. Ample evidence of important actions of estrogen in the male, from whatever source, has accumulated over the decades since the early work following the identification of the sex hormones. The seminal report on estrogen insensitivity in an adult man with an inactivating mutation of ERα [27] generated heightened interest in estrogen receptors in the male and provided the impetus for growth of investigations on this topic. An extensive literature on the effects of estrogens in the male developed subsequently and has been the subject of many reviews [e.g. 8].

History of Aromatase

The need to include aromatase in any discussion of testosterone metabolism, in males in particular, was made more obvious by reports on men with mutations of the cytochrome P450 aromatase gene (*CYP19*) [13]. With the full determination of the chemical structure of the sex hormones in the 1930s it became evident that testosterone and the estrogens were closely related. The true nature of that relationship was first suggested to Bernhard Zondek in 1934 when he was astonished to find that stallion's urine contained even more estrogen than that of pregnant mares. [28]. He was even more surprised to find a high concentration of estrogens in the testes of stallions [29]. From these observations he concluded that the estrogen which was present naturally in stallions had to be a metabolite of androgens. The subsequent endeavours leading to the establishment of the relationship between androgens and estrogens have been incorporated recently into an engaging review provided by some of the participants in these studies (History of Aromatase: Saga of an Important Biological Mediator and Therapeutic Target) [30].

A few major steps are deserving of mention and are sufficient for the purposes of this chapter. Firstly, Zondek was shown to be prescient in the conclusion he drew when a few years later an increase in estrogenic activity in urine was noted after the administration of testosterone propionate to men [31]. Studies of estrogen biosynthesis received an added stimulus when 19-OH-androstenedione was isolated in1955 from incubation of androstenedione with bovine adrenals [32] and shown to be converted to estrone by endocrine tissues [33]. This was suggested to be the first step of an enzymatic process leading to the removal of the C19 methyl group and the desaturation of the A ring of an estrogen. Further work indicated that19-oxo-androstenedione was an intermediary compound between 19-OH-androstenedione and estrogen. Definitive proof for the conversion of a non-aromatic steroid to an estrogen was demonstrated by the use of a radiolabeled steroid (4-C^{14}-testosterone) as substrate [34]. Thus, the following scheme was proposed: testosterone → 19-OH-androstenedione → 19-oxo-androstenedione → estrogen. A strict requirement for oxygen and for reduced nicotinamide adenine dinucleotide phosphate (NADPH) was noted for the formation of estrogen from both C19-oxygenated compounds. It was not until the 1980s when a pure preparation of an enzyme was finally achieved [35] that the "aromatization process" was found to be the action of a single enzyme rather than a multienzyme system. The last step in aromatization also required an oxidation that was shown to occur at C1 with the loss mainly of 1β-tritium from samples of androstenedione labeled with ^3H at C1 in either the α or β position [36]. To conclude this section it is interesting to note that a one-step radiometric assay for aromatase activity was developed, from the more basic study, in which tritium release from a 1β-tritium-labeled substrate was measured as tritiated water (^3H_2O) [37]. Soon this assay was being applied with great success in studies on breast cancer and especially in studies on the development of aromatase inhibitors.

Aromatase Properties and Structure

Cytochrome P450 aromatase (P450arom) is a member of the cytochrome P450 superfamily which is a large and diverse group of enzymes whose function is mostly to catalyze the oxidation of organic substances. They function mainly in the metabolism of xenobiotic substances such as drugs and other toxic chemicals but are also important in the biosynthesis and metabolism of lipids and steroid hormones. While most cytochromes P450 act as monooxygenases to insert one atom of oxygen into an organic substrate, P450arom characteristically operates as a single enzyme in a series of oxidation steps to accomplish an androgen → estrogen conversion.

$$RH + O_2 + 2H^+ + 2e^- \rightarrow ROH + H_2O$$

P450arom is the only P450 enzyme in vertebrates known to catalyse the biosynthesis of all estrogens from androgens. In a three-step process, each step requires one mole of oxygen, one mole of NADPH, coupled with its redox partner cytochrome P450 reductase, for every mole of androgenic steroid substrate. The first two steps are C19-methyl hydroxylation steps while the third involves the aromatization of the steroid A-ring, a property unique to P450arom—setting it apart from other P450s. The human enzyme is a monomeric protein existing as a single polypeptide chain of 503 amino-acid residues (molecular mass about 55 kDa) and comprising principally a heme group, a specific substrate binding element and an amino terminal transmembrane domain anchoring it to the endoplasmic reticulum. Early studies on human placental aromatase suggested its presence in mitochondria also; however, later work concluded that the enzyme activity was the result of contamination of the preparation by microsomal P450arom. The subject of mitochondrial metabolism with respect to the methyl group at C19 is the subject of discussion in a later section of this chapter.

Whereas the human placental P450arom has been the most studied and is the enzyme against which aromatase preparations from other tissues (e.g. ovaries, adipose tissues) and from other species are compared, it may be noted that Osawa and colleagues [38] proposed that a second form of the enzyme was present in the placenta. Subsequent work with the pig provided evidence of the existence of distinct, intraspecies isoforms of P450arom, the first described in any species [39]. More than one isoform has also been reported in equine preparations [40] and in several species of fish [41]. These findings suggest that some species possess a unique mechanism for regulating androgen metabolism whose biological significance remains to be more fully explored.

Proper understanding of the mechanism of aromatase action has been hindered by the inability to achieve a high degree of purity in the final product to allow its crystallization. A major difficulty stems from the fact that a portion of the enzyme is embedded in the endoplasmic reticulum membrane. Efforts have finally been crowned with the successful crystallization of the enzyme by a group of investigators in Buffalo, NY [42] who recently reported on the crystal structure of human placental aromatase, the only natural mammalian, full-length P450 in hormone biosynthetic pathways to be crystallized so far. When crystals of P450arom were formed with its natural substrate androstenedione the enzyme's androgenic specificity and unique catalytic mechanism were revealed—showing why membrane anchoring is necessary for the lipophilic androgen substrates to gain access to the active site.

Aromatase Distribution and Regulation

While the biosynthesis of estrogens in mammalian species is principally associated with the ovaries, testes and placenta it is not restricted to these tissues. Even within the gonads and placenta the detection of the *CYP19* gene and its product P450arom is not restricted to one cell type. Moreover, the formation of estrogens occurs in other sites within the reproductive system of both male and females that point to important responses to estrogens that are not determined by a gonadal source of the hormone. A role for aromatase activity may even include a protection from excessive exposure to testosterone in some situations. Beyond the reproductive system the distribution of the *CYP19* gene and P450arom has now been demonstrated for an impressive list of organs and tissues [43]. These sites of local estrogen production include adipose tissue, bone (osteoblasts and chondrocytes), muscle (vascular endothelial and aortic smooth muscle) and numerous sites in the brain. It is important to recognize that while the amounts of estrogen formed are small—and do not have much effect on the level of estrogens in the blood circulation—the concentration can be high within the site of production and have biological significance for the tissues in a paracrine role. The case of the adrenal glands is somewhat special insofar as the biosynthesis of estrogens is relatively moderate under normal circumstances but the manner of their production differs to a degree, as will be discussed later in this chapter.

The level of aromatase activity depends initially on the expression of the *CYP19* gene to generate the P450arom enzyme. After the human *CYP19* gene was cloned more than twenty years ago [44] an expansive literature has developed that embraces the study of the coding region of a number of vertebrate species and the 5′-untranslated region of the transcript upstream from the start of translation. Suffice to note that variations in the promoter regions of the transcripts, even within a species, largely determine the specificity of expression of P450arom for the different sites of estrogen production. Because the base sequence comprising the promoter differs the regulation of the gene in each site is dependent on different agents (e.g. cAMP, gonadotrophins, cytokines). Thus the regulation of estrogen biosynthesis is unique for each tissue type, including differences in the mode of regulation among the principal sources (gonads and placenta).

Aromatase in Testicular Cells

(a) *Leydig Cells.* From the early discovery by Zondek in 1934 of high concentrations of estrogens in the testes of the stallion [29] it was assumed that the Leydig cells were the source. In both the stallion and boar testes the remarkable abundance of interstitial tissue, with a preponderance of Leydig cells [45], seemed the most likely source of the extremely high concentrations of estrogens in the urine [28, 46] and plasma of the mature animals [3, 47]. Many decades after Zondek's findings it was shown that testicular interstitial tissue was the major site of estrogen biosynthesis in the human testes [48]. Direct evidence for the location of aromatase activity was only possible when purified Leydig cell preparations were made from adult rats [49], immature pigs [50] and mature boars [51], with a marked increase after LH/hCG exposure in each case. Moreover, the location of the aromatase enzyme has been determined by immunocytochemistry in the testes of several species (rat, sheep, equine). In human subjects the immunostain was always associated with the Leydig cells and was absent from Sertoli cells [52]. Aromatase activity was measured by a biochemical assay for validation and the results were found to be significantly correlated with the immunostain intensity.

(b) *Sertoli Cells.* The above assumption concerning the Leydig cells as sole source of estrogens from the testes was challenged when pure preparations of rat Sertoli cells became available in1974. Sertoli cells isolated from 18-20-day-old rats synthesized low but detectable amounts of estradiol from testosterone as substrate and a dramatic increase was observed when Follicle-Stimulating Hormone (FSH) had been added to the medium [53]. Dorrington reviewed the early studies that led to the proposal of a two-cell, two-gonadotrophin model for the synthesis of testicular estradiol in the immature rat; however, the model was applicable only for a limited time-span in the young rat as the Sertoli cells ceased aromatase activity which thereafter resided in the adult Leydig cells. Unfortunately, the erroneous assumption that the Sertoli cells are the principal source of estrogen biosynthesis in the adult testes of rats and other species has been difficult to eradicate—despite several studies revealing the absence or relatively limited capability of Sertoli cells for aromatase activity [49, 54].

(c) *Germ Cells.* Although sex steroid binding to spermatozoa had been suggested from several studies in the past, specific binding of estradiol to human spermatozoa was demonstrated, in 1981, using the radiolabelled steroid [55]. A similar property may be seen in stallion spermatozoa where multiple washes (>10x) were unable to completely remove the small amounts of estrone detected by radioimmunoassay [56]. Furthermore, the binding of [^{3}H]-estrone sulphate (the principal estrogen in stallion semen) could not be displaced fully (about 20% reduction) by the presence of >100-fold excess of non-radioactive estrone sulfate (unpublished data). These findings, however, do not address the question of the source of the estrogens bound to spermatozoa. Do the germs cells in the male have the capacity for estrogen biosynthesis?

Germ cells of the mouse testes were the first to be shown to express P450arom [57]. The first observation that human ejaculated spermatozoa contain active P450arom was soon followed by several reports for the human subject. Two recent reviews on the subject of aromatase, estrogens and male reproduction have provided a timely account of current knowledge concerning the possible significance of estrogen biosynthesis by the germ cells [58, 59]. Suffice to say that a strong case is made for the importance of aromatase activity in the testes and germ cells in relation to spermatogenesis. Together with increasing knowledge on the distribution and regulation of ERs in the germ cells and reproductive tract future studies on P450arom activity should make a major contribution to a better understanding of the development and maturation of spermatozoa.

Aromatase in the Reproductive Tract

A comprehensive review of estrogens in the physiology of the efferent ductules and epididymis has recently been provided [60]. The effect of estrogens on the male reproductive tract was clearly shown by their regulation of reabsorption of luminal fluid from the head of the epididymis of the rat [6]. High concentrations of estrogens found in the rete testes fluid are derived from the testes; the spermatozoa may continue to be a source of estrogen as they enter the epididymis [61]. However, the presence of the *CYP19* gene is apparent in the caput epididymal epithelium itself in the monkey, human and rat [62-64] and could serve in the local synthesis of estrogen for the ERs present in the epididymis. The interplay among the potential sources of estrogen and the role of the ERs remains to be explored more fully in the regions of the reproductive tract in terms of maturation and maintenance of the spermatozoa.

Sulfotransferase activity within the epididymis is an added feature that has possible implications for modifying the exposure of spermatozoa to estrogens and for regulation of the physiological functions of the epididymis in support of the spermatozoa. The expression of the enzyme is remarkably high in the boar [23] and stallion (e 1), where the suggestion of regional differences along the tract was noted. The presence of the enzyme has also been shown in the epididymal epithelium of the boar by immunohistochemistry [65]. Similar evidence was obtained for the mouse and bovine epididymis [66, 67] as well as some sulfatase present in the boar [65] and equine tissues [68].

Table 1. Conjugation of Estrogens by the Male Reproductive Tract (%)*

	Boar				Stallion	
	Estrone		Estradiol		Estrone	Estradiol
	boar 1	boar 2	boar 1	boar 2		
Epididymis Caput	83.6	89.7	88.8	87.1	93.5 (2)	95.1 [95.4]
Corpus	83.4	-	77.9	-	91.4±4.8 (3)	-
Cauda	77.1	-	71.0	-	88.8±5.7 (6)	88.9 [93.4]
Vas deferens	82.4	81.9	84.5	79.9	85.7±5.2 (6)	78.1 [96.3]

*Percentage of total estrogens in incubation media. ( ) number of animals; [ ] present as sulfates.

Aromatase in Brain

The effects of testosterone on the brain depend partly on its metabolism in the tissues throughout the brain. In fact, the principal hormone masculinizing the brain is not testosterone but its metabolite, estradiol. Aromatization is required for both sexual differentiation of the brain and the display of adult sexual behaviour [69]. However, it is clear that androgens regulate the transcription or stability of aromatase mRNA in specific brain areas in the rat and may account for the higher levels of aromatase activity in the brain of males [70]. Based on the quantification of ^3H_2O formed from [1α/β-^{3}H]-androstenedione this sensitive assay has been used to quantify aromatase activity in discrete brain nuclear regions in the rat [71]. Improvements in quantitative methods of immunocytochemical assays will enhance the application of the sensitive biochemical assay to localize and measure P450arom and its activity in discrete cell populations in the brain.

Regions of particular interest for estrogen action in the brain include sites of regulation of gonadotrophin production and release, and sexual behaviour. Both aspects have spawned an extensive literature across vertebrate species and well beyond the focus of this chapter on androgen conversion to estrogens—which is mainly directed to the male. The question of the role of estrogens from the gonads relative to local biosynthesis of estrogen in the brain is posed, to the greatest degree, by the very large amounts of estrogens produced by the testes of the stallion and boar. To some extent the estrogen 'load' in these males may be mitigated by the estrogens in the peripheral blood being largely in a sulfoconjugated form and predominantly as the weaker estrogen, estrone [3, 47]. Nonetheless, it was possible to demonstrate that estradiol or estrone exerted a synergistic effect on libido when administered with testosterone to boars that had been castrated after reaching maturity [7].

Aromatase Isoforms

Until 1994 it was held that P450arom in all vertebrate species examined was encoded by a single gene and was represented by a single gene product similar to human placental P450arom—the most completely characterized aromatase enzyme [43]. Expression occurs in many tissues and control is exerted in a tissue-specific manner largely by differences in the promoter region. However, a study in the pig revealed the presence of at least two active forms of P450arom [39]. The pig had shown a wide range of tissues expressing the enzyme and, when a difference was found in its activity between a gonadal and a placental source, further investigation led to evidence for the existence of two isoforms of P450arom. As added support, not only were the rates of conversion of androgen → estrogen different but the isoforms responded differently to specific P450arom inhibitors. At the same time a report on a novel aromatase was suggested for the transient production of estrogens by peri-implantation blastocysts in the pig [40]. Further work established that multiple enzymes of porcine aromatase are encoded by three distinct genes (type I, ovary; type II, placenta; type III, embryo/blastocyst) [72]. The active form of P450arom expressed in the adrenal glands and testes of fetal and newborn pigs resembles the isoform expressed in the ovary rather than being an additional type [73]. A general review of mammalian aromatases has been provided by Conley and Hinshelwood [74]; an interesting discussion of the adaptive evolution of mammalian aromatases, based on pigs, peccaries and other Suiformes, appeared subsequently [75]. Although less attention has been given to other vertebrates it is clear that isoforms of P450arom occur. Two distinct isozymes of P450 arom were demonstrated for the brain and ovary in several species of fish [76]. In contrast the porcine hypothalamic aromatase was shown to be the gonadal form (designated "gonadal/hypothalamic") and, interestingly, its expression is regulated differently in the hypothalamus than in the testes [77].

Aromatase Metabolism of Testosterone and Androstenedione

Part 2

Non-aromatizing Action of P450arom

The first step in aromatization is a C19-methyl hydroxylation to form C19-hydroxy-testosterone or C19-hydroxy-androstenedione. These intermediate compounds are known to be released from the active site of the enzyme. Indeed it has been shown in the rat brain that 19-hydroxylation of androgens greatly exceeds aromatization and the 19-hydroxy- and 19-oxo-androgen products accumulate in the media in quantities 5 times greater than the estrogens [78]. Similarly, rat ovaries produce 19-oxygenated androgens in quantities exceeding those of estrogens [79]. The identification of 19-hydroxy-androstenedione as a principal metabolite of androstenedione by porcine granulosa cells has also been noted [80, 81]. 19-Hydroxy-androgens have been identified in incubation studies with equine testicular tissues [82, 83] and found as endogenous steroids in testicular tissue of the horse [84]. That they are distinct metabolites of androgens, and not merely trapped transient aromatization intermediates, is clear from the identification of 19-hydroxy-testosterone and 19-hydroxy-androstenedione from testicular venous blood of mature pigs as well as from the incubation of purified preparations of porcine Leydig cells [85]. The secretion of 19-hydroxy-androgens raises questions concerning a physiological role beyond that of intermediates in the biosynthesis of norandrogens and estrogens. In the rat, a potent sodium-retaining and hypertensinogen action has been demonstrated for 19-hydroxyandrostenedione [86]. In dog adrenal glands, the activity of 19-hydroxylase towards androstenedione is much greater than that of aromatase, thereby accounting for the much greater secretion of 19-hydroxy-androstenedione from the glands [87]. In human subjects ACTH and angiotensin II can induce its release from the adrenal glands [88]. Whether two distinct enzymes exist for the 19-hydroxylation and aromatase actions on androstenedione is still uncertain in some situations.

An ability to catalyze hydroxylation at C19, as well as more typically at C11, has been demonstrated for the highly purified $P450_{11\beta}$ system of adrenal cortex mitochondria [89]. This enzyme showed further 19-oxidase activity and demethylation at the 10-position to give C_{18}-steroids, estrone (aromatase activity) and 19-norandrostenedione (nonaromatizing C10-19 lyase activity). In this way the adrenal enzyme is similar to the human placental P450arom but differs in having C11-hydroxylating activity as its predominant role in the formation of C_{21} and C_{19} steroids in the adrenals. It is interesting to note that more than fifty years ago, the testes in some fish species (salmonids) were first shown to produce an 11-oxygenated steroid (11-keto-testosterone) as the male hormone [90]. Later, evidence was presented that a mammalian species also secretes 11-hydroxylated androgens from the gonads—11β-hydroxy-testosterone and 11β-hydroxy-androstenedione were isolated from testicular vein blood of the domestic pig [21]. Recently it was shown that an 11β-hydroxylase enzyme was induced by human chorionic gonadotrophin (hCG) in Leydig cells of the mouse and caused the production of 11-keto-testosterone [91]. Since both 19-hydroxy-androgens and 11-hydroxy-androgens are secreted by the testes of the boar, it is possible that two separate enzymes in the Leydig cells are involved—one microsomal (P450arom) and one mitochondrial (11β-hydroxylase). Both are capable of forming estrogens and so express a complement of enzyme activities (Figure 3). Their relative contribution to the high amounts of estrogens produced by the boar is unknown. These and other similar findings have been discussed recently in the context of evolution of mammalian aromatases [75].

One further interesting product of the P450arom enzyme in the boar testes, 1-hydroxy-testosterone, belongs in the category of nonaromatizable androgens [92]. The amounts produced were almost equal in proportion to those for estradiol. This novel metabolite could not be formed by the porcine placental P450arom, or serve as substrate for aromatization with both of the porcine enzymes and with bovine and human P450arom. Its presence in testicular vein blood of the boar was also noted. Added support for its secretion in the boar comes from our earlier observations (unpublished) where a major peak from HPLC of venous blood extracts yielded 1, 4-androstadien-3-one-17β-ol (Δ^1-testosterone) at GC/MS analysis—the inference being that dehydration of 1α/β (or 2α/β)-OH-testosterone had occurred. A physiological role for 1β-OH-testosterone has yet to be defined but its action *in vitro* on prostatic cell lines, in comparison with 5α-dihydrotestosterone, has been described [92].

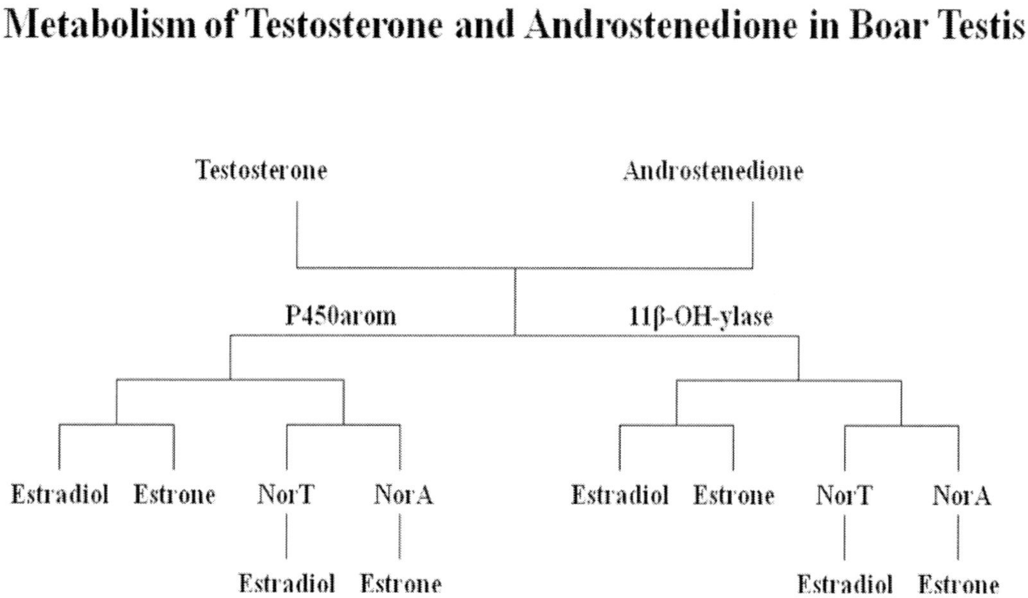

Figure 3. Possible pathways in the biosynthesis of C_{18} steroids.

Table 2. Aromatizing and Non-aromatizing Reactions in Steroidogenic Organs

	Human		Equine		Porcine	
	Ar	Non-Ar	Ar	Non-Ar	Ar	Non-Ar
Testes	+	±	+	+	+	+
Ovary	+	±	+	+	+	+
Placenta	+	±	+	+	+	+
Adrenal	+	±	±	±	+	±

Ar, aromatizing; Non-Ar, non-aromatizing; ±, not determined definitively.

C19 Anabolic Steroids: Nortestosterone and Norandrostenedione

Biosynthesis

Known sources for the biosynthesis of norandrogens include the ovary [11, 12], testis [24], adrenal [87] and placenta [93, 94], with the degree of participation from the various sources being dependent upon the species—insofar as data are available on human, equine and porcine species (Table 2). The extent to which P450arom is the principal, or sole, agent producing the norandrogens remains largely unresolved. Moreover, it has yet to be established in most cases whether the norandrogens are intermediates or by-products in the biosynthesis of estrogens. Their presence in testicular vein blood indicates that they are secretory products in certain cases, as noted above.

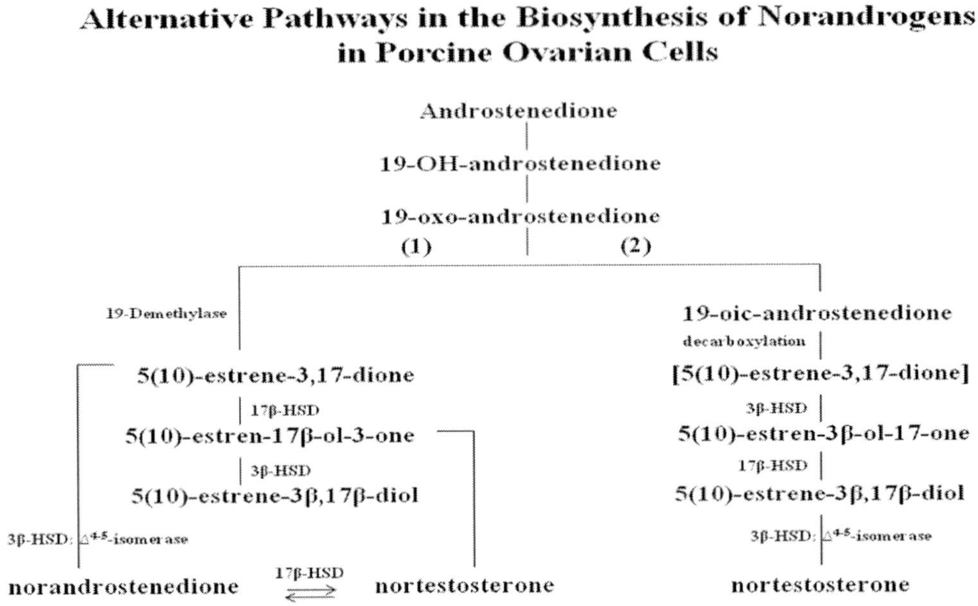

Figure 4a. Pathways proposed for the biosynthesis of norandrogens.

5(10)-estrene-3β,17β-diol 3, 17-dioxo-4-androsten-19-oic acid

Figure 4b. Intermediate compounds in the formation of C_{18} neutral steroids.

The pathway proposed for the metabolism of androstenedione by porcine ovarian granulosa cells has been a subject of dispute (Figure 4a). In one laboratory, production of estrone *in vitro* was accompanied by formation of a novel 19-norandrogen, which led to 19-norandrostenedione as a major end-product—through further metabolism of the intermediate compound by the 3β-hydroxy/$\Delta^{4,5}$-isomerase enzyme [80]. On the other hand, in a second investigation a hypothesis was formulated for the production of C_{18} neutral steroids through the intermediacy of 19-oic-androstenedione (Figure 4b) which appeared as a major metabolite of aromatase activity in porcine granulose cells in culture [81]. Furthermore, it was contended that the 19-norandrostenedione reported in the earlier studies could have been derived as an artifact from 19-oic-androstenedione as a result of degradation in storage and during the isolation procedure. However, this view seems to have ignored the fact that the intermediate, estrenediol had been isolated in both studies.

In the testes a proposed mechanism for the formation of C_{18} neutral steroids was presented from a study of *in vitro* metabolism of C_{19} substrates with minced testicular tissues from stallions [82]. After the second hydroxylation at C19 by aromatase the loss of the carbon at that site as formic acid, via a reverse aldol-type condensation, yielded an intermediate compound (3, 5(10)-estradiene) that by alternate sites of protonation could give rise either, (a) directly to a norandrogen or (b) through a 5(10)-3-oxo-steroid—followed by isomerase and reduction steps—to form a stable metabolite, 5(10)-estrene-3,17-diol. This latter compound does not permit aromatization of the A-ring and was detected in significant amounts as a sulfated steroid in the stallion testicular tissues. Based on this study and on those of a series from the same laboratory on the origin of C18 neutral steroids isolated from extracts of urine from the male horse, it was suggested that 19-norandrostenedione and 19-nortestosterone could arise from C19-oic-steroids as chemical artifacts of the analytical procedure [84]. The possible occurrence of 19-norandrostenedione as a sulfoconjugated steroid (an "enol-sulfate") was examined but dismissed in favour of the excretion of a 19-carboxylic acid form (Figure 4b) which is a compound sufficiently polar to appear in the urine and in the conjugate fraction of the urinary extracts. After its isolation the identification was later established [95] by LC-MS and GC-MS, with the mass spectrum corresponding to that given earlier for the 19-carboxylic acid of androstenedione found in porcine ovarian follicular fluids [81]. The conclusion drawn was that whereas the 19-oxo-androgens are good substrates for P450arom, the 19-oic acids are poor substrates. It is likely that decarboxylation takes place as an artifact of the methodology; however, it seems possible that an enzymatic step may also occur to some degree in a manner analogous to the removal of the $-CH_3$ groups at C4 in the biosynthesis of cholesterol. Both the artifactual and natural synthesis could proceed to the formation of the 19-norandrogens as suggested in the following scheme (Figure 5).

Whether a similar situation applies to the actions of aromatase in the adrenal glands remains to be determined. It may be noted that 19-oic-11-deoxycorticosterone is a product of a P450 enzyme which through 19-OH- and 19-oxo- intermediates in the adrenal glands, is then converted to the 19-nor- form of 11-deoxycorticosterone by other tissues in the body [96]. Perhaps, a similar pathway may account for the production of 19-norandrostenedione—alongside that for estrone—by mitochondrial preparations of bovine adrenal cortex [89]; no evidence of 19-oic-androstenedione was reported; rather a nonaromatizing 10-demethylase, or C10-19-lyase reaction, was implied.

Without any doubt, the placental P450arom has been the centre of major attention over several decades and remains the focus of intensive investigation. Much of the incentive for the work on the enzyme stems from the need for a better understanding of the mechanism by which the series of three monooxidative steps are coupled to convert androstenedione to estrone—to aid in development of an irreversible inhibitor of aromatase for the prevention and treatment of human breast cancer. Significant progress has been made as seen in two recent reports. The crystal structure of aromatase was solved for the first time—using the enzyme purified from term human placenta in complex with its natural substrate androstenedione [42]. The aromatase has a relatively small androgen-specific cleft that binds the androstenedione molecule snugly and suggests the existence of a single site rather than multiple active sites. In the second paper [97], a kinetic analysis of the three-step aromatase reaction of human cytochrome P450arom revealed that the enzyme is distributive, that is, with the sequential reaction allowing free dissociation of the intermediates. This is in accord with the secretion of C19-hydroxyandrogens. While the subject of the regulation of P450arom has implications beyond clinical interests, it is not within the range of topics appropriate for discussion in this chapter.

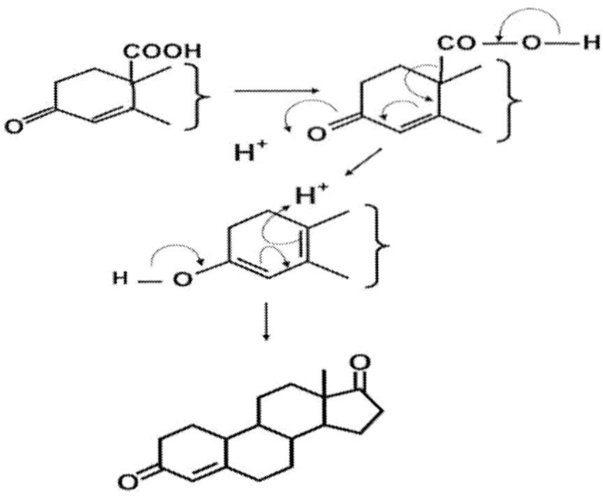

Figure 5. Mechanism of decarboxlation of the 3-oxo-4-ene-19-carboxylic acid. [Reprinted from E.Houghton *et al.: Analytica Chimica Acta*, 2007 586, 196-207, with the permission of the authors and publishers, Elsevier.]

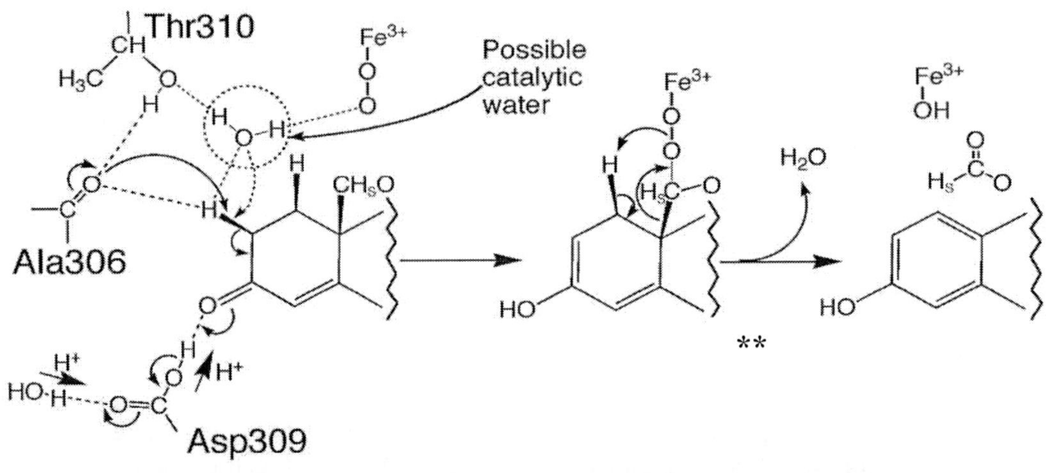

Figure 6. Presence of a putative enol (**) intermediate from P450arom activity that might enable formation of a sulfated steroid. [Reprinted from D. Ghosh *et al.*: *Nature* 457:219–223, 2009 (295), with the permission of the authors and publisher].[Reproduced from D. Ghosh *et al.*: *Nature* 457:219–223, 2009 (295) with permission from Nature Publishing Group.]

One further site for the biosynthesis of 19-norandrogens, however, presents an interesting addition. The preimplantation blastocysts (or conceptuses) have been identified as a significant source of steroids. Blastocysts from several species are known to produce estrogens, especially those of the pig and horse. An isozyme of P450arom is present in the porcine blastocyst which shows catalytic differences from the placental form and exhibits a much higher production of 19-nortestosterone than estradiol from testosterone as substrate [94]. The product ratio of estradiol/nortestosterone was 6: 94 for the blastocyst form and 6: 94 for the placenta; the site that is responsible for the catalytic differences between the two forms remains to be determined. Activity of the blastocyst form is limited to a very short period (1-2 days) at an early stage in development of the pig embryo [98] but extends for much longer in the horse [99]. Our studies on steroids in the equine yolk-sac fluid indicate that 19-

norandrostenedione appears to be present in greater concentrations than other steroids, including estrone which had been assumed to be the major product [100]. Moreover, the 19-norandrogen was found in much higher amounts in the conjugate fraction and was assumed to exist in an enol form, as a sulfate. From the studies cited above there remains the possibility that it occurs as 19-oic-androstenedione. This seems unlikely because our work included extraction from samples stored at -20^{0}C for 1-3 years by which time degradation of the 19-oic steroids would have resulted largely in their disappearance from the conjugated fraction. An enol form of an intermediate (Figure 6) has not yet been established for the material in the equine yolk-sac fluid that gives rise to the norandrostenedione isolated in our investigations. Regardless of the biochemistry it is nonetheless tempting to speculate on a role for a potential anabolic steroid (19-norandrostenedione) in the development of the conceptus.

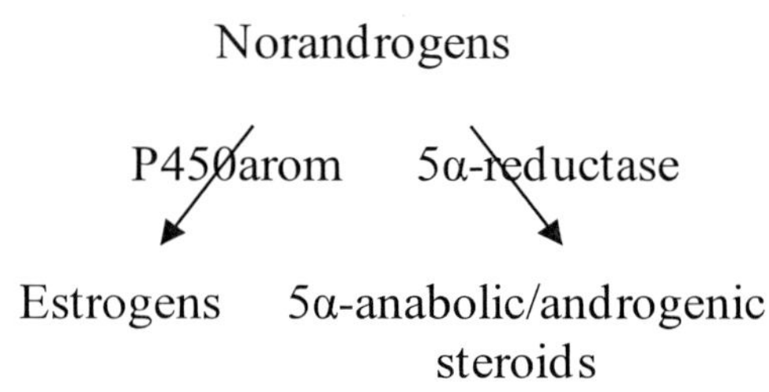

Figure 7. Biologically active products from metabolism of norandrogens.

Metabolism

The fate of the 19-norandrogens produced in the body is also the focus in this chapter—rather than what happens to them after their administration as an exogenous source of an anabolic steroid. More particularly an interest lies in determining the extent to which P450arom can produce biologically important products—estrogens and anabolic/androgens. Other enzymes in the liver and elsewhere can influence the availability of the estrogens and anabolic steroids being formed from the 19-norandrogens but their actions are of lesser concern in this chapter.

Aromatization of 19-norandrogens in the stallion testis was demonstrated in a series of studies [83, 94]. Two aromatizing enzyme systems seemed to exist: one system was less productive but more specific for 19-norandrogens. With equine testicular microsomes it was shown that aromatization occurred through the loss of 1β, 2β hydrogen atoms. In a second species known for its high production of estrogens in the testes, it was found that the amounts of estrogen synthesized by purified preparations of porcine Leydig cells was essentially equal from androstenedione and 19-norandrostenedione as substrates (Figure 8 and [101]).

Evidence for aromatase activity on 19-norandrogens is limited in other species but may be present to a minor extent in the human placenta [102]. The presence of a cytochrome P450 enzyme in the human liver that can act on 19-norandrogens to generate a phenolic ring A has been proposed as responsible for the appearance of gynecomastia where excessive doses of anabolic steroid products have been used by bodybuilders. No literature seems to exist on other sites of aromatization (e.g. adipose tissue) as to whether norandrogens are indeed formed or metabolized to estrogens.

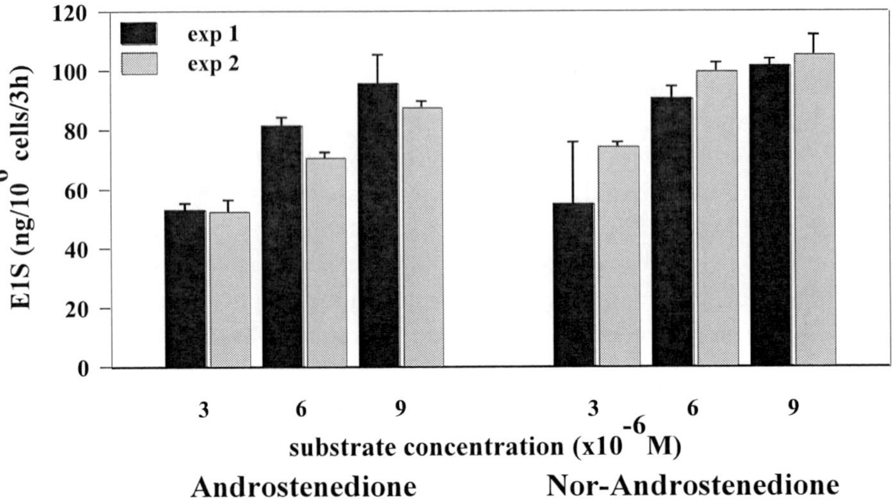

Figure 8. Estrone sulfate (E1S) formation from androstenedione and norandrostenedione by porcine Leydig cells in culture for 3 hours.

Because 5α-reductase activity results in a more active androgen (5α-dihydrotestosterone) than testosterone, it might be suggested that the enzyme could alter the biological activity of the 19-norandrogens. In fact many efforts have been made to block the enzyme's reducing action on the anabolic steroids to control the androgenic side-effects that otherwise might follow. To the contrary, it has been reported that 5α-reduction of 19-nortestosterone resulted in lower androgenicity—the opposite effect from reduction of testosterone [103]. However, the focus in this chapter is on the position of P450arom in the scheme of steroid metabolism of androgens and, therefore, discussion of 5α-reductase is limited to evidence for a possible relationship to aromatase. One such case was demonstrated with porcine Leydig cells where use of a 5α-reductase inhibitor led to a significant increase in estrogen secretion [104]. The increase was seen to be made at the expense of production of 5α-estrane-3β, 17β-diol and 3β-hydroxy-5α-estran-17-one—two major metabolites that were both present almost exclusively in the sulfo-conjugated steroid fraction, implying that further reduction of the 3-oxo- group in the latter compound led to 3-sulfate formation. A similar pattern in metabolism of androstenedione, the parent compound, had been observed earlier [54]. It may be noted that isomers of estrane-3, 17-diol, as sulfates, are present in extracts of normal urine of the male horse [95].

Other enzymes that might be involved in the metabolism of 19-norandrogens have received little attention. The action of 17β-hydroxysteroid dehydrogenases can be inferred; and the production of 6α-hydroxy-norandrostenedione and 11β-hydroxy-norandrostenedione has been shown for porcine Leydig cells [105]. It would be interesting to know whether a 4-hydroxy-norandrogen is formed naturally in view of the action of 4-hydroxy-androstenedione as an aromatase inhibitor. To conclude this section, the potential participation of a 3-reductase in 19-norandrogen metabolism is raised. The tissue specificity of the anabolic steroid, 19-nor-4-androstene-3β, 17β-diol, has been examined in rats [106]. Increases in muscle and bone mass without significant stimulation of prostate growth were reported from administration of the steroid in silastic capsules. Whether the steroid is a natural product of 19-nortestosterone metabolism in the body and may undergo metabolism by 5α-reduction—or even be restored again by oxidation to 19-nortestosterone—remains to be demonstrated. The 3α-isomer, 19-nor-4-androstene-3α, 17β-diol ("estren") was under investigation as a nongenomic selective activator of the estrogen receptor for use in prevention of osteoporosis [107] but was shown to have weakly estrogenic action in the uterus [108]. Furthermore, it was suggested that it might induce nuclear ERα- and AR-mediated responses—the latter action would infer that estren could have been converted to 19-nortestosterone by oxidation. The biological actions of the 19-norandrogens and their neutral and phenolic metabolites are not addressed as being inappropriate for this chapter.

Conclusion

A key role for P450arom in both sexes appears to be in maintaining a balance between androgenic and estrogenic actions in the body. Furthermore, the ability of the aromatase to produce C19-norandrogens in some cases can contribute to a balance for androgenic/anabolic actions. Although the liver is the major site of steroid metabolism it is clear that the presence of P450arom activity in various tissues can have significant consequences. Very limited data are available to-date but it is important to note a large variation amongst species in the ratio of androgen/estrogen production in the gonads as well as in the local metabolism of the gonadal steroids. Several questions await further study such as what are the biological implications of estrogen formation by the male germs cells. Are nortestosterone and norandrostenedione formed locally by P450arom where it is actively producing estrogens in peripheral tissues (e.g. brain, adipose)? As a final comment, the position of endogenous anabolic steroids (norandrogens) in general still remains poorly investigated in spite of the discovery of their existence in ovarian follicular fluids over sixty years ago [11].

Acknowledgment

The assistance of Heather Christie in the preparation of this chapter is greatly appreciated.

References

[1] Zhu, BT; Conney, AH. Functional role of estrogen metabolism in target cells: review and perspectives. *Carcinogenesis,* 1998 19, 1-27.

[2] Farnsworth, WE; Brown, JR. Testosterone metabolism in the prostate. *National Cancer Institute Monograph,* 1963 12, 323.

[3] Raeside, JI. Seasonal changes in the concentration of estrogens and testosterone in the plasma of the stallion. *Animal Reproduction Science,* 1978/1979 1, 205-211.

[4] Simpson, ER; Zhao, Y; Agarwal, VR; Michael, MD; Bulun, SE; Hinshelwood, MM; Graham- Lorence, S; Sun, T; Fisher, CR; Zin, K; Mendelson, CR. Aromatase

expression in health and disease. *Recent Progress in Hormone Research*, 1997 52, 185-213.

[5] Risbridger, GP; Ellem, SJ; McPherson, SJ. Estrogen action on the prostate gland: a critical mix of endocrine and paracrine signaling. *Journal of Molecular Endocrinology,* 2007 39, 183-188.

[6] Hess, RA; Bunick, D; Lee, KH; Bahr, J; Taylor, JA; Korach, KS; Lubahn, DB. A role for oestrogens in the male reproductive system. *Nature,* 1997 390, 509-512.

[7] Joshi, HS; Raeside, JI. Synergistic effects of testosterone and oestrogens on accessory sex glands and sexual behaviour of the boar. *Journal of Reproduction and Fertility,* 1973 33, 411-423.

[8] Lindzey, J; Korach, KS. Estrogen actions in males: Insights through mutations in aromatase and estrogen-receptor genes. In: Bagatell C, Bremner WJ, editors. *Contemporary Endocrinology: Androgens in health and disease.* Totowa, NJ: Humana Press Inc; 2009; 89- 102.

[9] Ruokonen, A; Vikho, R. Steroid metabolism in testis tissue: concentrations of unconjugated and sulphated neutral steroids in boar testis. *Journal of Steroid Biochemistry*, 1974 5, 33-38.

[10] Dumasia, MC; Houghton, E; Jackiw, M. Steroids in equine testis: the identification of endogenous 19-hydroxy and 19-nor neutral steroids by gas-chromatography- mass spectrometry. *Journal of Endocrinology*, 1989 120, 223-229.

[11] Short, RV. Identification of 19-norandrostenedione in follicular fluid. *Nature,* 1960 189, 232.

[12] Khalil, MW; Walton, JS. Identification and measurement of 4-oestren-3,17-dione (19-norandrostenedione) in porcine ovarian follicular fluid using high performance liquid chromatogreaphy and capillary mass gas chromatography. *Journal of Endocrinology*, 1985 107, 375-381.

[13] Carani, C; Qin, K; Simoni, M; Faustini-Fustini, M;Serpente, S; Boyd, J; Korach, KS; Simpson, ER. Effect of testosterone and estradiol in a man with aromatase deficiency. *New England Journal of Medicine,*1997 337, 91-95.

[14] Bilezikian, JP; Morishima, A; Bell, J; Grumbach, MM. Increased bone mass as a result of estrogen therapy in a man with aromatase deficiency. *New England Journal of Medicine,* 1998 339, 599-603.

[15] Russell, D; Wilson, JD. Steroid 5α-reductase: Two genes/two enzymes. *Annual Review of Biochemistry*, 1994 63, 25-61.

[16] Jacobi, GH; Wilson, JD. The formation of 5-alpha-androstane-3-alpha,17-beta-diol by dog prostate. *Endocrinology*, 1976 99, 602-610.

[17] Oliveira, AG; Coelho, PH; Guedes, FD; Mahecha, GAB; Hess, RA; Oliveira, CA. 5α-Androstane-3β,17β-diol (3β-diol), an estrogenic metabolite of 5α-dihydrotestosterone, is a potent modulator of estrogen receptor ERβ expression in the ventral prostrate of adult rats. *Steroids*, 2007 72, 914-922.

[18] Velle, W. Isolation of oestrone and oestradiol from the urine of adult boars. *Acta Endocrinologica*, 1958 28, 255-261.

[19] Dorfman, RI; Ungar, F. Metabolism of Steroid Hormones. New York, NY: Academic Press; 1965.

[20] Idler, DR; Schmidt, PJ; Ronald, AP. Isolation and identification of 11-ketotestosterone in salmon plasma. *Canadian Journal of Biochemistry and Physiology*, 1960 38, 1053-1057.

[21] Raeside, JI; Renaud, RL; Friendship, RM. Isolation of 11β-hydroxylated androgens from testicular vein blood of the mature boar. *Biochemical and Biophysical Research Communications*, 1989 162, 1194-1199.

[22] Raeside, JI; Christie, HL; Renaud, RL. Steroid metabolism in the epididymis and vas deferens of the stallion. *Reproduction,* 2001 27(Suppl.), Abstract No. 68.

[23] Raeside, JI; Christie, HL; Renaud, RL. Androgen and estrogen metabolism in the reproductive tract and accessory sex glands of the domestic boar (*Sus Scrofa). Biology of Reproduction*, 1999 61, 1242-1248.

[24] Ruokonen, A; Laatikainen, T; Laitinen, EA; Vihko, R. Free and sulfate-conjugated neutral steroids in human testis tissue. *Biochemistry*, **1972** *11*, 1411–1416.

[25] Burrows, H. Biological Actions of Sex Hormones. Second Edition. Cambridge: Cambridge University Press; 1949.

[26] David, KG; Dingemanse, E; Freud, J; Laqueur, E. Über krystallinisches mannliches Hormon aus Hoden (Testosteron) wirksamer als aus harn oder aus Cholesterin bereitetes Androsteron. *Hoppe Seylers Zeitschrift Physiologische Chemische*, 1935 233-281.

[27] Smith, EP; Boyd, J; Frank, GR. Estrogen resistance caused by a mutation in the estrogen- receptor gene in man. *New England Journal of Medicine*, 1994 331, 1056-1061.

[28] Zondek, B. Oestrogenic hormone in the urine of the stallion. *Nature*, 1934 133, 209-210.

[29] Zondek, B. Professor Bernhard Zondek: An interview. *Journal of Reproduction and Fertility*, 1966 12, 3-19.

[30] Santen, RJ; Brodie, H; Simpson, ER; Siiteri, PK; Brodie, A. History of Aromatase: Saga of an important biological mediator and therapeutic target. *Endocrine Reviews*, 2009 30, 343-375.

[31] Steinach, E; Kun, H. Transformation of male sex hormones into a substance with the action of a female hormone. *Lancet,* 1937 230, 845.

[32] Meyer, AS. Conversion of 19-hydroxy-4-androstene-3,17-dione to estrone by endocrine tissue. *Biochimica Biophysica Acta*, 1955 17, 441-442.

[33] Meyer, AS; Hayano, M; Lindberg, MC; Gut, M; Rodgers, OG. The conversion of 4-androstene-3,17-dione-4-C14 and dehydroepiandrosterone by bovine adrenal homogenate preparations. *Acta Endocrinologica*, 1955 18, 148-168.

[34] Baggett, B; Dorfman, RI; Engel, LL; Savard, K. The conversion of testosterone-3-C14 to C14-estradiol-17β by human ovarian tissue. *Journal of Biological Chemistry*, 1956 221, 931-94.

[35] Hall, PF; Chen, S; Nakajin, S; Shinoda, M; Shively, JE. Purification and characterization of aromatase from human placenta. *Steroids*, 1987 50, 37-50.

[36] Brodie, HJ; Hayano, M; Gut, M. The stereochemical course of catalytic hydrogenation of ring A unsaturated steroids. *Journal of the American Chemical Society*, 1962 84, 3766-3767.

[37] Thompson Jr, EA; Siiteri, PK. The involvement of human placental microsomal cytochrome P-450 in aromatization. *Journal of Biological Chemistry*, 1974 249, 5373-5378.

[38] Osawa, Y; Yoshida, N; Fronckowiak, M; Kitawaki, J. Immunoaffinity purification of aromatase cytochrome P-450 from human placental microsomes, metabolic switching from aromatization to 1β and 2β-monohydroxylation, and recognition of aromatase isozymes. *Steroids*, 1987 50, 11-28.

[39] Corbin, CJ; Khalil, MW; Conley, AJ. Functional ovarian and placental isoforms of porcine aromatase. *Molecular and Cellular Endocrinology*, 1996 113, 29-37.

[40] Choi, I; Simmen, RC; Simmen, FA. Molecular cloning of cytochrome P450 aromatase complementary deoxyribonucleic acid from preimplantatio porcine and equine blastocysts identifies multiple 5′-untranslated exons expressed in embryos, endometrium and placenta. *Endocrinology*, 1996 137, 1457-1467.

[41] Tchoudakova, A; Callard, GV. Identification of multiple CYP19 genes encoding different ` cytochrome P450 aromatase isozymes in brain and ovary. *Endocrinology*, 1998 139, 2179- 2189.

[42] Ghosh, D; Griswold, J; Erman, M; Pangborn, W. Structural basis for androgen specificity and oestrogen synthesis in human aromatase. *Nature*, 2009 457, 219-223.

[43] Simpson, ER; Clyne, C; Rubin, G; Boon, WC; Robertson, K; Britt, K; Speed, C; Jones, M. Aromatase−A brief overview. *Annual Review of Physiology*, 2002 64, 93-127.

[44] Means, GD; Mahendroo, MS; Corbin, CJ; Mathis, JM; Powell, FE; Mendelson, CR; Simpson, ER. Structural analysis of the gene encoding human aromatase cytochrome P-450, the enzyme responsible for estrogen biosynthesis. *Journal of Biological Chemistry*, 1989 264, 19385-19391.

[45] Fawcett, DW; Burgos, MH. Studies on the fine structure of the mammalian testis. II. The human interstitial tissue. *American Journal of Anatomy*, 1960 107, 245-269.

[46] Velle, W. Urinary oestrogens in the male. *Journal of Reproduction and Fertility*, 1966 12, 65-73.

[47] Schwarzenberger, F; Toole, GS; Christie, HL; Raeside, JI. Plasma levels of several androgens and estrogens from birth to puberty in domestic male pigs. *Acta Endocrinologica*, 1993 128, 173-177.

[48] Payne, AH; Kelch, RP; Musich, S; Halpern, ME. Intertesticular site of aromatization in the human. *Journal of Clinical Endocrinology*, 1976 42, 1081-1087.

[49] Valladeres, LE; Payne, AH. Induction of testicular aromatization by luteinizing hormone in mature rats. *Endocrinology*, 1979 105, 431-436.

[50] Saez, JM; Benahmed, M; Reventos, J; Bommelaer, MC; Monbriel, C; Haour, F. Hormonal regulation of pig Leydig cells in culture. *Journal of Steroid Biochemistry*, 1983 19, 375-384.

[51] Raeside, JI; Renaud, RL. Estrogen and androgen production by purified Leydig cells of mature boars. *Biology of Reproduction*, 1983 28, 727-733.

[52] Inkster, S; Yue, W; Brodie, A. Human testicular aromatase: immunocytochemical and biochemical studies. *Journal of Clinical Endocrinology and Metabolism*, 1995 80, 1941- 1947.

[53] Dorrington, JH; Armstrong, DT. Follicle-stimulating hormone stimulates estradiol-17β synthesis in cultured Sertoli cells. *Proceedings of the National Academy of Science USA*, 1975 72, 2677-2681.

[54] Raeside, JI; Lobb, DK. Metabolism of androstenedione by Sertoli cell enriched preparations and purified Leydig cells from boar testes in relation to estrogen formation. *Journal of Steroid Biochemistry*, 1984 20, 1267-1272.

[55] Cheng, C Y; Boettcher, B; Rose, RJ; Kay, DJ; Tinneberg, HR. 1981 The binding of sex steroids to human spermatozoa: An autoradiographic study. *International Journal of Andrology*, 1981 4, 1-17.

[56] Raeside, JI; Christie, HL. Estrogen concentrations in semen of the stallion. *Animal Reproduction Science*, 1997 48, 293-300.

[57] Nitta, H; Bunick, D; Hess, RA; Janulis, L; Newton, SC; Millette, CF; Osawa, Y; Shizuta, Y; Toda, K; Bahr, JM. Germ cells of the mouse testis express P450 aromatase. *Endocrinology*, 1993 132, 1396–1401.

[58] Carreau, S; Hess, RA. Oestrogens and spermatogenesis. *Philosophical Transactions of the Royal Society B*, 2010 365, 1517-1535.

[59] Carreau, S; Wolczynski, S; Galeraud-Denis, I. Aromatase, oestrogens and human male reproduction. *Philosophical Transactions of the Royal Society B*, 2010 365, 1571-1579.

[60] Joseph, A; Shur, BD; Hess, RA. Minireview: Estrogen, efferent ductules, and the epididymis. *Biology of Reproduction,* 2011 84, 207–217.

[61] Carreau, S; Genissel, C; Bilinska, B; Levallet, J. The oestrogen sources in the testis and the reproductive tract of the male. *International Journal of Andrology*, 1999 22, 211-223.

[62] Pereyra-Martinez, AC; Roselli, CE; Stadelman, HL; Resko, JA. Cytochrome P450 aromatase in testis and epididymis of male *rhesus* monkeys. *Endocrine*, 2001 16, 15-19.

[63] Carpino, A; Romeo, F; Rago, V. Aromatase immunolocalization in human ductuli efferentes and proximal ductus epididymis. *Journal of Anatomy*, 2004 204, 217-220.

[64] Wiszniewska, B. Primary culture of the rat epididymal epithelial cells as a source of oestrogen. *Andrologia*, 2002 34, 180-187.

[65] Hoffmann, B; Rostalski, A; Mutembei, HM; Goericke-Pesch, S. Testicular steroid hormone secretion in the boar and expression of testicular and epididymal steroid sulphatase and estrogen sulphotransferase activity. *Experimental and Clinical Endocrinolology and Diabetes*, 2010 118, 274-280.

[66] Tong, MH; Song, W-C. Estrogen sulfotransferase: discrete and androgen-dependent expression in the male reproductive tract and demonstration of an in vivo function in the mouse epididymis. *Endocrinology*, 2002 143, 3144-3151.

[67] Frenette, G; Leclerc, P; D'amours, O; Sullivan, R. Estrogen sulfotransferase is highly expressed along the bovine epididymis and is secreted into the intraluminal environment. *Journal of Andrology*, 2009 30, 580-589.

[68] Lemazurier, E; Seralini, GE. Evidence for sulfatase and 17-beta-hydroxysteroid dehydrogenase type 1 activities in equine epididymis and uterus. *Theriogenology*, 2002 58, 113-121.

[69] MacLusky, NJ; Naftolin, F. Sexual differentiation of the central nervous system. *Science*, 1981 211, 1294-1302.

[70] Roselli, CF. Brain aromatase: roles in reproduction and neuroprotection. *Journal of Steroid Biochemistry and Molecular Biology*, 2007 106, 143-150.

[71] Weisz, J. In vitro assays of aromatase and their role in studies of estrogen formation in target tissues. *Cancer Research (Suppl.)*, 1982 42, 3295s-3298s.

[72] Graddy, LG; Kowalski, AA; Simmen, FA; Davis, SL; Baumgartner, WW; Simmen, RC. Mutiple isoforms of porcine aromatase are encoded by three distinct genes. *Journal of Steroid Biochemistry and Molecular Biology*, 2000 73, 49-57.

[73] Conley, A; Corbin, J; Smith, T; Hinshelwood, M; Liu, Z; Simpson, E. Porcine aromatases: studies on tissue-specific, functionally distinct isozymes from a single gene? *Journal of Steroid Biochemistry and Molecular Biology*, 1997 61, 407-413.

[74] Conley, A; Hinshelwood, M. Mammalian aromatases. *Reproduction*, 2001 121, 685-695.

[75] Conley, AJ; Corbin, CJ; Hughes, AL. Adaptive evolution of mammalian aromatases: Lessons from Suiformes. *Journal of Experimental Zoology*, 2008 309A, 1-12.

[76] Callard, GV; Tchoudakova, A. Evolutionary and functional significance of two CYP19 genes differentially expressed in both brain and ovary of goldfish. *Journal of Steroid Biochemistry and Molecular Biology*, 1997 61, 387-392.

[77] Corbin, CJ; Berger, T; Ford, JJ; Roselli, CE; Sienkiewicz, W; Trainor, BC; Roser, JF; Vidal, JD; Harada, N; Conley, AJ. Porcine hypothalamic aromatase cytochrome P450: isoform characterization, sex-dependent activity, regional expression and regulation by enzyme inhibition in neonatal boars. *Biology of Reproduction*, 2009 81, 388-395.

[78] Hahn, EF; Miyairi, S; Fishman, J. 19-Hydroxylation of androgens in the rat brain. *Proceedings of the National Academy of Science USA*, 1985 82, 2728-2730.

[79] Norton, BI; Miyairi, S; Fishman, J. 19-Hydroxylation of androgens by rat granulose cells. *Endocrinology*, 1988 122, 1047-1052.

[80] Khalil, MW; Morley, P; Glasier, MA; Armstrong, DT; Lang, T. Formation of 4-oestrene- 3,17-dione (19-norandrostenedione) by porcine granulosa cells *in vitro* is inhibited by the aromatase inhibitor 4-hydroxyandrostenedione and by the cytochrome P-450 inhibitors aminoglutethimide phosphate and ketoconazole. *Journal of Endocrinology*, 1989 120, 251- 260.

[81] Garrett, WM; Hoover, DJ; Shackleton, CHL; Anderson, LD. Androgen metabolism by porcine granulosa cells during the process of luteinization *in vitro*: Identification of 19-oic- androstenedione as a major metabolite and possible precursor for the formation of C_{18} neutral steroids. *Endocrinology*, 1991 129, 2941-2950.

[82] Smith, SJ; Cox, JE; Houghton, E; Dumasia, MC; Moss, M. In-vitro biosynthesis of C_{18} neutral steroids in horse testes. *Journal of Reproduction and Fertility,* 1987 35 (Suppl.), 71-78.

[83] Silberzahn, P; Gaillard, J-L; Quincey, D; Dintinger, T; Al-Timimi, I. Aromatization of testosterone and 19-nortestosterone by a single enzyme from equine testicular microsomes. Differences from human placental aromatase. *Journal of Steroid Biochemistry,* 1988 29, 119-125.

[84] Dumasia, MC; Houghton, E; Jackiw, M. Identification of endogenous C_{18} neutral steroids in stallion testis tissue by GC-MS. *Journal of Endocrinology,* 1985 107 (Suppl.), Abstract No. 135.

[85] Raeside, JI; Renaud, RL; Friendship, RM; Khalil, MW. Secretion of 19-hydroxy-androstenedione and 19-hydroxytestosterone by porcine Leydig cells in vitro and in vivo. *Journal of Endocrinology*, 1993 137, 281-289.

[86] Sekihara, H. 19-Hydroxyandrostenedione: evidence for a new class of sodium-retaining and hypertensinogenic steroids. *Endocrinology,* 1983 113, 1141-1148.

[87] Osawa, Y; Yarborough, C. Non-aromatising androgen C10-19 lyase: biosynthesis of 19- norandrostenedione by dog adrenal. *Endocrinology,* 1983 112 (Suppl.), Abstract No. 664.

[88] Sekihara, H; Torii, R; Osawa, Y; Takaku, F. Angiotensin II induces the release of 19-hydroxyandrostenedione in man. *Journal of Clinical Endocrinology and Metabolism,* 1985 61, 291-296.

[89] Suhara, K; Ohashi, K; Takahashi, K; Katagiri, M. Aromatizing and non-aromatizing 10- demethylase activity of adrenal cortex mitochondria P-450 11β. *Archives of Biochemistry and Biophysics,* 1988 267, 31-37.

[90] Idler, DR; Macnab, HC. The biosynthesis of 11-ketotestosterone and 11β-hydroxy-testosterone by Atlantic salmon tissues *in vitro. Canadian Journal of Biochemistry and Physiology, 1967 45, 581-589.*

[91] Yazawa, T; Uesaka, M; Inaoka, Y; Mizutani, T; Sekiguchi, T; Kajitani, T; Kitano, T; Umezawa, A; Miyamoto, K. Cyp11b1 is induced in the murine gonad by Luteinizing Hormone/Human Chorionic Gonadotropin and involved in the production of 11-ketotestosterone, a major fish androgen: conservation and evolution of the androgen metabolic pathway. *Endocrinology*, 2008 149, 1786-1792.

[92] Corbin, CJ; Mapes, SM; Marcos, J; Shackleton, CH; Morrow, D; Safe, S; Wise, T; Ford, JJ; Conley, AJ. Paralogues of porcine aromatase cytochrome P450: A novel hydroxylase activity is associated with the survival of a duplicated gene. *Endocrinology*, 2004 145, 2157- 2164.

[93] Dintinger, T; Gaillard, JL; Moslemi, S; Zwain, I; Silberzahn, P. Androgen and 19-norandrogen aromatization by equine and human placental microsomes. *Journal of Steroid Biochemistry*, 1989 33, 949-954.

[94] Kao, YC; Higashiyama, T; Sun, X; Okubo, T; Yarborough, C; Choi, I; Osawa, Y; Simmen, FA; Chen, S. Catalytic differences between porcine blastocyst and placental aromatase isozymes. *European Journal of Biochemistry*, 2000 267, 6134-6139.

[95] Houghton, E; Teale, P; Dumasia, MC. Studies related to the origin of C18 neutral steroids isolated from extracts of urine from the male horse: The identification of urinary 19-oic acids and their decarboxylation to produce estr-4-en-17β-ol-3-one (19-nortestosterone) and estr-4-ene-3,17-dione (19-norandrost-4-ene-3,17-dione) during sample processing. *Analytica Chimica Acta*, 2007 586, 196-207.

[96] Gomez-Sanchez, CE; Gomez-Sanchez, EP; Shackleton, CHL; Milewich, L. Identification of 19-hydroxydeoxycorticosterone, 19-oxo-deoxycorticosterone, and 19-oic- deoxycorticosterone as products of deoxycorticosterone metabolism by rat adrenals. *Endocrinology*, 1982 110, 384-389.

[97] Sohl, CD; Guengerich, FP. Kinetic analysis of the three-step steroid aromatase reaction of human cytochrome P450 19A1. *Journal of Biological Chemistry*, 2010 285, 17734-17743.

[98] Choi, I; Collante, WR; Simmen, RCM; Simmen, FA. A developmental switch in expression from blastocyst to endometrial/placental-type cytochrome P450 aromatase genes in the pig and horse. *Biology of Reproduction*, 1997 56, 688-696.

[99] Heap, RB; Hamon, M; Allen, WR. Studies on oestrogen synthesis by the preimplantation equine embryo. *Journal of Reproduction and Fertility*, 1982 32 (Suppl.), 343-352.

[100] Raeside, JI; Christie, HL. The presence of 19-norandrostenedione and its sulphate form in yolk-sac fluid of the early equine conceptus. *Journal of Steroid Biochemistry and Molecular Biology*, 2008 108, 149-154.

[101] Raeside, JI; Renaud, RL; Friendship, RM. Aromatization of 19-norandrogens by porcine Leydig cells. *Journal of Steroid Biochemistry*, 1988 32, 729-735.

[102] Townsley, JD; Brodie, HJ. Studies on the mechanism of estrogen biosynthesis. 3. The stereochemistry of aromatization of C19 and C18 steroids. *Biochemistry*, 1968 7, 33-40.

[103] Toth, M; Zakar, T. Relative binding affinities of testosterone, 19-nortestosterone and their 5 alpha-reduced derivatives to the androgen receptor and to other androgen-binding proteins: a suggested role of 5 alpha-reductive steroid metabolism in the dissociation of "myotropic" and "androgenic" activities of 19-norandrostenedione. *Journal of Steroid Biochemistry*, 1982 17, 653-660.

[104] Raeside, JI; Renaud, RL; Marshall, DE. Effect of a 5α-reductase inbititor on the metabolism of 19-norandrogens by porcine Leydig cells. *Biochemical and Biophysical Research Communications*, 1992 183, 1254-1259.

[105] Raeside, JI; Renaud, RL; Marshall, DE. Hydroxylation of 19-norandrogens by porcine Leydig cells. *Journal of Steroid Biochemistry and Molecular Biology*, 1992 42, 637-641.

[106] Page, ST; Marck, BT; Tolliver, JM; Matsumoto, AT. Tissue selectivity of the anabolic steroid, 19-nor-4-androstenediol-3β,17β-diol in male Sprague Dawley rats: selective stimulation of muscle mass and bone mineral density relative to prostate mass. *Endocrinology*, 2007 49, 1987-1993.

[107] Kousteni, S; Chen, JR; Bellido, T; Han, L; Ali, AA; O'Brien, CA; Plotkin, L; Fu, Q; Mancino, AT; Wen, Y; Vertino, AM; Powers, CC; Stewart, SA; Ebert, R; Parfitt,

[108] AM; Weinstein, RS; Jilka, RL; Manolagas, SC. Reversal of bone loss in mice by nongenotropic signaling of sex steroids. *Science*, 2002 298, 843-846.

[109] Hewitt, SC; Collins, J; Grissom, S; Hamilton, K; Korach, KS. Estren behaves as a weak estrogen rather than a nongenomic selective activator in the mouse uterus. *Endocrinology*, 2006 147, 2203-2214.

In: Testosterone
Editor: Konstantin Chichinadze

ISBN 978-1-62100-492-9

Chapter V

Testosterone Suppression due to Stress: Possible Mechanisms and Reproductive Consequences

María del Socorro Retana-Márquez
Departamento Biología de la Reproducción, Universidad Autónoma Metropolitana-Iztapalapa, México City C.P., México

Abstract

In mammals, chronic exposure to stressors of different nature, strength or quality has long been recognized as a profound disruptive factor in reproductive function. In males, stress suppresses testosterone secretion, spermatogenesis and sexual arousal. Severe suppression of reproduction appears to be caused by several hormones that are secreted when the hypothalamic-pituitary-adrenal (HPA) axis is activated during stress. Since Hans Selye suggested in 1946 that chronic stress increases activity in the HPA axis and at the same time suppresses activity in the hypothalamic-pituitary-gonadal (HGA) axis, there has been much work demonstrating this opposite relationship. Corticotropin releasing hormone (CRH), corticotrophin (ACTH), β-endorphins, and glucocorticoids can inhibit HGA axis function. The centrally mediated inhibition of Gonadotropin Releasing Hormone (GnRH) by the hormones of the HPA and the recently discovered Gonadotropin inhibitory hormone (GnIH), the decrease in pituitary responsiveness to GnRH, and the direct effects of stress-hormones on testis leading to the reduction in testosterone secretion are discussed. This chapter focuses on the suppression of testicular testosterone caused by stress, as well as its reproductive consequences in fertility and sexual behavior in males.

Introduction

Testosterone is the main and most important androgen in male vertebrates. In mammals, this sexual steroid is synthesized by Leydig cells in the interstitial compartment of the testis, estimated to be approximately 500 million [1]. Testosterone synthesis is under the control of the pulsatile release of the pituitary gonadotropin luteinizing hormone (LH), which, in turn, is controlled by the episodic release of the gonadotropin releasing hormone (GnRH) from the hypothalamus. Both the medial preoptic area (MPOA) and the arcuate nucleus (ARC) in the medial basal region of the hypothalamus, contain important centers for the control of gonadotropin secretion. Peptidergic neurons in this region secrete the decapeptide GnRH, also called luteinizing hormone–releasing hormone (LHRH), in a pulsatile fashion [2]. Neurons from other regions of the brain make synapses in this area and influence both the frequency and the amplitude of GnRH secretory pulses through catecholamine-related, dopamine-related, and endorphin-related mechanisms [3]. This hormone is released into the hypophyseal-portal system, and transported to the gonadotrophs of the anterior pituitary where it binds to high-affinity receptors coupled to G proteins [4] on the plasma membrane of pituitary gonadotrophs, stimulating the synthesis and release of luteinizing hormone (LH) and follicle stimulating hormone (FSH) [5]. Slow-frequency GnRH pulses favor FSH secretion, whereas frequent pulses favor LH secretion [6]. LH is released to the bloodstream from the anterior pituitary gonadotrophs and reaches the testis, where it interacts with specific LH receptors on the surface of testicular Leydig cells [7].

In the testis, receptor activation is coupled primarily to Gs proteins, leading to stimulation of adenylate cyclase and the formation of cAMP, which binds to the regulatory subunit of a protein kinase and causes dissociation of the regulatory subunit and activation of the catalytic subunit [3]. The activated protein kinase operates through unidentified steps to stimulate the synthesis of testosterone biosynthesis enzymes [8]. The signal is terminated by endocytosis and degradation of the LH-receptor complex [9].

Cholesterol is the substrate for all steroid biosynthesis, and testosterone is synthesized by a sequence of enzymatic reactions that converts cholesterol to the first steroid produced: pregnenolone, and then, through a number of steroid intermediates, to testosterone [10]. Leydig cells utilize two separate pathways in the synthesis of androgens, the type of pathway usually being species specific. The Δ4 pathway (cholesterol → pregnenolone → progesterone → androstenedione → testosterone) is found in most rodents including the rat and mouse [11]. The Δ5 pathway (cholesterol → pregnenolone → 17a-hydroxypregnenolone → dehydroepiandrosterone → androstenedione → testosterone) is found in dogs [12], rabbits [13], pigs [14], humans and higher primates [15, 16]. Testosterone biosynthesis in Leydig cells occurs with the conversion of cholesterol to pregnenolone, when the side chain is cleaved by enzyme cytochrome P450 in the inner mitochondrial membrane. Pregnenolone diffuses out of the mitochondria to the microsomal compartment where, if the 5-ene pathway is used, pregnenolone is converted to 17α-hydroxypregnenolone by the enzyme cytochrome P450 17α-hydroxylase/17,20 lyase and eventually to dehydroepiandrosterone by the same enzyme. If the 4-ene pathway is used, pregnenolone is converted to progesterone through the action of 3-β-hydroxysteroid dehydrogenase (3β-HSD) and then to 17α-hydroxyprogesterone and androstenedione by cytochrome P450 17α-hydroxylase/17,20 lyase. Androstenedione is then converted to testosterone by the action of 17-ketosteroid reductase. Testosterone can also be converted to dihydrotestosterone in target tissues by 5α-reductase enzyme or to estradiol by aromatase. In general, the cholesterol side chain cleavage cytochrome P450 is found in the mitochondria and the rest of the enzymes are found in the microsomal compartment of steroidogenic cells, although 3β-HSD can also be found in the mitochondria of some species and some tissues (See [1] for review). The testosterone synthesized by Leydig cells is secreted into the blood, and it can be metabolized to its 5α-reduced and highly active metabolite, dihydrotestosterone or aromatized to 17β-estradiol in peripheral tissues [10], as shown in Figure 1. Although virtually all steroid production occurs in the interstitial compartment of the testis, Sertoli cells contain significant levels of aromatase activity that can convert androgen substrates into estrogens [17].

Androgens produced by Leydig cells are responsible for the development and maintenance of male sexual characteristics in the body such as the internal sex organs and external genitalia of the male reproductive system, male secondary sexual characteristics, muscular and skeletal systems, and for the maintenance of spermatogenesis, as well as for the expression of sexual behavior [18].

These two last aspects of masculine reproduction will be considered in this review, as well as the effects of chronic stress on them.

In the males of many species of vertebrates, testosterone levels, sexual behavior, and spermatogenesis are reproductive functions that are impaired during stress. Consequently, there have been a number of studies in relation to the effects of stress on reproduction, both in males and females in several animal species, including human beings.

Homeostasis, Stress and Adaptive Response to Stress

Living organisms maintain a dynamic equilibrium called homeostasis through adjustments in the internal medium controlled by biological systems. Homeostasis is constantly threatened by internal or external adverse forces, which are called stressors [19,20]. Thus, stress has been defined as a state of threatened homeostasis, which is re-established as a result of complex behavioral and physiological adaptive responses by the organism [19]. The adaptive responses to stress depend on the characteristics of the stressor, which can be emotional or physical, acute or chronic; the intensity of the stressor must also be considered [21]. The stress response is mediated by the stress system, which involves the Central Nervous System (CNS) and peripheral components (see [19, 22] for review). The hypothalamus and the brain stem are the central components of the stress system, and it includes the parvocellular neurons which release corticotropin-releasing hormone (CRH); the arginine vasopressin (AVP) neurons of the paraventricular nuclei (PVN) of the hypothalamus; the CRH neurons of the paragigantocellular and parabrachial nuclei of the medulla, and the locus coeruleus (LC); and other mostly noradrenergic (NE) cell groups in the medulla and pons (LC/NE system). The peripheral components of the stress system include the peripheral components of the hypothalamic-pituitary-adrenal (HPA) axis; the efferent sympathetic-adrenomedullary system; and components of the parasympathetic system [20, 22, 23]. In the CNS, the stress response includes facilitation of neural pathways that promote acute, time limited adaptive functions, such as arousal, alertness, vigilance, improved cognition and focused attention, and inhibition of neural pathways that control acutely vegetative, nonadaptive functions, such as eating, growth, and reproduction. In addition, stress related changes lead to increased oxygenation and nutrition of the brain, heart and skeletal muscles, which are all organs crucial to the central coordination of the stress response and the 'fight or flight' reaction [19]. Coordination of the endocrine response to chronic stress by the CNS includes the participation of the HPA axis, which is an important regulator of homeostatic functions [24]. The stress response is associated with increases in the levels of plasma glucocorticoids. The secretion of glucocorticoids from the adrenal cortex is under the control of adrenocorticotropin (ACTH), which in turn, is released from the anterior lobe of the pituitary. ACTH secretion is regulated by CRH and to a minor extent by Arginine Vasopressin (AVP) [19, 21, 22, 25, 26]. Glucocorticoids play an important role in the regulation of basal activity of the HPA axis, as well as in the termination of the stress response by acting on extrahypothalamic centers, the hypothalamus and the pituitary gland. The negative feedback of glucocorticoids on the secretion of CRH and ACTH serves to limit the total duration of tissue exposure of the organism to glucocorticoids, thus minimizing the catabolic, lipogenic, antireproductive, and the immunosuppressive effects of these hormones (Figure 2). A dual-receptor system exists for glucocorticoids in the CNS, which includes the glucocorticoid receptor type I or mineralocorticoid receptor (MR) that responds to low concentrations of glucocorticoids, and the classic glucocorticoid receptor (GR) type II that responds to both basal and stress concentrations of glucocorticoids. The negative feedback control of the CRH and ACTH secretion after exposure to stress or during the circadian and ultradian peaks is mediated through type II glucocorticoid receptors [20, 22, 23]. Corticosterone exerts negative feed back on the HPA-axis through GR activation in the PVN in a genomic fashion [27]. However, corticosterone also regulates HPA-axis activity through non-genomic actions [28] in the hypothalamus, pituitary and hippocampus through membrane located receptors [29, 30].

Consequences of Stress on Reproductive Function

Chronic exposure to stressors increases HPA axis activity and concomitantly reduces Hypothalamic-Pituitary-Gonadal (HPG) axis activity [31], the severe suppression of reproduction during stress has been corroborated in many studies. Males under chronic stress exhibit suppression of testosterone secretion [32, 33, 34], spermatogenesis [35, 36, 37], fertility [38] and sexual behavior [34, 39, 40, 41]. Since the system responsible for reproduction is directly linked to the stress system [42, 43], suppression of reproduction is caused by the HPA axis hormones secreted during stress, such as CRH, ACTH, β-endorphins, and glucocorticoids on HPA axis function [44-48]. These components of the HPA axis inhibit the reproductive axis at all levels. In the hypothalamus, GnRH release from neurons of the MPOA is suppressed by CRH, directly, through synaptic connections between CRH neurons and GnRH neurons in the MPOA [49] or indirectly, through β-endorphins from arcuate POMC neurons [21, 22, 46, 50]. In the pituitary, LH secretion decreases as a result of glucocorticoid-mediated reduction in its responsiveness to GnRH [45]. Glucocorticoids also exert direct gonadal effects, with subsequent alterations in sex steroid output [51,52,53]. Likewise, glucocorticoids induce target tissue resistance to gonadal sex steroids [54]. These pathways are shown in Figure 3.

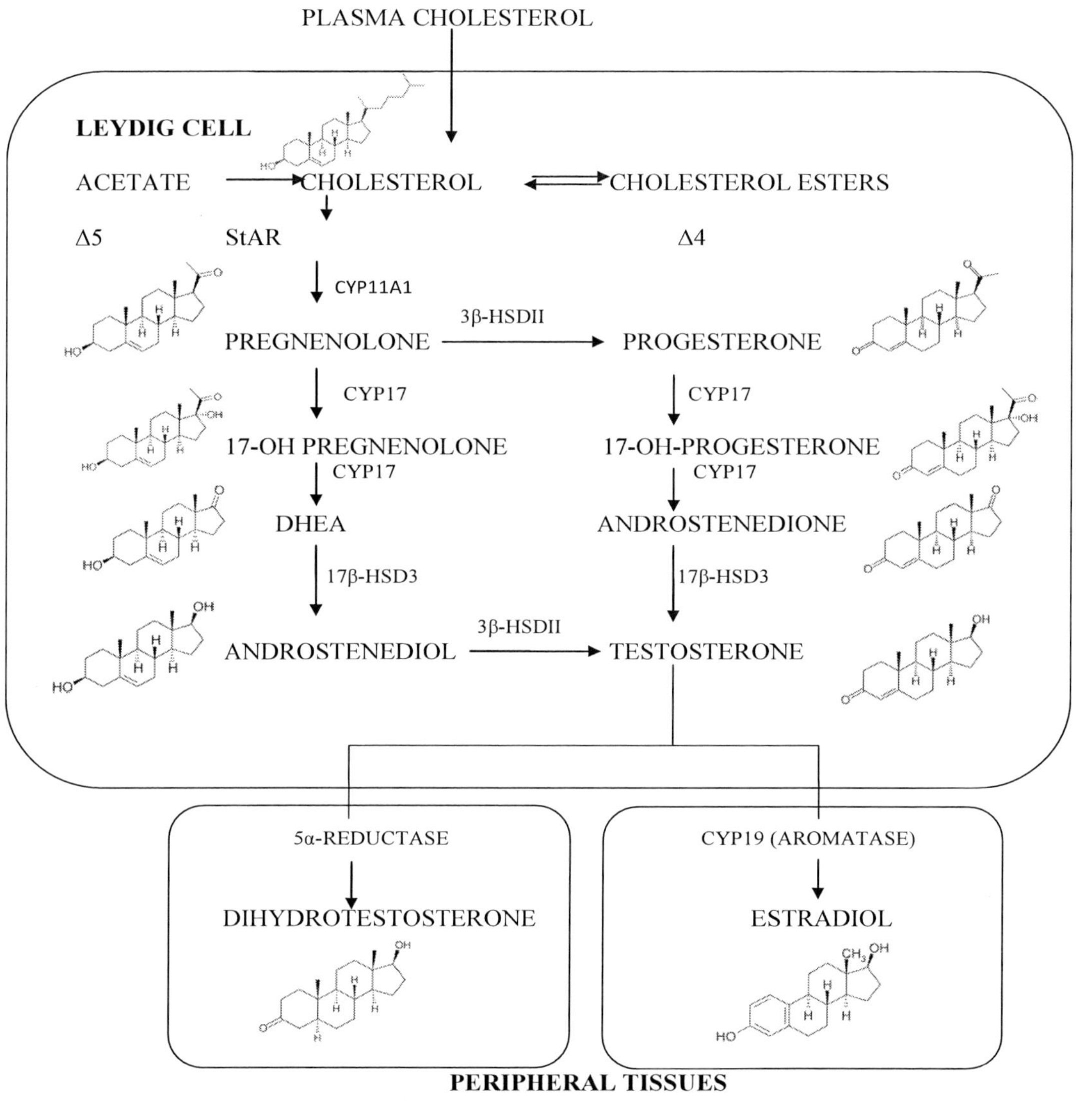

Figure 1. Pathways of testosterone synthesis in testis. Cholesterol for testosterone synthesis can come from three sources: (1) plasma cholesterol, (2) cholesterol newly synthesized within the Leydig cell, and (3) cholesterol stored as cholesterol esters in Leydig cells. The arrival of cholesterol to the inner mitochondrial membrane for side-chain cleavage to pregnenolone is the rate-limiting reaction and is under control of the luteinizing hormone. Conversion of pregnenolone to testosterone can take place by two pathways: one in which reduction of the 17-keto group is accomplished before A-ring oxidation and the other in which this sequence is inverted. CYP11A1= Cytochrome P450, cholesterol side chain cleavage enzyme; CYP17= Cytochrome P450 enzime, 17α-hydroxylase; DHEA=dehydroepiandrosterone; HSD=hydroxysteroid dehydrogenase; StAR=steroidogenic acute regulatory protein [3].

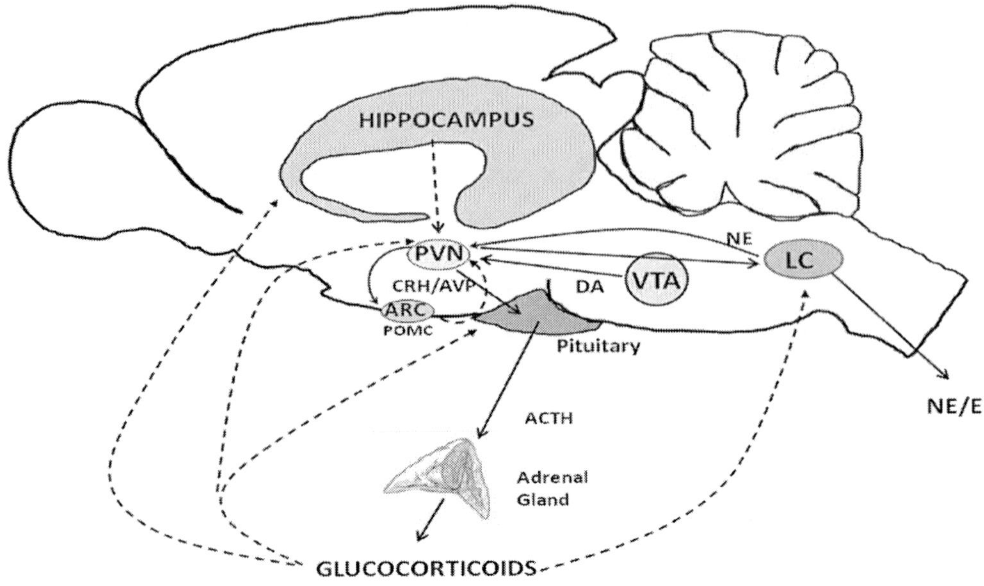

Figure 2. Central and peripheral structures involved in the stress system. During stress, corticotrophin releasing hormone (CRH) and arginine vasopresine (AVP) pulsations increases, resulting in the increase of adrenocorticotropin hormones (ACTH) secretion from the anterior pituitary, which in turn, stimulates the secretion of glucocorticoid hormones by the adrenal cortex. The CRH/AVP neurons and the neurons of the locus coeruleus/norepinephrine (LC/NE) system are reciprocally innervated and activate each other. Glucocorticoids are the final effectors of the HPA axis and participate in the control of whole body homeostasis. They play a key regulatory role on the basal activity of the HPA axis and onthe termination of the stress response by acting at extra-hypothalamic centers such as the hippocampus, the hypothalamus and the pituitary gland.

Opioids and the HPG Axis during Stress

Suppression of testosterone plasma levels caused by chronic stress can be attenuated by naltrexone (NTX), which suggests that the effects of stress on testosterone levels could be partially mediated by endogenous opioids, mainly β-endorphins, aside from CRF and glucocorticoid [55]. The inhibitory effects of both peptides could be exerted directly in the testis, inhibiting androgen synthesis, and by decreasing GnRH release from the MPOA. Both CRF and β-endorphins can exert effects on the HPG axis by inhibiting GnRH release from the hypothalamus [56-58], inhibiting LH release from the pituitary [56-62], and inhibiting testosterone synthesis directly in Leydig cells [63-68], thus decreasing testosterone in plasma. All these effects caused by CRF, opioids and stress can be reverted or prevented by the administration of the opioid antagonists naloxone or naltrexone, thus increasing GnRH [58], as well as plasma levels of LH [69] and testosterone [67, 68].

Aside from its known antireproductive functions in the brain and the hypothalamus, CRF acts as a direct and indirect (β-endorphin mediated) anti-reproductive peptide in the testis, where both peptides function as negative regulators of gonadotropin actions [63, 70, 71]. CRF secretion in Leydig cells is stimulated by serotonin through 5HT2 receptors [72], and it has been proposed that, during stress, serotonin is released and stimulates CRF secretion in Leydig cells [63]. Testosterone synthesis can be suppressed, not only by glucocorticoids [52, 53, 73] but also by endogenous opioid peptides, both of which inhibit the enzymes involved in steroidogenesis [66-68]. The inhibition of testicular steroidogenesis by local opioids, specifically β-endorphin, can be prevented by the infusion of opioid antagonists such as naloxone and naltrexone methobromide (a peripheral opioid antagonist), suggesting that these effects are mediated, at least in part, by the opioid μ-receptor subtype [66-68]. When rats are treated with NTX the decrease in plasma testosterone due to stress is attenuated [51]. NTX and NTX methobromide can stimulate an increase in testicular testosterone, as well as in pituitary LH in male rats [65, 66], and rhesus monkeys [74]. The stimulatory effect of NTX in control males could be due to the stimulation of LH release from the pituitary, as well as to stimulation of testicular testosterone secretion by increasing the activity of the enzymes involved in testosterone biosynthesis [66-68]. All this evidence supports the idea that the inhibitory effects of stress on testicular steroidogenesis are mediated, at least to some extent, by opioids. More studies, however, will be necessary to demonstrate opioid release in brain structures, pituitary, and testis in the male rat during stress.

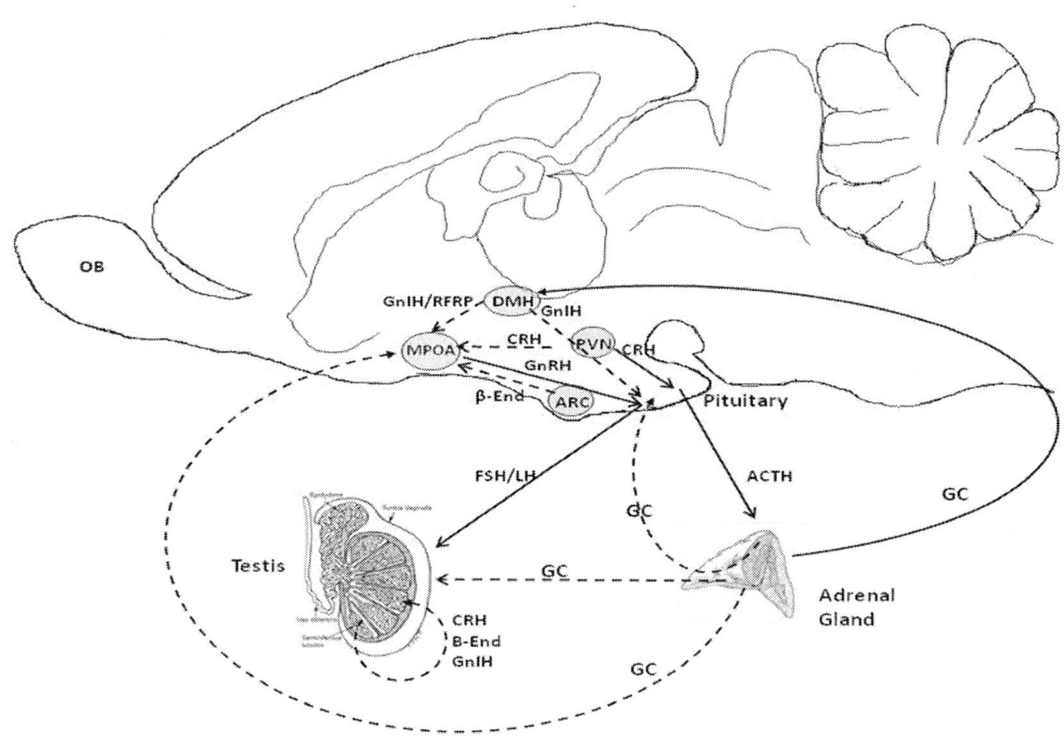

Figure 3. Neuroendocrine pathways involved in the suppression of HPG axis by HPA axis. During stress CRH neurons in PVN activate and stimulate the secretion of ACTH in the anterior lobe of the pituitary. This hormone stimulates synthesis and secretion of glucocorticoids in the adrenal cortex. HPG axis is inhibited at all levels by HPA axis. GnRH release from MPOA is inhibited by CRH, β-endorphins, and GnIH/RFRP directly in the hypothalamus. Glucocorticoids decrease the responsiveness of gonadotrophs to GnRH, reduce steroidogenesis in testis, and inhibit GnRH release directly and indirectly through GnIH/RFRP. Solid lines = stimulation. Dashed lines = inhibition.

GnIH/RFRP Hormone and HPG Axis during Stress

Other hormones, however, are also implicated in the inhibition of the HPG axis, both in physiological conditions, as well as during stress. Recent research in the context of reproduction control involves the participation of a recently identified peptide in the brain of birds. This peptide acts directly on the pituitary to inhibit gonadotropin release

in quail, so it was named gonadotropin-inhibitory hormone (GnIH) [75]. GnIH homologues have been identified in a number of other vertebrates, including mammals and are named RFamide related peptides (RFRPs) [76]. This peptide was discovered in the hypothalamus [77] and is expressed in RFRP neurons within the dorsomedial nucleus (DMH) in rats, with fibers extending both to the median eminence and to the preoptic area, making putative contact with GnRH neurons within the hypothalamus [78-80], and GnIH receptors are expressed on GnRH-I and -II neurons in birds [81]. As in birds, mammalian GnIH homologues (RFRP) act to inhibit pituitary synthesis of the gonadotrophin subunits α and β [82] as well as gonadotropin release in several mammalian species, such as rats [83], hamsters [84], sheep [85], and humans, [84]. Furthermore, RFRP and its receptor have been demonstrated both in avian and mammalian gonads. This means that RFRP can act directly at multiple levels: within the brain, on the pituitary, and in the gonads [81]. This evidence indicates that GnIH and its related peptides are important modulators of reproductive function at the level of GnRH neurons, the gonadotroph and the gonads.

RFRP is also involved in the negative regulation of the HPG axis during stress, as both acute and chronic immobilization stress leads to an up-regulation of RFRP expression in the dorsomedial hypothalamus (DMH) of adult male rats [87]. Current findings provide a novel mechanism by which HPA axis activation can influence reproductive function. The mechanism through which the HPA axis inhibits the HPG axis involves adrenal glucocorticoids. These steroid hormones, released during the stress response, act on glucocorticoid receptors (GR) in hypothalamic RFRP neurons, causing increased transcription of the RFRP gene, thus increasing RFRP expression in the DMH [87]. RFRP released from this hypothalamic area inhibits GnRH release through a direct postsynaptic mechanism, causing hyper polarization in GnRH neurons [88, 89], and decreases pituitary sensitivity to GnRH [87, 90], thus contributing to hypothalamic suppression of reproductive function.

Glucocorticoid and HPG during Stress

Glucocorticoid is considered the "stress hormone" because its concentration in plasma rises sharply in response to stress, and it also exerts an inhibitory effect on GnRH neurons [21, 91]. It decreases responsiveness of the pituitary gonadotroph to GnRH, resulting in decreased LH secretion [45, 92]; it has direct effects on gonads, decreasing the sensitivity of Leydig cells to LH, or decreasing testicular receptors to this hormone [93], with subsequent alteration in sex steroid output [51-53]. Besides, it renders target tissues of gonadal steroids resistant to these hormones [42, 50, 54, 94, 95].

Suppression of gonadal function secondary to chronic activation of the HPA axis has been demonstrated in males of different species. Chronic stress by immobilization [32,33,96], intermittent electric foot shock [34, 55, 97], prolonged exercise [98], constant illumination

[99], forced swimming in cold water [34, 55, 58], noise, fasting [100], surgery [101], crowding and social stress [102, 103] in rats, causes a decrease in hypothalamus CRH content, an increase in plasma levels of ACTH and glucocorticoids, as well as a general inhibitory effect on the HPG axis, through decreasing LH and testosterone. The same results have been observed in hamsters [104]. In humans, highly trained athletes of both genders [105] and ballet dancers [106], prolonged physical stress due to exercise [107] or military training [108], as well as sleep deprivation [107], increases plasma levels of cortisol and ACTH, with a concomitant decrease in LH and testosterone.

GLUCOCORTICOIDS AND TESTOSTERONE

The reduction in testosterone during chronic stress has been long attributed to glucocorticoids, since the increase in these hormones during stress is associated with testicular involution and a significant drop in testosterone secretion, as well as diminished libido and fertility [109]. Additionally, it has been observed that glucocorticoids directly inhibit testosterone synthesis by Leydig cells *in vitro* [52,110]. Glucocorticoid receptors are expressed in primary spermatocytes, peritubular myoid cells, and in Leydig cells [111, 112, 113], suggesting that these hormones can directly affect spermatogenesis and steroidogenesis in the testis. The underlying mechanisms of steroidogenic inhibition in Leydig cells by glucocorticoids during stress include the inhibition of the transcription of genes encoding testosterone biosynthetic enzymes [52, 114], as well as the reduction in the levels of steroidogenic enzymes, including 20-22 lyase, 3β-hydroxysteroid dehydrogenase, and 17α-hydroxylase/C17-20 lyase [8, 51, 52, 115]. The extent of glucocorticoid activity in Leydig cells depends on whether the steroid is metabolized or not. Intracellular levels of corticosterone (CORT) are regulated by 11β-hydroxysteroid dehydrogenase (11βHSD), which has two known isoforms: type I, which is an oxidoreductase, which catalyzes the interconversion of 11β-hydroxyl steroids, such as CORT and 11-keto steroids, such as 11-dehydrocorticosterone (11DHC) in rats. Type II 11βHSDH is a unidirectional oxidase that inactivates CORT through conversion to 11DHC [109]. The inhibition of steroidogenesis in Leydig cells, directly mediated by glucocorticoids during stress occurs when the activity of the enzyme (11βHSD1) that dehydrogenates and inactivates intracellular corticosteroid is low [53,103,116]. GLucocorticoids can also directly inhibit testosterone biosynthesis in Leydig cells through a nongenomic mechanism, reducing the production of cytoplasmic cAMP during acute stress [73].

Stress-mediated increase in glucocorticoids levels is also involved in the initiation of Leydig cell apoptosis [117, 118], potentially contributing to suppression of circulating testosterone levels [109]. As is known, apoptosis (programmed cell death) is characterized morphologically by shrinkage of total cell volume, increased cell density and compaction of cell organelles [119, 120]. During apoptosis there is a double-strand, endonuclease-specific cleavage of nuclear DNA at the linker regions between nucleosomes, leading to the production of oligonucleosomal fragments that are multiples of 180 DNA base pairs [121].

Immature and adult Leydig cells treated with 100nM CORT for either 4 or 24 h *in vitro* showed increased frequencies of apoptosis compared with untreated controls. Ultra structural analysis confirmed the signs of apoptosis, including nuclear fragmentation and formation of apoptotic bodies [117]. Administration of CORT in vivo at doses ranging from 2.5-7.5 mg/100g BW in male rats increased Leydig cell apoptosis after 24 h of treatment. At the same time, 11HBSD in Leydig cells decreased concurrently with decreased serum testosterone levels [117]. CORT administration induces Leydig cell apoptosis through the activation of the Fas system, which activates proteolytic machinery, causing target cells apoptosis within hours [122]; cleavage of procaspase-3, responsible for the proteolysis of a large number of protein substrates and cell disassembly during the execution phase of apoptosis [123-125]; and loss of mitochondrial membrane potential, causing cytochrome C and other proteins to leak from the mitochondria causing activation of caspases [126], and the respiratory chain becomes uncoupled from ATP synthesis giving rise to reactive oxygen species (ROS) generation and further potentiating the death process [127]. Together all of these events are implicated in the process of corticosterone-induced Leydig cell apoptosis [109, 118]. The decline in testosterone resulting from Leydig cell apoptosis during stress is mediated through direct stimulation of Leydig cells by glucocorticoid [52, 117, 118, 128, 129], or through combined changes in serum glucocorticoid and LH levels [34].

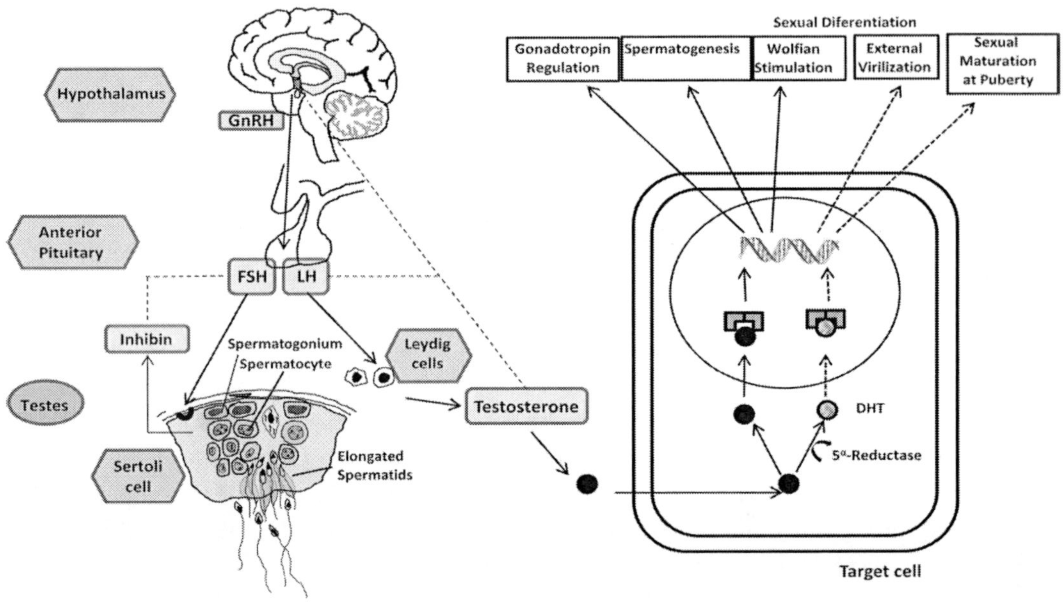

Figure 4. The neuroendocrine control of Hypothamo-pituitary- testicular axis involves the secretion of GnRH from MPOA in the hypothalamus. This hormone stimulates the release of FSH and LH from the pituitary. FSH promotes spermatogenesis and LH stimulates the interstitial Leydig cells to produce testosterone. Secreted testosterone binds to the androgen receptors in its target cells, either directly or after conversion to dihydrotestosterone (DHT). DHT binds more tightly than testosterone. Androgens induce several effects, which are mediated either by testosterone (solid lines) or by dihydrotestosterone (broken lines). Solid lines = stimulation. Dashed lines = inhibition.

The suppression of testosterone, due to steroidogenic inhibition and apoptosis of Leydig cells during stress, has been proposed to be the main factor for the impairment of spermatogenesis and male sexual behavior. These are very important issues concerning reproductive problems observed in males of several species of vertebrates in which infertility and/or diminished sexual motivation are problems induced by stress that impair reproductive success.

Testosterone Role in Male Reproduction

Testosterone is important for the initiation and regulation of male reproductive events, which include formation of the male phenotype during sexual differentiation, promotion of sexual maturation at puberty, regulation of gonadotropin secretion by the hypothalamic-pituitary system, initiation and maintenance of spermatogenesis, control of sexual behavior and erectile function in males [3]. Testosterone enters cells by passive diffusion and is converted to dihydrotestosterone (DHT) by 5α-reductase in cells expressing this enzyme. Testosterone, or its 5α-reduced metabolite dihydrotestosterone (DHT), bind to cytosolic androgen receptors (ARs) which subsequently dimerize, translocate to the nucleus, and bind to androgen response elements (AREs) in the promoters of androgen-responsive genes [130, 131] to modulate gene transcription in a so-called "genomic" pathway of action to initiate biologic responses [3, 132]. The testosterone-receptor complex regulates gonadotropin secretion and virilization of the wolffian ducts during male sexual differentiation. The DHT-receptor complex controls external virilization during embryogenesis and the development of most male secondary sexual characteristics during puberty, including androgen-mediated hair growth and loss (Figure 4). Testosterone is the active hormone involved in the control and maintenance of spermatogenesis, although DHT may play a role in human spermatogenesis [133, 134].

Stress, Sexual Dysfunctions, Spermatogenesis and Male Infertility

Stressful situations can provoke erectile dysfunction as well as decrease in both libido and fertility in men. Even though stress is not the only factor in the etiology of infertility, it is considered an additional risk factor for idiopathic infertility [135], and there are several studies supporting this hypothesis. Sperm quality decreases in men after a natural disaster, such as an earthquake [136]. In the same way, emotional stress related to work or the depressive reaction to infertility or its therapy, causes decreased semen quality [137]. Psychological stress also has a negative influence on semen volume, sperm motility [138], sperm concentration [139], and on sperm morphology, increasing sperm abnormalities, both in healthy [140-142] and subfertile men [143]. Severe psychological stress brought on by the death of a relative or spouse consistently lowers sperm count [144], in some cases leading to oligospermia or azoospermia [145, 146]. This potential reduction in fertility is most likely caused by the stress induced decline of testosterone [145, 147], although it is possible that there are also direct effects of stress on the seminiferous epithelium, impairing spermatogenesis [142].

Male fertility depends on the continuous daily production of millions of spermatozoa. Spermatogenesis is a highly complex process and requires 6 to 9 weeks for completion, with autocrine, paracrine and endocrine factors controlling the entire process (see [148] for review). During spermatogenesis, immature germ cells (diploid spermatogonia) undergo mitotic division, differentiation and meiosis to give rise to haploid round spermatides, which transform, without further division, into highly specialized elongated spermatids [149]; this process is called spermiogenesis. The final step of spermatogenesis is spermiation, and involves removal of spermatid cytoplasm to yield the streamlined spermatozoa capable of motility, and its release into the tubule lumen [150]. Spermatogenesis occurs within the seminiferous tubules of the testis, in close association with the Sertoli cells. At the completion of spermatogenesis, spermatozoa released into the seminiferous tubule lumen proceed to the rete testis, and then they enter the epididymis. In adult males, spermatogenesis is mainly regulated by FSH and testosterone, acting through specific receptors in Sertoli cells, which provide factors necessary for the successful progression of spermatogonia into spermatozoa [148, 151]. Testosterone binds with intracellular ARs, which are expressed in Sertoli cells, Leydig cells, and peritubular myoid cells of the testis [152-157]. Testosterone is implicated in the initiation of spermatogenesis in rodent models, via actions as a germ cell survival factor [158, 159], probably in synergy with FSH and LH [160], as well as in the promotion of spermiogenesis [161].

The actions of testosterone include maintenance of earlier germ cell populations, an essential function at meiosis, and maintenance of germ cell viability particularly at stage VII of the spermatogenic cycle, as well as major effects on spermiogenesis [148,151]. Hence, changes in testicular testosterone levels result in large changes in sperm output. Spermatogenesis in intact rats is suppressed when testicular testosterone reduces to 4% of normal, but it can be maintained if the testosterone level is held at 8% of normal [162], with FSH levels remaining at 60% to 80% of normal. Therefore, an intratesticular testosterone level of approximately 20 ng/ml is sufficient for the maintenance of quantitatively complete spermatogenesis [163,164], which is fivefold less than in the normal testis. However, this concentration of testosterone is still approximately four- to eightfold greater than serum levels.

Surprinsingly, testosterone is not required for spermatogonial development [165], and high testicular T concentrations may be detrimental to spermatogonial development [166], and the suppression of testicular testosterone levels is needed to promote spermatogonial development [167]. However, two key sites of androgen action are evident, specifically in meiosis [168-171] and spermiogenesis [162, 172-174]. Of these, the completion of meiosis during the onset of spermatogenesis appears to be remarkably sensitive to testosterone [168, 170] wherein exogenous testosterone administration, resulting in intratesticular testosterone concentrations 40% of normal, markedly promoted meiotic progression from preleptotene through to pachytene spermatocytes [171]. Progression of meiotic spermatocytes through stages VII and VIII is decreased when intratesticular testosterone levels are severely suppressed using a combination of gonadotropin suppression plus the anti-androgen flutamide to eliminate residual androgen action [175-177]. Thus, it seems likely that testosterone facilitates meiotic progression, at least in part, by promoting the survival of meiotic spermatocytes through the hormone sensitive stages VII and VIII.

Testosterone, along with FSH and LH are known to influence the fate of germ cells, since their suppression induces germ cell apoptosis [151]. Following testosterone reduction, preferential germ cell death in stages VII–VIII, particularly meiotic and postmeiotic cells is reported [178-180]. Ethane dimethanesulphonate (EDS) provokes the selective destruction of Leydig cells when administered, which reduces intratesticular testosterone, and provokes degeneration of pachytene spermatocytes and round spermatids in stage VII [178]. Testosterone replacement suppresses the appearance of apoptotic cells in this stage [180]. Similar studies in EDS-treated rats have demonstrated that testosterone induces apoptosis in most stages of the spermatogenic cycle, but that testosterone appears to promote apoptosis of pre-meiotic cells in stage XII [181], is perhaps a reflection of inhibitory effects of testosterone on spermatogonia as described above. Hence, as observed during the initiation of spermatogenesis, testosterone acts to support spermatogenesis in the adult through mechanisms that regulate germ cell viability particularly, but not exclusively, at stage VII and perhaps stage VIII of the spermatogenic cycle. Testosterone is necessary for initiation [171], maintenance [182] and restoration [172, 174] of all phases of spermiogenesis. Testosterone alone can initiate and maintain the production of round spermatids from pachytene spermatocytes and their subsequent elongation [171]. The conversion of round to elongated spermatids is another particular site in spermiogenesis at which testosterone action is required [172, 174, 183-185]. The most marked changes are in round spermatids at stage VIII (i.e., step 8 round spermatids) that virtually disappear from the epithelium. Succeeding studies demonstrated that suppression of intratesticular testosterone impairs the conversion of step 7 to step 8 round spermatids due to the premature detachment of step 8 round spermatids from the epithelium [148, 151, 173]. Recent studies in mice lacking LH-R, which have testicular testosterone levels only 2% of normal, showed that the conversion of round spermatids to elongated spermatids was abolished by the administration of the AR antagonist flutamide, suggesting that mid-spermiogenesis requires only very low testosterone levels in this model [186].

Androgens possibly regulate adhesion between Sertoli cells and step 8 round spermatids [161, 173, 187], though definitive in vivo proof for this propositionhas not been found [183]. Androgen suppression does not appear to disturb the structure of the ectoplasmic specialization [187], which is a Sertoli cell-specific junctional complex [188]. Cell adhesion molecules such as members of the cadherins may be important, since in vitro studies show that N-cadherin antibodies block the androgen-stimulated adhesion between rat Sertoli cells and isolated round spermatids, and N-Cad production by Sertoli cells in vitro is stimulated by androgens [189].

While testosterone is likely to act directly on the AR to support spermatogenesis in the normal adult rat, the 5α-reduction of testosterone to DHT is important for androgen action on the seminiferous epithelium when intratesticular testosterone levels are reduced. The ability of testosterone to restore spermatogenesis, as evidenced by round and elongated spermatid populations and an assessment of the androgen-dependent conversion of step 7 to 8 round spermatids, was compromised by administration of a 5α-reductase inhibitor [173, 176]. High doses of testosterone block the effect of the enzyme inhibition, presumably due to the restoration of intratesticular testosterone levels that can then interact directly with the AR [190]. Maintenance of low levels of spermatogenesis in men who fail to achieve azoospermia in response to T-based contraception has a greater 5αR activity [191, 192], suggesting increased androgenic support via higher levels of DHT.

Testicular Germ Cell Death Induced by Stress

Considering that spermatogenesis is a process highly dependent on testosterone, which has been widely demonstrated to be suppressed during chronic stress, it can be expected to be significantly impaired in stressful conditions, as has been reported in a number of studies.

Chronic stress by 6 h-immobilization for 60 days causes a significant reduction in the amount of mature spermatids in the testis and spermatozoon concentration in the cauda epididymis in male adult rats [31]. The same was observed with a different stress paradigm, consisting of forced swimming for 3 min in water at 32°C daily for 15 days [193]. This reduction in spermatogenesis is associated with low plasma levels of LH and testosterone, which causes atrophy in seminal vesicles [31]. These results confirm the importance of testosterone during spermatogenesis in the conversion of round spermatids from stage VII to stage VIII of the spermatogenic cycle [186].

One of the proposed mechanisms to explain the reduction in germ cells and therefore in spermatogenesis, due to stress is the germ cell death by apoptosis. Testicular germ cell death occurs spontaneously throughout spermatogenesis [194] and is a constant feature in a variety of mammalian species [195,196]. Nonetheless, several studies have provided evidence that the degeneration of germ cells involves apoptosis in response to stress and testosterone withdrawal [159]. Repeated exposure to immobilization during 2 hours for 7 days is capable of inducing DNA fragmentation and apoptosis in spermatogonia and primary spermatocytes. These changes were associated with a transient increase in serum CORT and a decrease in serum testosterone [197,198]. When adult male rats are treated with EDS, an agent which leads to testosterone withdrawal by the selective destruction of Leydig cells, the occurrence of germ cell loss by apoptosis increases remarkably [199], demonstrating that cell death in the seminiferous epithelium is due to testosterone decrease. A single exposure of rat testes to heat (43°C for 15 minutes) results in selective but reversible damage to the seminiferous epithelium through increased germ cell apoptosis. Heat–induced germ cell apoptosis predominantly occurs in pachytene spermatocytes and early round spermatids at stages I-IV and pachitene, diplotene, and dividing spermatocytes at stages XII-XIV stages, which are the most susceptible to heat. Intratesticular testosterone plays a fundamental role in protecting germ cells against heat induced cell death [200]. Similar results were observed with heat exposure of monkey testes, with transient decrease in serum testosterone [201]. Germ cell apoptosis due to testicular heat shock is followed by transient sub fertility [202]. Mild hypothermia of the testis (10°C for 30 minutes) causes apoptosis in methaphasic spermatocytes; secondary spermatocytes and spermatogonia at stages XII and XIV were the most sensitive cells to hypothermia [203]. Stress by cooling (4°C for 60 minutes) rat testes results in apoptotic germ cell loss within 8 hours. Pachitene spermatocytes at stages XII-I were the cells most sensitive to cooling, and germ cell lost was accompanied by a decrease in testosterone [204].

Glucocorticoid can, not only impair spermatogenesis and fertility through decreasing testosterone concentration, but also seems to act directly in testis causing apoptosis of testicular germ cells, as has been demonstrated by studies in which the administration of an exogenous glucocorticoid such as dexamethasone (Dex) in a dose of 7 mg/Kg BW during 7 days induced apoptosis in spermatogonia [205]. It is proposed that the molecular mechanisms of glucocorticoid-induced apoptosis include the regulation of transcription of genes mediated by the glucocorticoid receptor which might be tentatively grouped into three classes: (i) genes directly implicated in death and survival decisions; (ii) genes whose (de)regulation might lead to cellular distress, and (iii) genes not causal in the death response [206].

The latest evidence in the study of mechanisms regulating spermatogenesis in testes is the finding that RFRP/GnIH and its receptor are present both in testis and accessory reproductive organs of birds such as quail [207] and mammals, such as the hamster [208]. This hormone is located in the testicular interstitial cells and germ cells, such as spermatocytes and elongated spermatids; receptors for this hormone have been identified in spermatocytes, and round and elongated spermatids [207, 208]. These findings highlight a possible novel autocrine and/or paracrine role for RFRP in Syrian hamster testis, potentially contributing to the differentiation of spermatids during spermiogenesis.

Additionally, there is evidence that the administration of GnIH to mature birds induces testicular apoptosis and decreases spermatogenic activity. Spermatocytes, spermatogonia, and Sertoli cells are the most vulnerable cell types [78, 209]. The same is observed in the testis of starlings during seasonal testicular regression [210]. In many species of mammals and birds it is considered that the decrease in circulating testosterone is the main cause of testicular apoptosis [211]. As testosterone is a known testicular cell-survival factor in rodents [159, 212], it is likely that apoptotic cell death in the testis is a result of a RFRP/GnIH-induced decrease in testicular testosterone [84].

Molecular Mechanisms of Germ Cell Apoptosis

Survival of a cell is dependent on the regulation of specific pro- and anti- apoptotic gene products. The expression of Bcl-2, an anti-apoptotic gene, which promotes cell survival, reduces after testes are exposed to heat [213]. Other members of the Bcl-2 family, including Bax, Bak, Bcl-xs and Bad, can block the ability of Bcl-2 to inhibit apoptosis and subsequently promote cell death [214]. The proapoptotic Bax protein increases after mild testicular hyperthermia in rats [215] and monkeys [201], leading to germ cell death. On the other hand, the expression level of Fas, which is involved in intercellular transmission of the death signal, and p53 protein, a potent inducer of apoptosis, increases significantly [213]. The Fas-FasL system has been recognized as a key physiological regulator of apoptosis in germ cells of the human testis [216]. Fas is a transmembrane receptor localized especially in spermatocytes and spermatids, both in rats and mice testes [217, 218]. To transmit the death cell signal inside cells, Fas must be activated by binding its ligand FasL, a membrane-bound form, initiating a cascade of protease (caspase) activity [219, 220]. FasL is mainly found in Sertoli cells, in pachytene spermatocytes, and in round spermatids [218]. The Fas system in the testis has been identified as one paracrine signaling system by which Sertoli cells, expressing FasL, can initiate killing of Fas-expressing germ cells [217].

Other mechanisms involved in germ cell apoptosis due to stress have been identified, besides testosterone withdrawal. Apoptosis in germ cells is also mediated by the induction of heme oxigenase-1 (HO-1) in Leydig cells, which is a carbon monoxide (CO)-generating inducible enzyme. This enzyme suppresses the activity of P450 monooxygenases responsible for testosterone synthesis in Leydig cells. In addition, the CO generated by HO-1 could be bound directly to the prosthetic heme of P450 cytochromes and thereby inhibit testosterone synthesis in Leydig cells [221]. CO has been proposed to serve as a signaling molecule, acting in Sertoli cells to trigger Fas/FasL-mediated apoptosis in germ cells, specifically spermatogonia and spermatocytes. However, the possibility that CO could directly stimulate germ cell apoptosis is not excluded. All of these mechanisms have been demonstrated in rats by exposure to cadmium chloride ($CdCl_2$), a stressor causing oligozoospermia [221].

A variety of cellular mechanisms such as DNA repair [222], the heat shock response [223], apoptosis [224], and the oxidative stress response [225] are triggered in the testes after exposure to different types of stressors. At least 73 genes related to stress response are expressed in germ cells during spermatogenesis [226], and many of the genes that are involved in yhe stress response are known to express in testes of infertile animal models and humans [227]. The differential expression of stress response genes during spermatogenesis contributes to the different susceptibility of germ cells to stress. During germ cell development, different spermatogenic cell types show remarkable variation in their susceptibility to stressful stimuli. Spermatogonia are more sensitive to damage caused by x-ray irradiation [228], whereas round spermatids are highly sensitive to alkylating agents such as cyclophosphamide [229]. A differential response to heat stress has been reported, with spermatogonia and spermatozoa being the most resistant, whereas spermatocytes and early spermatids showed the highest degree of sensitivity [230].

Oxidative Stress in Testes

Reactive oxygen species (ROS), including the superoxide anion and hydrogen peroxide are not always toxic to the human spermatozoa. Evidence suggests that small amounts of ROS are necessary for spermatozoa to acquire fertilizing capabilities [231-234]. Low levels of ROS can enhance the ability of human spermatozoa to bind with the zonae pellucida; this effect is reversed by vitamin E [235]. Other studies show that low concentrations of hydrogen peroxide (H_2O_2) stimulate sperm capacitation, hyperactivation, acrosome reaction, and oocyte fusion [236]. Other ROS such as nitric oxide and superoxide anion ($O2^{\bullet -}$) have also been shown to promote sperm capacitation and acrosome reaction [237].

However, high levels of these species can be deleterious and cause oxidative damage to Leydig and germ cells in testis [238, 239]. Therefore, oxidative stress is considered a major factor in the etiology of male infertility. ROS can induce lipid peroxidation and DNA fragmentation in isolated spermatozoon [240], disrupting both the motility of these cells [241], and their ability to support normal embryonic development [231, 242]. In testes, oxidative stress disrupts both steroidogenesis in Leydig cells [243] and spermatogenesis in the germinal epithelium [244]. Additionally, a correlative relationship between male infertility and evidence of oxidative stress in the ejaculate has been reported in clinical studies [245, 246].

Oxidative stress occurs when the production of (ROS) or nitrogen species (RNS) exceed their efficient removal by the available antioxidant systems [239]. The most prominent ROS are superoxide anion ($O_2^{\bullet -}$), hydrogen peroxide (H_2O_2) and the hydroxyl ion ($OH^{\bullet}$), peroxyl ($RO_2^{\bullet}$), hydroxiperoxyl ($HO_2^{\bullet}$). NRS include: nitrogen dioxide ($NO_2^{\bullet}$), nitric oxide ($NO^{\bullet}$), which can also act as a potent oxidizing agent, such as peroxynitrite ($ONOO^-$), through its interaction with superoxide radicals [247, 248] and can play a role in amplifying cellular injury. Oxidative damage can occur to many classes of molecules, including lipids, proteins, nucleic acids, and sugars; consequently, cell, nuclear, and mitochondrial membranes, structural and cytoplasmic proteins, complex carbohydrates, RNA, and DNA are all potential targets of oxidative stress [247]. In a tissue like the testis, with its high rates of metabolism and cell replication, oxidative stress can be especially damaging, which makes the antioxidant capacity of the tissue very important [239]. Both spermatogenesis [249] and Leydig cell steroidogenesis [250, 251] are vulnerable to oxidative stress, therefore, the presence of antioxidant enzymes and free radical scavengers to ensure that spermatogenic and steroidogenic functions of this organ are not impacted by oxidative stress is crucial [238].

The major antioxidant enzymes in mammals are superoxide dismutase (SOD), which converts superoxide to hydrogen peroxide [252, 253]; glutathione/glutathione peroxidase (GPX), which reduce hydrogen peroxide to yield water and reduced glutathione. Hydrogen peroxide can also be reduced by catalase to produce oxygen and water [247]. All of these antioxidant enzymes are expressed in the testis [254, 255]. A number of nonenzyme factors also function as antioxidants in the testis. Among them, vitamin C [256], vitamin E [257], resveratrol [258], and melatonin [259] have each proven efficacious in reducing testicular oxidative stress under different circumstances.

During spermatogenesis, developing germ cells must migrate progressively from the basal to the adluminal compartment of the seminiferous epithelium, where elongated spermatids are eventually released into the tubular lumen at spermiation [260]. This process, per se, requires extensive tissue restructuring in the seminiferous epithelium, resulting in the production of reactive ROS and RNS. If left unchecked, these radicals can induce cell damage and eventually death [252]. The antioxidant defense systems in testis includes SOD [261], which is expressed in both in Sertoli and germ cells [262], GPX, highly expressed in both spermatogenic and Leydig cells [238, 262] and catalase, expressed primarily in peritubular and interstitial cells [263] although it is of limited importance in the testes [238). Despite the antioxidant systems present in testis in order to support its dual functions of steroidogenesis and sperm production, a wide variety of endogenous and exogenous factors are known to perturb these defenses and generate a state of oxidative stress. Cryptorchidism [264], testicualr torsion [265], varicocele [266], hyperthyroidism [267], diabetes [268], infection [269], physical exercise [270, 271], reproductive imbalance [272, 273], retinoids [274], and xenobiotics [275, 276] are some of the factors that are known to cause oxidative stress in the testes. Additionaly, oxidative stress is also caused in brain by restraint stress and corticosterone administration [277], which could contribute indirectly to the impairment in the control of HPG axis.

Associated to oxidative stress in the testis is the reduction in testicular testosterone production in a number of conditions such as cryptorchidism [278], aging [279], and ischemia reperfusion (IR) injury [280]. On the other hand, steroidogenesis itself produces ROS, largely from mitochondrial respiration and the catalytic reactions of the steroidogenic cytochrome P450 enzymes [281]. The ROS produced by spermatogenesis, if unchecked by intracellular antioxidants, can also damage mitochondrial membranes and contribute to the inhibition of subsequent steroid production [282].

Germ Cell Apoptosis as a Consequence of Oxidative Stress

Oxidative stress in the testis is one of the major factors that induce apoptosis in Leydig cells [283] and germ cells, as has been demonstrated in numerous studies. In vitro [284] or in vivo [285] heat stress, chemicals [286], sexual hormones such as estradiol [273], or testosterone [287], ischemia [288], as well as CORT administration [118, 289] cause oxidative stress inducing apoptosis in both in Leydig and germ cells. Spermatids and spermatocytes are the most affected. At the same time, lipid peroxidation and levels of hydrogen peroxide increase, while SOD and catalase activities decrease, indicating that physiological processes of oxidative stress have a direct linkage to the extent of germ cell apopotosis in the seminiferous epithelium [288]. After heat stress, the expression of hypoxia-inducible factor 1 alpha (HIF1A) mRNA increases and HIF1A protein is translocated to the germ cell nucleus, which is consistent with hypoxic stress. Increased expression of heme oxygenase 1 (Hmox1) and the antioxidant enzymes glutathione peroxidase 1 (GPX1) are consistent with oxidative stress response. Concomitantly, germ cell death is associated with an increase in the expression of the effector caspase cleaved caspase 3 and a decrease in the expression of the protein inhibitor of caspase-activated DNase (ICAD). Reduced expression of ICAD contributes to increased activity of caspase-activated DNAse and is consistent with the increased rates of DNA fragmentation, which can be detected by TUNEL staining. Thus, transient mild testicular hyperthermia results in temperature-dependent germ cell death, and elevated temperature results in a complex stress response, including induction of genes associated with oxidative stress and hypoxia [285].

Although the molecular mechanisms of apoptosis induction by oxidative stress in testis have not been completely elucidated, some of the pathways involved have been obtained from in vitro studies in which germ cells were exposed to H_2O_2 [290]. Induction of germ cell apoptosis is directly associated with a significant increase in lipid peroxidation and a concomitant decrease in SOD and catalase activity. Apoptotic signaling pathways include increased expression of Fas, FasL, Bid, Bak, Bad, Bax (proapoptotic), and caspase-8 and caspase-9 markers, as well as p53 (inducer of apoptosis), along with a simultaneous decrease in the Bcl-2 (antiapoptotic) protein at the highest concentration of H_2O_2 exposure. Both, c-jun N-terminal kinase and p38 phosphorylated forms were found to be up-regulated. Interestingly, up-regulation of the nuclear transcription factor kappa B was also observed. The respective transcripts for many of the above proteins followed an identical trend. Caspase-3 activity was also estimated to be 30-fold higher. Taken together, these data indicate that testicular germ cells are prone to apoptosis at very low concentrations of H_2O_2, the mechanism of which involves extrinsic and intrinsic, as well other regulatory pathways [290]. The proposed extrinsic and intrinsic pathways for testicular germ cell apoptosis [290] are shown in figure 5.

Reactive oxygen species act in chain reaction: a compound carrying an unpaired electron will react with another compound to generate an unpaired electron, in such a manner that "radical begets radical." Therefore, the basic problem is to break this chain reaction by the formation of nonradical end products [291, 292].

Apoptosis caused by oxidative stress in germ cells and Leydig cells, as well as spermatozoa have shown to be prevented by treatment with antioxidants, mainly Vitamin E (α-tochopherol) [271, 287, 293], and N-acetyl cysteine [294]. Vitamin E is an important nonenzymatic antioxidant that elevates scavenger enzyme activity [295].

Thus, it induces significant restoration of testicular SOD, CAT, GPX, and GST activities and glutathione content. The protection in testicular steroidogenesis and gametogenesis by α-tocopherol may be due to less production of free radicals as well as less lipid peroxidation [296]. Restoration of testicular steroidogenic and gametogenic function can be attributed to intracellular free radical scavenging, which increases with the incorporation of vitamin E

[297]. Chain-breaking antioxidants such as α-tocopherol inhibit lipid peroxidation (LPO) in membranes by scavenging peroxyl (RO•) and alkoxyl (ROO•) radicals. The ability of α-tocopherol to maintain peroxyl radical reduction in the plasma membrane depends on the recycling of α-tocopherol by external reducing agents such as ascorbate or thiols [298]. Hence, α-tocopherol is able to function again as a free radical chain-breaking antioxidant, even though its concentration is low [291, 299].

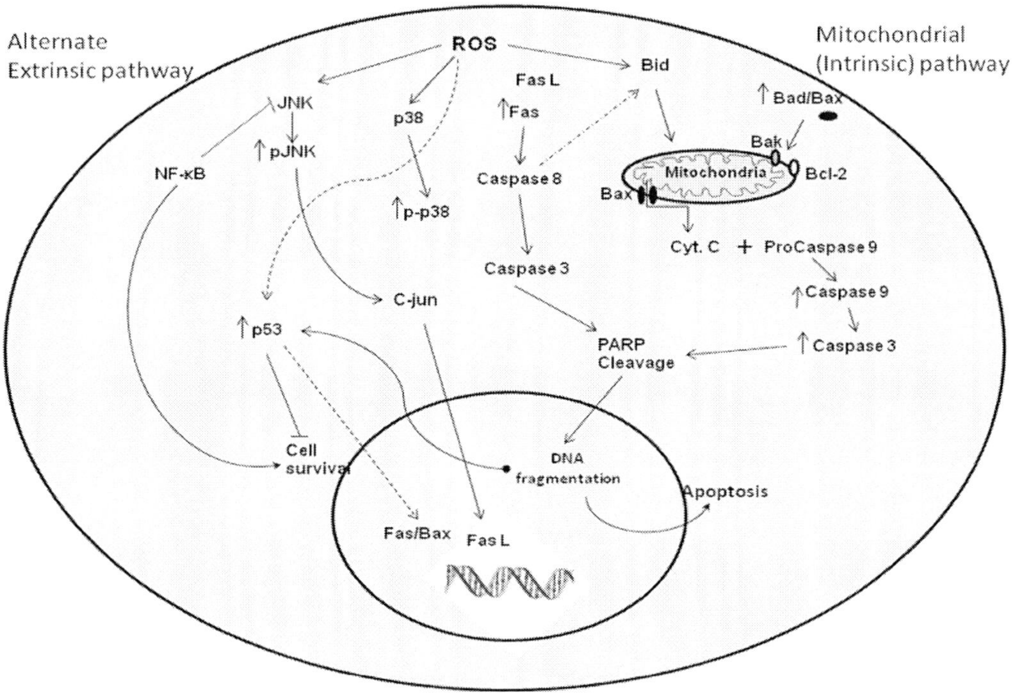

Figure 5. Pathways involved in testicular germ cell apoptosis induced by oxidative stress. Apoptosis follows both extrinsic and intrinsic pathways. The extrinsic pathway involves the activation of death receptors, namely Fas. Following the binding of FasL with Fas, activation of caspase-8 occurs, ensuring the direct activation of executioner caspases-3, 6, 7 and, subsequently, apoptosis. The intrinsic or the mitochondrial pathway involves pro-apoptotic Bid/Bax/Bad (Bcl-2 family members), which move from the cytosol to the outer mitochondrial membrane leading to changes in the mitochondrial membrane permeability and release of cytochrome c into the cytosol. Cytochrome c association with the apoptotic protease activating factor-1 and procaspase-9 promotes the activation of caspase-9, followed by downstream events leading to apoptosis. At the same time, the antiapoptotic protein Bcl-2 decreases. p53-induced apoptosis results from cellular redox alterations. The nuclear transcription factor NF-κB proteins exert pro-apoptotic effects on germ cells, inducing elevated expression of death effector genes such as p53 oxidative stress may also be responsible for activation of JNK and p38 MAP kinases which are important mediators of stress-inducing leading to apoptosis. Poly(ADP-ribose) Polimerase (PARP), an enzyme has a role in polymerizing ADP-ribose in DNA repair is cleavaged by caspase 3, leading to DNA fragmentation and apoptosis. Solid lines = stimulation. Dashed lines = inhibition. Adapted from [290].

Oxidative stress has also been associated with apoptosis in ejaculated spermatozoa [300-304]. Apoptosis in spermatozoa is related with an increase in the levels of ROS, cytochrome c, and caspases 9 and 3, which in turn, correlate negatively with semen variables (motility, concentration and morphology) in infertile men [291, 304]. The reduction of sperm motility related with ROS [305] may be due to a decrease in axonemal protein phosphorylation and sperm immobilization, resulting in a reduction in membrane fluidity necessary for sperm–oocyte fusion [236, 291, 306]. Apoptosis induced in spermatozoa by ROS can be due to the disruption of mitochondrial membranes, which release cytochrome c protein from the mitochondria and activate the caspases to induce apoptosis [291]. Apoptosis in sperm may also be initiated by ROS-independent pathways involving the cell surface protein Fas [307]. When Fas ligand binds to Fas, apoptosis occurs [308]. In men with abnormal semen parameters, the percentage of Fas-positive spermatozoa can be as high as 50%.

The presence of spermatozoa that possess apoptotic markers such as positive Fas and DNA damage indicates that in men with abnormal semen parameters, such as abnormal morphology, abnormal biochemical functions, and nuclear DNA damage, a named "failed apoptosis" has occurred [309], due to problems in activating Fas mediated apoptosis, as well as failure to clear spermatozoa marked for elimination by apoptosis [309]. These findings suggest a major role for apoptosis in human male infertility; therefore, future research should be directed toward defining the mechanisms of regulation of apoptosis as a key mediator of abnormal human sperm production [291].

Stress, Testosterone and Sexual Behavior

Sexual behavior in males is possibly the most vulnerable aspect of male reproduction. Studies in animal models indicate that chronic stress attenuates both motivational and consummatory components of sexual behavior [310], thus diminishing the likelihood of reproductive success. The inhibition of masculine sexual behavior has been studied mainly in the context of social stress. In Talapoin monkeys, subordinate males subjected to chronic social stress show no increase in aggression or sexual behavior [311]. In mice, repeated attacks of conspecifics during several days, impair [312] or even abolish [313] all aspects of male sexual behavior. Utilizing different experimental paradigms, it has been shown that chronic exposure to either cold water immersion or electric foot shocks results in prolonged mount, intromission, and ejaculation latencies and a decrease in the frequencies of ejaculations [34, 55, 314]. Male rats exposed to several weeks of mild, unpredictable stressors, exhibit altered mounting behavior [315, 316], as well as prolonged latencies to achieve their first intromission and ejaculation [316]. Repeated exposure to physical stressors with a psychogenic component, such as restraint, also increases latencies to achieve ejaculation [314]. In the same way, psychological stress induced in rats exposed for 10 weeks to the sounds and smells of other rats that were being repeatedly shocked also causes decreased mounting behavior and prolonged intromission and ejaculation latencies [317]. Together, these reports indicate that sexual behavior of male rodents can be altered by chronic psychological, as well as chronic systemic stressors. In studies modeling post traumatic stress disorder (PTSD), exposure to a single traumatic event, followed days later by reminders of the event, decreases sexual motivation indicated by prolonged mount and intromission latencies [318]. These findings are similar to sexual dysfunction observed in war veterans diagnosed with PTSD, who report hypoactive sexual desire [319, 320].

Sexual activity in humans is also vulnerable to disruption by stressors. Individuals diagnosed with either generalized anxiety disorder or obsessive compulsive disorder frequently report reductions in sexual desire [321], while those with major depressive disorder [322] or post traumatic stress disorder (PTSD) [319, 320] are at greater risk for experiencing physiological impairments in their sexual functioning in addition to reductions in desire, less sexual activity and erectile difficulties [323]. Diminished sexual desire (libido) and erectile dysfunction have also been observed in men with chronic illness and troubles in work or with their partner [324].

Testosterone and/or its metabolites, estradiol (E2) and DHT, promote the display of mating behavior in adult males of all mammals studied [325]. Consequently, testosterone suppression resulting from neuroendocrine alterations caused by stress is expected to impair not only spermatogenesis, as has been demonstrated, but also sexual behavior, directly or indirectly. However, despite the evidence that the secretion of gonadotropins and gonadal steroids decreases in males in response to different stressors, only in a few reports has a relation between the increase of adrenal corticosteroid and the suppression of testosterone and sexual behavior been established. Subordinate male monkeys subjected to chronic social stress do not display sexual behavior; this has been associated with a decrease in plasma LH and testosterone [311]. The impairment of sexual behavior in male rats caused by physical stress is associated with increases in plasma CORT and concomitant decreases in plasma testosterone [34, 55]. This finding suggests that the inhibition of masculine sexual behavior could be attributed, at least in part, to the diminution of androgens, which in turn might be due to biochemical and apoptotic effects of CORT in Leydig cells, as has been discussed above (see section on glucocorticoid and testosterone). However, even when testosterone decreases with chronic stress, this androgen does not seem to be directly responsible for the effects of stress on sexual behavior, since the administration of testosterone to castrated males does not attenuate the effects of stress on this behavior [34]. This implies that other mechanisms are also involved, making the panorama more complex. Mechanisms underlying the effects of stress on sexual behavior seem to involve the participation of almost all of the components of the HPA axis.

The increase in glucocorticoid secretion is the distinctive response to stress, as has been confirmed in numerous studies, in which it has been observed to be associated with a decrease in testosterone. Increases in adrenal corticosteroid during stress, or corticosteroid administration suppress circulating androgens as well as territorial and courtship behaviors in amphibians [326], reptiles [327], birds [328], baboons [329] and stallions [330]. Nevertheless, the impairment of sexual behavior can hardly be attributed to a direct effect of CORT, since administration of different doses (0.5-4 mg) of this glucocorticoid to sexually experienced male rats during 4 or 8 consecutive days does not replicate the effects of stress as none of the copulatory parameters is modified. Plasma testosterone is not modified by CORT administration either [331]. These findings might be explained by the relatively low doses administered, since larger doses of CORT (5-7.5 mg/100g BW) are needed in order to induce apoptosis in testis, for example [117, 205]. Another factor that must be considered to explain the lack of effect of corticosterone on sexual behavior is the sexual experience of males, since this factor modifies the extent to which stressful situations alter testis functionality and sexual behavior. Stress induces more severe alterations on sexual parameters, such as mount and ejaculation latencies, as well as ejaculatory frequency in naive males compared to sexually experienced males [55]. In the same way, sexual experience can influence an individual's response to acute stress. Males engaging in sexual interactions prior to predator odor exhibited reduced risk assessment behavior and increased hippocampal cell proliferation [332, 333]. On the other hand, the effects of stressors on sexual behavior are not always associated to an increase in glucocorticoid levels as shown by studies in which motivational and consummatory aspects of masculine sexual behavior are severely affected in male rats exposed to electric foot shocks [34, 55], but no increase in plasma CORT is associated to these effects.

Sexual behavior in males is controlled by a complex central neuronal network which is closely influenced by sexual steroids and its metabolites. Main central structures involved in the control of sexual behavior include olfactory bulbs, amygdala, MPOA, PVN, bed nucleus of the stria terminalis (BNST), ventromedial hypothalamus (VMH) and ventral tegmental area (VTA) [325]. Environmental cues are gated in the olfactory bulb and sent to the amygdala and then to the MPOA, directly or through BNST. MPOA integrates the internal (i.e. endocrine status of the male) and external (i.e. the presence of a receptive female) information, and sends efferent information to the motor system through the VTA, thus initiating sexual motor patterns [325]. Steroid hormones activate mechanisms of sexual motivation by directing the synthesis of enzymes and receptors for several interactive neurochemical systems. These include dopamine (DA), norepinephrine (NE), melanocortin (MC), opioids and oxytocin (OT) systems acting in hypothalamic and limbic regions, of the brain to stimulate sexual arousal [333], as well as acetylcholine (Ach), Gamma-amino butyric acid (GABA), serotonin (5-HT), NE, opioids and DA acting on structures involved in the initiation of motor patterns [325].

Central neuronal circuitry related to stress can directly inhibit the motivational component of sexual behavior [335], and two of the main neuronal peptides that inhibit masculine sexual behavior participate in the central response to stress. These peptides are CRH and β-endorphins, which can inhibit sexual motivation by acting directly on central structures regulating sexual motivation [335-337]. CRH is the main mediator released in the hypothalamus during neuroendocrine response to stress, and is part of the inhibitory central mechanisms involved in the suppression of sexual behavior due to stress [338]. Intraventricular injection of this neuropeptide inhibits all parameters of masculine sexual behavior in rats: significantly long mount, intromission and ejaculation latencies and lower ejaculation frequencies. All these inhibitory effects are blocked by co-administration of the opioid antagonist naloxone [337]. Furthermore, the suppression of masculine sexual behavior due to psychological stress can also be partially recovered with the administration of astressin, which is a CRH antagonist [339]. These findings suggest that during the stress response CRH, might inhibit sexual behavior acting on the hypothalamic MPOA, which is a brain structure of central importance for the display of masculine sexual behavior in males [325], and where GnRH neurons are located. This inhibition can be through direct synaptic connections between CRH neurons and GnRH neurons in that structure [49], or indirectly through the release of proopiomelanocortin (POMC), from which β-endorphins are derived. POMC neurons, are located in the arcuate nucleus [335], and project to the MPOA, Further evidence shows that CRH has been detected in the MPOA, and stress induces a diminution of CRH in that structure, probably due to its release in that site [340].

OPIOIDS AND MASCULINE SEXUAL BEHAVIOR

The endogenous opioid system is activated in response to a number of stressors, both physical and psychological, such as immobilization, cold-water immersion, and electric foot shocks [341]; and plasma β-endorphins increase with these stressors [340,342]. These stressors also cause an increase in POMC synthesis rate, as well as β-endorphin release from the arcuate nucleus in the hypothalamus [343]. In men, social or psychological chronic stress causes erectile dysfunction, increases plasma levels of β-endorphins, and decreases sexual motivation (libido). Treatment with the opioid antagonist naltrexone (NTX) improves these symptoms and increases penile blood flow and the number of sexual acts in a dose-dependent manner [324]. In healthy sexually active men, NTX increases the number and intensity of orgasms; this suggests that endogenous opioids modulate orgasmic response and the perceived intensity of sexual arousal and orgasm in men [344]. The inhibition of sexual behavior caused by stress can be blocked by the opioid antagonist NTX administered before exposure to stressors. These findings indicate that endogenous opioids could be involved in the effects of stress on sexual behavior [55]. Endogenous opioids, specifically β-endorphins, are released from the hypothalamus and pituitary during stress, with a concomitant increase of these opioids in plasma [335, 343, 345, 346], Furthermore, the increase in β-endorphins caused by stress is much higher at the onset of the dark phase of the light/dark cycle [347], during which rats display sexual activity. Endogenous opioid peptides are commonly accepted as having an inhibitory role in male sexual behavior (see [348] for review). These inhibitory effects of opioid peptides are apparently mediated by μ-opioid receptors, since the administration of selective μ-receptor agonists into the MPOA of rats delays the initiation of male copulatory behavior [349, 350], and opioid receptor antagonists, such as naloxone and naltrexone, prevent these effects [325, 335, 351].

The hypothalamic PVN is another area where endogenous opioids and/or opioid μ receptor agonists can also inhibit male sexual behavior by preventing dopamine receptor agonists and oxytocin induced penile erection [352, 353], and must be considered to explain the effects of stress and naltrexone on stressed males. Endogenous opioid peptides exert a dual effect on sexual behavior. On the one hand, they facilitate the anticipatory phase of sexual behavior by improving sexual arousal and motivation, acting in the ventral tegmental area to increase the activity of the mesolimbic dopaminergic system [348, 354, 355]. On the other hand, they inhibit the consummatory phase of sexual behavior, impairing sexual performance, by acting in the MPOA [335, 356]. Therefore, it is possible that some of the alterations in sexual parameters observed in stressed males might be due to the action of endogenous opioids in the MPOA and PVN. Most hypothalamic endogenous opioids are located in POMC neurons situated in the arcuate nucleus, which project to the MPOA, a brain structure of central importance for the display of sexual behavior in males [325]. This is one of the central structures that expresses μ-receptors [357] and is commonly recognized as a brain area in which opioid peptides act to inhibit male sexual behavior [354], mainly through opioid receptors of the μ type [349]. Therefore, prevention of the inhibitory effects of stress on sexual behavior by NTX administration suggests that the effects of stressors are mediated, at least partially, by endogenous opioids, mainly β-endorphins, probably acting on μ-opioid receptors, since NTX is an antagonist of μ-opioid receptors [342, 358]. Some of the neural pathways mediating central and peripheral structures mediating masculine sexual behavior are shown in figure 6.

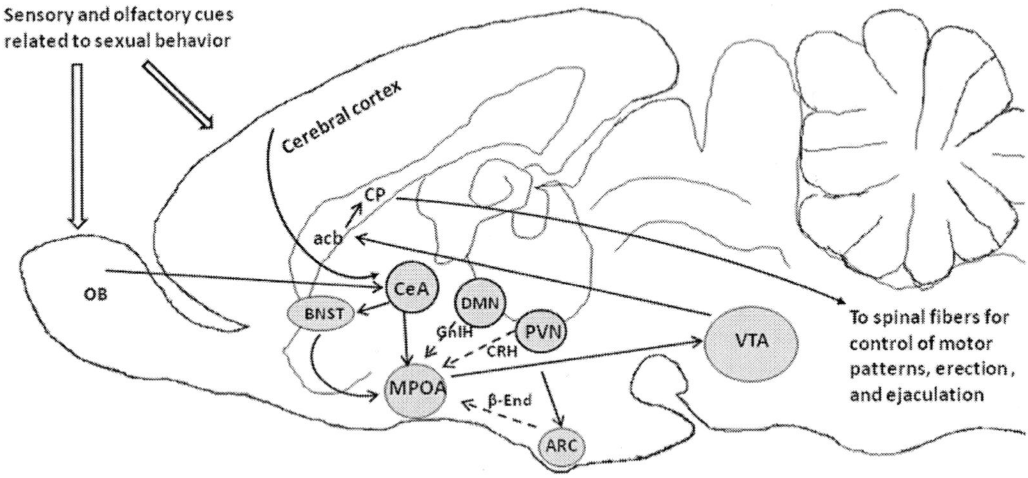

Figure 6. Some of the neural pathways regulating male copulatory behavior in the rat are shown. Environmental cues are received in the cerebral cortex and olfactory bulb (OB) and lead to the activation of central amygdala (CeA). The signals reach medial preoptic area (MPOA) directly or through the bed nucleus of stria terminalis (BNST). The medial preoptic area (MPOA) integrates both internal (endocrine status) and external information (the presence of a receptive female, for example) and send efferent signals to the striatal motor system through the ventral tegmental area (VTA), thus initiating motor patterns of sexual behavior. MPOA activity can be suppressed by inhibitory factors such as gonadotrropin inhibitory hormone/RFamide-related peptide (GnIH/RFRP) from dorsomedial nucleus (DMN), as well as CRH from paraventricular nucleus (PVN) and β-endorphins from arcuate nucleus (ARC). Solid lines = stimulation. Dashed lines = inhibition.

RFRP AND MASCULINE SEXUAL BEHAVIOR

Aside from opioids, RFRP (GnIH) should also be considered among the mechanisms by which sexual behavior is impaired by stress. Although evidence is scarce, there are studies showing that intracerebroventricular (ICV) RFRP administration in adult rats suppresses sexual behavior, with increased mount, intromission and ejaculation latencies with a concomitant reduction in ejaculation frequency [83]. In birds, central GnIH administration reduces the frequency of copulation solicitation display, which is a GnRH-dependent behavior in male [359] and female [360, 361] sparrows. However, much more research of the effects of RFRP in this important aspect of reproductive physiology of males and females is needed. Likewise, the precise physiological mechanisms of GnIH/RFRP action in the brain and the differences between genders and possibly species will be the focus of future studies.

CONCLUSION

The stress system coordinates the stress response in order to re-establish homeostasis through physiological and behavioral adaptive responses [22, 19]. Both central (CRH, AVP, and β-endorphins) and peripheral (glucocorticoids, epinephrine and norepinephrine) effectors of the stress system provoke behavioral and peripheral changes that permit the organism to adapt and survive. The reproductive system is closely related to the stress system and is directly influenced by its effectors, thus suppressing reproductive function in response to stress [21, 22].

The consequences of stress on reproductive function have been observed at all levels of the HPG axis and are mediated mainly by glucocorticoids [362, 363], which are known as the stress hormones for that reason. These adrenal steroids induce the expression of GnIH/RFRP, which decreases GnRH release in the hypothalamus [85], reduces pituitary LH secretion by reducing its responsiveness to GnRH [45], and inhibit testicular steroidogenesis [51, 52, 53]directly, and indirectly by inducing apoptosis of Leydig cells [109, 118]. Likewise, glucocorticoids decrease spermatogenesis by causing apoptosis directly on testicular germ cells [205], or indirectly through the decrease of testosterone secretion due to apoptosis in Leydig cells [109, 118]. Apoptosis in germ cells, Leydig cells [284-288] and spermatozoa [291, 294] is caused by oxidative stress.

As a result of the actions of the HPA axis on the HPG axis function during stress, the impairment of sexual behavior, as well as infertility have been observed in males of different species of vertebrates, thus decreasing reproductive success. Therefore, the involvement of GnIH/RFRP, CRH, β-endorphins and glucocrticoids in the HPA-HPG interaction should be pertinent to most vertebrates. As has been demonstrated by the extensive literature, HPA axis activation is implicated in a number of causes of infertility and reproductive dysfunction related to stress [87, 364, 365], and may significantly influence the efficacy of assisted reproductive procedures in humans [135, 366, 367]. In addition, chronic stress is of primary concern in captive breeding programs as well as in agricultural breeding programs [368]. The recent findings about GnIH/RFRP as part of the mechanisms involved in the HPA-HPG interaction during stress is crucial for understanding the mechanisms underlying one of the most common suppressors of HPG activity [85]. Also, assessment of oxidative stress in testes and semen in captive animals will help to understand and propose antioxidant treatments for the improvement of captive breeding programs, as well as assisted reproduction in humans.

The discovery of GnIH in the avian brain and its role in the neuroendocrine control of reproduction [75, 86] opens new approaches to the study of reproductive neuroendocrinology across species. Now it is known that GnRH is not the only hypothalamic neurohormone controlling reproduction in vertebrates. Future research will elucidate the interactions of GnRH with GnIH and kisspeptin, as well as the role of GnIH on reproductive function in vertebrates.

REFERENCES

[1] D.M.Stocco and M.J. McPhaul, *Physiology of testicular steroidogenesis*. Neil JD. Knobil and Neill's Physiology of Reproduction. Jimmy D. Neill, Ed, Elsevier, (2006), pp977-1016.

[2] A.J. Silverman, L.C. Krey and E.A. Zimmerman, *Biol Reprod*, 20, 98 (1979).

[3] J.E. Griffin and J.D. Wilson, *Disorders of the testes and the male reproductive tract*. Larsen PR, Kronenberg HM, Melmed S, Polonsky KS. Williams textbook of endocrinology (2003), pp709-769.
[4] B.E. Hawes and P.M. Conn, *Clin Chem*, 39, 325 (1993).
[5] J. D. Neill, J.M. Patton, R.A. Dailey, R.C. Tsou and G.T. Tindall, *Endocrinology* 101, 430, (1977).
[6] J.C. Marshall and M.L. Griffin, *Hum Reprod*, 8, 56, (1993).
[7] M. Ascoli, F. Fanelli and D.L. Segaloff, *Endocr. Rev*. 23, 141, (2002).
[8] A.H. Payne and G.L. Youngblood. *Biol Reprod*,; 52, 217, (1995).
[9] P.S. LaPolt, X.C. Jia and C. Sincich, *Mol Endocrinol*, 5, 397, (1991).
[10] A.H. Payne and P.J. O'Shaughnessy, Structure, function and regulation of steroidogenic enzymes in the Leydig cell. A. H. Payne, M. P. Hardy, and L. D. Russell, The Leydig Cell, A. H. Payne, M. P. Hardy, Eds. Cache River Press, Vienna, IL. (1996), pp259-286
[11] T.K. Kwan, A.K. Pertiwi, N.F. Taylor and D.B. Gower, *Biochim. Biophys. Acta*. 962, 214, (1988).
[12] K.B. Eik-Nes, *The Androgens of the Testis*, K. B. Eik-Nes, Eds, Dekker, New York. (1970).
[13] P.F. Hall, C.C. Sozer and K.B. Eik-Nes, *Endocrinology* 74, 35, (1964).
[14] W.D. Booth, *J. Reprod. Fertil. 42, 459, (1975).*
[15] J. Rajfer, S.C. Sikka and R.S. Swerdloff, *J. Clin. Endocrinol. Metab*. 64, 62, (1987).
[16] R. Rey, S. Campo, S. Ayuso, C. Nagle and H. Chemes, *Biol Reprod*. 52, 997, (1995).
[17] E.M. Ritzen, M.P. Van Damme, B. Froysa, C. Reuter, B. De La Torre and E. Diczfalusy, *J. Steroid Biochem*. 14, 533, (1981).
[18] R.S. Swerdloff and Wang, C. Clinical evalulation of Leydig cell function. A. H. Payne, M. P. Hardy, and L. D. Russell, Eds. The Leydig Cell, Cache River Press, Vienna, IL. (1996), pp663-694.
[19] G.P. Chrousos, *Nat.Rev.Endocrinol*.5, 375, (2009).
[20] G.P. Chrousos and P.W. Gold, *J. Am.Med. Assoc*. 267, 1244, (1992).
[21] E.O. Johnson, T.C. Kamilaris, G.P. Chrousos, P.W. Gold, *Neurosci. Biobeha. Rev*. 16,115, (1992)
[22] E. Charmandari, C. Tsigos and G.P. Chrousos, *Annu. Rev. Physiol*. 67, 259, (2005).
[23] K.E. Habib, P.W. Gold, G.P. Chrousos, *Endocrinol. Metab. Clin. North Am*. 30, 695, (2001).
[24] F.J. Tilders and F. Berkenbosch, *Acta Endocrinol. (Suppl.) (Copenh.),* 276, 63, (1986).
[25] A.B. Abou-Samra, J.P. Harwood, K.J. Catt and G. Aguilera, *Ann. NY Acad.Sci.*, 512, 67, (1987).
[26] A. Munk, P. Guyre and N. Holbrook. *Endocr. Rev.*, 5,25, (1984).
[27] E.R. de Kloet, E. Vreugdenhil, M.S.Oitzl, M. Joels. *Endocr.Rev.*, 19, 269, (1998).
[28] M.F. Dallman. *Front.Neuroendocr.*, 26, 103, (2005).
[29] H. Karst, S. Berger, M. Turiault, F. Tronche, G. Schutz, M. Joëls. *Proc. Nat.Acad.Sci.*, 102, 19204, (2005).
[30] F.L. Groeneweg, H. Karst, E.R. de Kloet, M. Joëls. *J Endocrinol.,*Feb 28. Epub ahead of print. (2011)
[31] H. Selye, *J.Clin.Endocrinol*. 6, 117, (1946).
[32] R. Collu, W. Gibb, and G.R. Ducharme, *Biol. Reprod*. 30, 416, (1984a).

[33] R. Collu, W. Gibb and G.R. Ducharme, *J. Endocrinol. Invest.* 7, 529, (1984b).

[34] S. Retana-Márquez, H. Bonilla-Jaime, G. Vázquez-Palacios, R. Martínez-García and J. Velázquez-Moctezuma, *Horm.Behav.*, 44, 327, (2003).

[35] S.A. Almeida, S.O. Petenusci, J.A. Anselmo-Franci, A.A. Rosa-e-Silva and T.L. Lamano-Carvalho, *Braz. J. Med. Biol. Res.*, 31, 1443, (1998).

[36] S.A. Almeida, S.O. Petenusci, J.A. Franci, A.A. Rosa e Silva and T.L. Carbalho, *Andrologia*, 32, 7, (2000).

[37] S.A. Almeida, W.G. Kempinas and T.L. Lamano Carvalho, *Braz. J. Med. Biol. Res.* 33, 1105, (2000b).

[38] D.M. Phillips, v. Lakshmi and C. Monder. *Endocrinology*, 125, 209, (1989).

[39] E.B. Keverne, *Ciba Found. Symp.* 63, 271, (1979).

[40] R.M. Sapolsky, Stress, social status, and reproductive physiology in free-living baboons. In: Crews, D. (Ed.), Psychobiology of reproductive behavior. Prentice-Hall, Englewood Cliffs. N.J, (1987). pp. 291–332,

[41] R. Sapolsky, L.C. Krey and B.S. McEwen,. *Endocr. Rev.*, 7, 622, (1986).

[42] G.P. Chrousos, D.J. Torpy and P.W. Gold, *Ann. Intern. Med.*, 129, 229, (1998).

[43] P. Tsigos and G.P Chrousos, *J. Psychosom. Res.*, 53, 865, (2002).

[44] P. Doerr and K.M. Pirke, *J.Clin.Endocrinol. Metab.*, 46, 622, (1976).

[45] N. Hagino, M. Watanebe and Goldzieher J, W. *Endocrinology*, 84, 308, (1969).

[46] C. Rivier and W. Vale, *Endocrinology*, 114, 914, (1984).

[47] D.J.S. Sirinatsinghji, L.H. Rees, J. Rivier and W. Vale, *Nature*, 305, 232, (1983).

[48] J.T.M. Vreeburg, W.J. De Greef, M.P. Ooms, P. Van Wouw and R.F.A. Weber RFA. *Endocrinology*, 115, 977, (1984).

[49] N. MacLusky, F. Naftolin and C. Leranth, *Brain Res*, 439, 391, (1988).

[50] C. Rivier, J. Rivier and W. Vale, *Science* 231, 607, (1986).

[51] T.E. Orr and D.R. Mann, *Horm.Behav.*, 24, 324, (1990).

[52] T.E. Orr, M.F. Taylor, A.K. Bhattacharyya, D,C, Collins and D.R. Mann, *J.Androl.*, 15, 302, (1994).

[53] M.P. Hardy and V.K. Ganjam, *J.Androl.*, 18, 475, (1997).

[54] D. Rabin, E.O. Johnson, D.D. Brandon, C. Liapi and G.P. Chrousos, *Biol.Reprod.*, 42, 74, (1990).

[55] S. Retana-Márquez, H. Bonilla-Jaime, G. Vázquez-Palacios and R. Martínez-García. *Physiol.Behav.*, 96, 333, (2009).

[56] T.J. Cicero. *Fed.Proc.*, 39, 2551, (1980).

[57]A. López-Calderón and M. González-Quijano, J. Tresguerres and C. Ariznavarreta. *J.Endocrinol.*, 124, 241, (1990).

[58] B. Bidzinska, F. Petraglia, S. Angioni, A.D. Genazzani, M. Riscuolo, G. Ficarra, A. Gallinelli, G.P. Trentini and A.R. Genazzani. *Neuroendocrinology*, 57, 985, (1993).

[59] O.F. Almeida, K.E. Nikolarakis and A. Herz. *Endocrinology*, 122, 1034, (1988).

[60] T.J. Cicero, E.R. Meyer, B.T. Miller and R.O. Bell. *J.Pharmacol.Exp.Ther.*, 246, 14, (1988).

[61] A. Barbarino, L. De Marinis, A. Tofani, S, Della Casa, C. D'Amico, A. Mancini, S.M. Corsello, R. Sciuto and A. Barini. *J.Clin.Endocrinol.Metab.*, 69, 523, (1989).

[62] K.T. O'Byrne, S.F. Lunn and A.F. Dixson. *Physiol. Behav.*, 45, 1077, (1989).

[63] M.L. Dufau, J.C. Tinajero and A. Fabbri. *FASEBS*, 7, 299, (1993).

[64] P.A. Kant and R.N. Saxena. Indian *J.Exp.Biol.*, 33, 165, (1995).

[65] M.L. Adams, B. Sewing, J.B. Forman, E.R. Meyer and T.J.Cicero. *J.Pharmacol.Exp.Ther.*, 266, 323, (1993).
[66] M.A. Akimbami, M.F. Taylor, D.C. Collins and D.R. Mann. *Neuroendocrinology*, 59, 343, (1994).
[67] T. Kostić, S. Andrić, R. Kovačević and D. Marić. *Steroids*, 62, 703, (1997).
[68] T. Kostić, S. Andrić, D. Marić and R. Kovačević. *J.Steroid Biochem.Mol.Biol.*, 66, 51, (1998).
[69] R. Norman and C. Smith. *Neuroendocrinology*, 55, 405, 1992.
[70] C.W. Bardin, C.L.C. Chen, P.L. Morris, I. Gerendai, C. Boitani, A.S. Liota AS, A. Margioris and D.T. Krieger. *Recent Prog.Horm.Res.*, 43, 1, (1987).
[71] N.L. Eskeland, C.J. Molineaux and B.S. Schachter. *Endocrinology*, 130, 1173, (1992).
[72] A. Fabri, J.C. Tinajero and M.L. Dufau. *Endocrinology*, 130, 1780, (1990).
[73] Q. Dong, A. Salva, C.M. Sottas, E. Niu, M. Holmes and M.P. Hardy. *J. Androl,* 25, 973, (2004).
[74] N.K. Mello, J.H. Mendelson, M.P. Bree and A. Skupny. Pharmacol.Biochem.Behav., 31, 683, (1988).
[75] K. Tsutsui, E. Saigoh, K. Ukena, H. Teranishi, Y. Fujisawa, M. Kikuchi, S. Ishii, P.J. Sharp. *Biochem. Biophys. Res. Commun.*, 275, 661, (2000).
[76] I.J. Clarke, Y. Qi, I. P. Sari and J.T. Smith. *Front.Neuroendocrinol.*, 30, 371, (2009).
[77] F.J.P. Ebling and S.M. Luckman. *Endocrinology*, 149, 899, (2008).
[78] F.J.P. Ebling. *Reproduction*, 129, 675, (2005).
[79] F.G. Revel, L. Ansel, P. Klosen, M. Saboureau, P. Pevet, J.D. Mikkelsen, V.Simmoneaux V 2007 *Rev. Endocr.Metab. Disord.*, 8, 57, (2007).
[80] J.T. Smith and I.J. Clarke. *Trend.Endocrinol.Metab.*, 21, 4, 255, (2010).
[81] G.E. Bentley, T. Ubuka, N.L. McGuire, R. Calisi, N. Perfito, L.J. Kriegsfeld, J. C. Wingfield and K. Tsutsui. *J.Neuroendocrinol.*, 21, 276, (2009).
[82] T. Ubuka, K. Ukena, P.J. Sharp, G.E. Bentley and K. Tsutsui. *Endocrinology*, 147, 1187, (2006).
[83] M.A. Johnson, K. Tsutsui and G.S. Fraley. *Horm Behav*. January ; 51(1): 171, (2007).
[84] K. Tsutsui, G.E. Bentley, G.Bedecarrats, T. Osugi, T. Ubuka and L.J. Kriegsfeld. *Front. Neuroendocrinol.*, 31, 284, (2010).
[85] I.J. Clarke, I.P. Sari, Y. Qi, J.T. Smith, H.C. Parkington, T. Ubuka, J. Iqbal, Q. Li, A.Tilbrook, K. Morgan, A.J. Pawson, K. Tsutsui, R.P. Millar and G.E. Bentley. *Endocrinology*, 149, 5811, (2008).
[86] T. Ubuka, K. Morgan, A.J. Pawson, T. Osugi, V.S. Chowdhury, H. Minakata, K. Tsutsui, R.P. Millar and G.E. Bentley. *Plos one*, 4, 1, (2009).
[87] E.D. Kirby, A.C. Geraghty, T. Ubuka, G.E. Bentley and D. Kaufer. *PNAS*, 106, 11324, (2009).
[88] M. Wu, I. Dumalska, E. Morozova, A.N. van den Pol and M. Alreja. *J. Physiol.*, 587, 1401, (2009).
[89] X-F. Li, J.S. Kinsey-Jones, Y. Cheng, A.M.I. Knox, Y. Lin, N.A.Petrou, A. Roseweir, S.L. Lightman, S.R. Milligan1, R.P. Millar and K.T. O'Byrne. *Plos One*, 4, 1, (2009).
[90] M. Murakami, T. Matsuzaki, T. Iwasa, T. Yasui, M. Irahara, T. Osugi and K. Tsutsui. *J.Endocrinol.*, 199, 105, (2008).
[91] S. Whirledge and J.A. Cidlowski. *Minerva Endocrinol.*, 35, 109, 2010).

[92] S. Ringstrom, D. Suter, J. D'Agostino, J. Hostetler and N. Schwartz. Effects of glucocorticoids on the hypothalamic-pituitary-gonadal axis. In: Genazzani A., Nappi G., Petraglia F., Martignoni E. (Eds.) Stress and related disorders: From adaptation to dysfunction. The Parthenon Publishing group. New Jersey, USA. (1991). pp: 297-305.
[93] G. Charpenet, Y. Taché, M. Bernier, J. Ducharme and R. Collu. *Biol. Reprod.*, 27, 6116, (1982).
[94] M.R. MacAdams, R.H. White and B.E. Chipps, *Ann. Intern. Med.*, 194, 104, (1986).
[95] N.C. Vamvakopoulos and G.P Chrousos, *J Clin Invest*, 92, 1896, (1994).
[96] M. González-Quijano, C. Ariznavarreta, A. Martin, J. Tresguerres and A. López-Calderón. *Neuroendocrinology*, 54, 447, (1991).
[97] M. Ishikawa, Ch. Hara, S. Ohdo and S. Ogawa. *Physiol. Behav.* 52, 475, (1992).
[98] T. Watanabe, A. Morimoto, Y. Sakata, M. Wada and N. Murakami, N. *J. Physiol.*, 439, 691, (1991).
[99] S. Persengiev, L. Kanchev and G. Vezenkova. *J. Pineal Res.* 11, 57, (1991).
[100] S. De Boer, S. Koopmans, J. Slangen, J.and J. Van Der Gugten. *Physiol. Behav.* 45, 989, (1989).
[101] G. Gray, E. Smith, D. Damassa, J, Ehrenkranz, J.and J. Davidson. *Neuroendocrinology*, 25, 247, (1978)
[102] P. Mormède, V. Lemaire, N. Castanon, J. Dulluc, M. Laval and M. Le Moal. *Physiol. Behav.*, 47, 1099, (1990).
[103] C. Monder, R.R. Sakai, Y. Miroff, D.C. Blanchard and R.J. Blanchard. *Endocrinology*, 134, 1193, (1994).
[104] T. Tsuchiya and I. Horii. *Psychoneuroendocrinology*, 20, 221, (1995).
[105] A. Luger, P.A. Deuster, S.B. Kyle, W.T. Gallucci and L.C. Montgomery, *N.Engl. J. Med.* 316, 1309, (1987).
[106] S.E. MacConnie, A. Barkan, R.M. Lampman, M.A. Schork and I.Z. Beitins, *N. Engl. J. Med.* 315, 411, (1986)
[107] K. Remes, K. Kuoppasalmi and H. Adlercreut. *Int. J. Sports Med.*, 6, 131, (1985).
[108] P.K. Opstad. *Eur. J. Endocrinol.,* 131, 56, (1994).
[109] M. P. Hardy, H-B. Gao, Q. Dong, R. Ge, Q. Wang, W. Ran Chai, X. Feng and C. Sottas. *Cell Tissue Res*, 322, 147, (2005).
[110] D.B. Hales and A.H. Payne. *Endocrinology*, 124, 2099, (1989).
[111] R. Schultz, J. Isola, M. Parvinen, J. Honkaniemi, A-C. Wikström, J-A. Gustaffson, and M. Pelto-Huikko. *Mol,Cel. Endocrinol.*, 95, 115, (1993).
[112] A. Stalker, L. Hermo, T. Antakly. *Am J Anat,*186, 369, (1989).
[113] A. Stalker, L. Hermo, T. Antakly. *Am J Anat*, 190, 19, (1991).
[114] A.H. Payne and L.L. Sha. *Endocrinology*, 129, 1429, (1991).
[115] B.M. Aguilar, A.M. Vingaard, and C. Vind. *J. Steroid. Biochem. Mol. Biol.*, 43, 565, (1992).
[116] G.X. Hu, H. Lin, C.M. Sottas, D.J. Morris, M.P. Hardy, and R.S. Ge. *J. Androl.*, 29, 345, (2008).
[117] H.B. Gao, M.H. Tong, Y.Q. Hu, Q.S. Guo, R.S. Ge, and M.P. Hardy. *Endocrinology*, 143, 130, (2002).
[118] H.B. Gao, M.H. Tong, Y.Q. Hu, H.Y. You, Q.S. Guo, R.S. Ge, and M.P. Hardy. *Mol Cell Endocrinol.* 199, 153, (2003).
[119] A.H. Wyllie, J.F.R. Kerr andA.R. Currie. *Int.Rev.Cytol.*, 68, 251, (1980).

[120] M.J. Arends, R.G. Morris and A.H. Wyllie. *Am.J.Pathol.*, 136, 593, (1990).

[121] A.H. Wyllie. *Nature*, 284, 555, (1980).

[122] Ashkenazi, A., Dixit, V.M., 1998. Death receptors: signaling and modulation. Science 281, 1305_/1308.

[123] G.M. Cohen. *Biochem.J.*, 326, 1, (1997).

[124] A.J. Polverino and S.D. Patterson. *J. Bio. Chem.*, 272, 7013, (1997).

[125] N.A. Thornberry and Y. Lazebnik. *Science* 281, 131, (1998).

[126] D.R. Green and J.C. Reed. Science, 281, 1309, (1998).

[127] M. Loeffler and G. Kroemer. *Exp. Cell Res.*, 256, 19, (2000).

[128] R.L. Norman RL. *Biol Reprod*, 49, 148, (1993).

[129] A. Tohei, T. Tomabechi, M. Mamada, M. Akai, G. Watanabe, and K. Taya. *J Vet Med Sci*, 59, 329, (1997).

[130] J. Lindzey, M.V. Kumar, M. Grossman, C. Young and D.J. Tindall. *Vitam. Horm.* 49, 383, (1994).

[131] M.J. Tsai and B.W. O'Malley. *Annu. Rev. Biochem*, 63, 451, (1994).

[132] R.M. Evans. *Science*, 240, 889, (1988).

[133] A.H. Payne, A. Kawano, and R.B. Jaffe. *J Clin Endocrinol Metab*, 37, 448, (1973).

[134] P. Price, J.A.H. Wass, and J.E. Griffin. *J Clin Invest*, 74, 1496, (1984).

[135] G. Collodel, E. Moretti, V. Fontani, S. Rinaldi, L. Aravagli, G. Saragò, S. Capitani, and C. Anichini. *Indian J Med Res*, 128, 254, (2008).

[136] M.Fukuda, K. Fukuda, T. Shimizu, W. Yomura, and S. Shimizu. *Hum Reprod*, 11, 1244, (1996).

[137] N.H. Hjollund, J.P. Bonde, T.B. Henriksen, A. Giwercman, and J. Olsen. *Epidemiology*, 15, 21, (2004).

[138] N. Schneid-Kofman and E. Sheiner. *Med Sci Monit*, 11, 11, (2005).

[139] M. Pook, B. Tuschen-Caffier, and W. Krause. *Hum Reprod*, 19, 954, (2004).

[140] J. Auger, F. Eustache, A.G. Andresen, D.S. Irvine, N. Jørgensen, N.E. Shakkebæk, J. Suominen, J. Toppari, M. Viruela and P.J. Jouannet. *Hum. Reprod.*, 16, 2710, (2001).

[141] P.T. Giblin, M.L. Poland, K.S. Moghissi, J.W. Ager, and J.M. Olson. *Fertil Steril*, 49, 127, (1988).

[142] A. Lenzi, F, Lombardo, P. Salacone, L. Gandini and E.A. Jannini. *J.Endocrinol.Invest.*, 26, 72, 2003)

[143] P.L. Bigelow, J, Jarrell and M.R. Young. *Fertil. Steril*, 69, 11, (1998).

[144] L. Fenster, D.F. Katz, A.J. Wyrobek, C. Pieper, D.M. Rempel, D. Oman, and S.H. Swan. *J Androl*, 18, 194, (1997).

[145] T. Theorell, R.A. Karasek and P. Eneroth. *J.Inter.Med.*, 227, 31, (1990).

[146] I. Gerhard, K. Lenhard, W. Eggert-Kruse and B. Runnebaum. *Hum.Reprod.*, 7, 830, (1992).

[147] L.E. Kreuz, R.M. Rose and R. Jennings. *Arch.Gen.Psychiatry.*, 26, 479, (1972).

[148] L. O'Donnell, S.J. Meachem, P.G. Stanton and R.I. McLachlan. Endocrine Regulation of Spermatogenesis. *Knobil and Neill's Physiology of Reproduction*, J. D. Neill (Ed), (2006), pp. 1017-1069. Elsevier, New York.

[149] D.M. de Kretser and J.B. Kerr. The cytology of the testis. In *The Physiology of Reproduction* (E. Knobil, and J. D. Neill, Eds.), Vol. 1, (1988). pp. 837–932. Raven Press, New York.

[150] Russell, L. Role in spermiation. In *The Sertoli Cell* (L. D. Russell and M. D. Griswold, Eds.), (1993). pp. 269–302. Cache River Press, Clearwater, FL.
[151] N. Sofikitis, N. Giotitsas, P. Tsounapi, D. Baltogiannis, D. Giannakis, N. Pardalidis. *J. Steroid Biochem. Mol. Biol.*, 109, 323, (2008).
[152] W.J. Bremner, M.R. Millar, R.M. Sharpe, and P.T. Saunders. *Endocrinology*, 135, 1227, (1994).
[153] S.W. Buzek and B.M Sanborn. *Biol.Repro*, 39, 39, (1988).
[154] C.M. Hill, M.D. Anway, B.R. Zirkin and T.R. Brown. *Biol. Reprod*, 71, 1348, (2004).
[155] X. Zhou, A. Kudo, H. Kawakami and H. Hirano. *Anat. Rec.*, 245, 509, (1996).
[156] G. Pelletier, C. Labrie and F. Labrie. *J. Endocrinol.* 165, 359, (2000).
[157] Q. Zhou, R. Nie, G.S. Prins, P.T. Saunders, B.S. Katzenellenbogen and R.A. Hess. *J. Androl.*, 23, 870, (2002).
[158] L.D. Russell, L.E. Alger and L.G. Nequin. *Endocrinology*, 120, 1615, (1987).
[159] J.S. Tapanainen, J.L. Tilly, K.K. Vihko, and A.J. Hsueh. *Mol. Endocrinol.* 7, 643, (1993).
[160] T. Matikainen, J. Toppari, K.K. Vihko and I. Huhtaniemi. *J. Endocrinol.* 141, 449, (1994).
[161] D.F. Cameron, K.F. Muffly and S.J. Nazian. *Proc. Soc. Exp. Biol. Med.* 202, 457, (1993).
[162] Y.T. Sun, N.G. Wreford, D.M. Robertson and D.M. de Kretser. *Endocrinology*, 127, 1215, (1990).
[163] B.R. Zirkin. *Semin. Cell. Dev. Biol. 9, 417, (1998).*
[164] C.A. Awoniyi, R. Santulli, R.L. Sprando, L.L. Ewing, and B.R. Zirkin. Endocrinology, 124, 1217, (1989).
[165] S. Meachem, V. von Schonfeldt S. and Schlatt. *Reproduction*, 121, 825, (2001).
[166] M.L. Meistrich and M. Kangasniemi. *J. Androl.* 18, 80, (1997).
[167] K. Matsumiya, M.L. Meistrich, G. Shetty, K. Dohmae, A. Tohda, A. Okuyama and Y. Nishimune. *Endocrinology*, 140, 4912, (1999).
[168] J. Singh, C, O'Neill and D.J. Handelsman, D. J. *Endocrinology*, 136, 5311, (1995).
[169] E. Steinberger. *Physiol. Rev.* 51, 1, (1971).
[170] D.J. Handelsman, J.A. Spaliviero, J.M. Simpson, C.M. Allan and J. Singh. *Endocrinology*, 140, 3938, (1999).
[171] M. Haywood, J. Spaliviero, M. Jimemez, N.J. King, D.J. Handelsman and C.M. llan. *Endocrinology*, 144, 509, (2003).
[172] L. O'Donnell, R.I. McLachlan, N.G. Wreford and D.M. Robertson. *Endocrinology*, 135, 2608, (1994).
[173] L. O'Donnell, R.I. McLachlan, N.G. Wreford, D.M. de Kretser, and D.M. Robertson. *Biol. Reprod.* 55, 895, (1996).
[174] R.I. McLachlan, N.G. Wreford, S.J. Meachem, D.M. De Kretser and D.M. Robertson. *Biol. Reprod*, 51, 945, (1994).
[175] A. El Shennawy, R.J. Gates and L.D. Russell. *J. Androl.* 19, 320, (1998).
[176] L. O'Donnell, K. Pratis, P.G. Stanton, D.M. Robertson and R.I. McLachlan. *J. Androl.* 20, 109, (1999).
[177] S.J. Meachem, N.G. Wreford, D.M. Robertson and R.I. McLachlan, R. I. *Int. J. Androl.* 20, 70, (1997).
[178] J.M. Bartlett, J.B. Kerr and R.M. Sharpe. *J. Androl.* 7,240, (1986).

[179] J.B. Kerr, S. Maddocks and R.M. Sharpe. *Cell. Tissue Res*. 268, 179, (1992).
[180] J.B. Kerr, M. Millar, S. Maddocks and R.M. Sharpe. *Anat. Rec*. 235, 547, (1993).
[181] K.Henriksen, H. Hakovirta and M. Parvinen. *Endocrinology*, 136, 3285, (1995).
[182] Y.T. Sun, D.C. Irby, D.M. Robertson and D.M. de Kretser. *Endocrinology*, 125, 1000, (1989).
[183] R.I. McLachlan, L. O'Donnell, S.J. Meachem, P.G. Stanton, D.M. de Kretser, K. Pratis and D.M. Robertson. *Recent Prog. Horm.Res*. 57, 149, (2002).
[184] C.A. Awoniyi, R. Santulli, R.L. Sprando, L.L. Ewing and B.R. Zirkin. *Endocrinology* 24, 1217, (1989).
[185] M.S. Mahendroo, K.M. Cala, D.L. Hess and D.W. Russell. *Endocrinology*, 142, 4652, (2001).
[186] F.P. Zhang, T. Pakarainen, M. Poutanen, J. Toppari and I. Huhtaniemi. *Proc. Natl. Acad. Sci. U S A*, 100, 13692, (2003).
[187] L. O'Donnell, P.G. Stanton, J.R. Bartles and D.M. Robertson. *Biol. Reprod*, 63, 99, (2000).
[188] A.W. Vogl, D.C. Pfeiffer, D. Mulholland, G. Kimel and J. Guttman. *Arch. Histol. Cytol*. 3, 1, (2000).
[189] K.J. Perryman, P.G. Stanton, K.L. Loveland, R.I. McLachlan and D.M. Robertson. *Endocrinology*, 137, 3877, (1996).
[190] P.B. Grino, J.E. Griffin and J.D. Wilson. *Endocrinology*, 126, 1165, (1990).
[191] R.A. Anderson, A.M. Wallace and F.C. Wu. *J. Clin. Endocrinol. Metab*. 81, 902, (1996).
[192] R.A. Anderson, R.W. Kelly and F.C. Wu. *J. Androl*. 18, 366, (1997).
[193] G.Z. Mingoti, R.N. Pereira and C.M.R. Monteiro. *Braz. J.Med.Biol. Res*., 36, 677, (2003).
[194] C. Huckins and E.F. Oakberg. *Anat. Rec*., 192, 519, (1978).
[195] D.J. Allan B.V. Harmon and S.A. Roberts. *Cell Prolif*., 25, 241, (1992).
[196] J.B. Kerr. *J. Reprod. Fertil*., 95, 825, (1992).
[197] H. Yazawa, I. Sasagawa, M. Ishigooka and T. Nakada. *Human Reprod*., 14, 1806, (1999).
[198] I. Sasagawa, H. Yazawa, Y. Suzuki and T. Nakada. *Arch.Androl*., 47, 211, (2001)
[199] L. Troiano, M.F. Fustini, E. Lovato, A. Frasoldati, W. Malorni, M. Capri, E. Grassilli, P. Marrama and C. Franceschi. *Biochem.Bioph.Res. Commun*., 202, 1315, (1994).
[200] Y.H. Lue, A.P. Sinha Hikim and R.S. Swerdloff. *Endocrinology*, 140, 1700, (1999).
[201] Y.H. Lue, B.L. Lasley, L.S. Laughlin, R.S. Swerdloff, A.P. Sinha, A. Leung, J.W. Overstreet and C. Wang. *J.Androl*., 23, 799, (2002).
[202] J.C. Rockett, F.L. Mapp, J.B. Garges, J.C. Luft, C. Mori and D.J. Dix. *Biol. Reprod*., 65, 229, (2001).
[203] J. Blanco-Rodríguez and C. Martínez-García. *J. Androl*., 18, 535, (1997).
[204] Z. Zhang, R.V. Short, T. Meehan, D.M. De Kretser, M.B. Renfree and K.L. Loveland. *J.Androl*., 25, 57, (2004)
[205] H. Yazawa, I. Sasagawa and T. Nakada. *Human Reprod*., 15, 917, (2000).
[206] S. Schmidt, J. Rainer, C. Ploner, E. Presul, S. Riml and R. Kofler. *Cell Death and Differentiation*, 11, S45, (2004).

[207] G.E. Bentley, T. Ubuka, N.L. McGuire, V.S. Chowdhury, Y. Morita, T. Yano, I. Hasunuma, M. Binns, J.C. Wingfield and K. Tsutsui. *Gen.Comp.Endocrinol.*, 156, 34, (2008).
[208] S. Zhao, E. Zhu, C. Yang, G.E. Bentley, K. Tsutsui and L.J. Kriegsfeld. *Endocrinology*, 151, 617, (2010).
[209] T. Ubuka, N.L. McGuire, R.M. Calisi, N. Perfito and G.E. Bentley. *Integ.Comp.Biol.*. 48, 560–569, (2008).
[210] K.A. Young, G.F. Ball and R.J. Nelson. *Biol.Reprod.*, 64, 706, (2001).
[211] K.A. Young and R.J. Nelson. *Reproduction*, 122, 677, (2001).
[212] I. Woolveridge, M. de Boer-Brouwer, M.F. Taylor, K.J. Teerds, F.C. Wu and I.D. Morris. *Biol.Reprod.*, 60, 461, (1999).
[213] M. Miura, I. Sasagawa, Y. Suzuki, T. Nakada and J. Fuji. *Fert.Steril.*, 4, 787, (2002).
[214] E. Yang, J Zha, J. Jokel, L.H. Boisel, C.B. Thompson and S.J. Korsmeyer. *Cell*, 80, 285, (1995).
[215] C.M. Yamamoto, A.P. Sinha Hikim, P.N. Huynh, B. Shapiro, Y.H. Lue, W.A. Salameh, C. Wang and R.S. Swerdloff. *Biol.Reprod.*, 63, 1683, (2000).
[216] V. Pentikainen, K, Erkkila and L. Dunkel. *Am.J.Physiol.*, 276, E310, (1999).
[217] J. Lee, J.H. Richburg, S.C. Younkin and K.Boekelheide. *Endocrinology*, 138, 2081, (1997).
[218] J. Lee, J.H. Richburg, E.B. Shipp, M.L. Meistrich and K. Boekelheide. *Endocrinology*, 140, 852, (1999).
[219] S. Nagata and P. Goldstein. *Science*, 267, 1449, (1995).
[220] S. Nagata. *Cell*, 88, 355, (1997).
[221] N. Ozawa, N. Goda, N. Makino, T. Yamaguchi, Y. Yoshimura and M.Suematsu. *J.Clin.Invest.*, 109, 457, (2002).
[222] A. Sancar A. *Annu. Rev.Genet.*, 29, 69, (1995).
[223] E.A. Craig EA. *Crit.Rev.Biochem.*, 18, 239, (1985).
[224] S. Cosulich and P. Clarke P. *Curr. Biol.*, 6, 1586, (1996).
[225] J.M. Gutteridge and B. Halliwell. *Ann. N Y Acad. Sci.*, 899, 136, (2000).
[226] A. Aguilar-Mahecha, B.F. Hales and B. Robaire. *Biol.Reprod.*, 65, 119, (2001).
[227] J.C. Rockett, P. Patrizio, J.E. Schmid, N.B. Hecht and D. Dix. *Mut.Res.*, 549, 225, (2004).
[228] W.J. Bremner and D.K. Clifton. *J.Androl.*, 4, 387, (1983).
[229] J.M. Trasler, B.F. Hales and B. Robaire. *Nature*, 316,144, (1985).
[230] W.C. Young. *J.Exp.Zool.*, 49, 459, (1927).
[231] R.J. Aitken. *J.Reprod.Fertil.*, 115, 1, (1999).
[232] C. Gagnon, A. Iwasaki, E. de Lamirande and N. Kovalski. *Ann.NY.Acad.Sci.*, 637, 436, (1991).
[233] E. de Lamirande, H. Jiang, A. Zini, H. Kodama and C. Gagnon. *Rev.Reprod.*, 2, 48, (1997).
[234] J.R. Drevet. *Mol.Cell.Endocrinol.*, 250, 70, (2006).
[235] R.J. Aitken, J.S. Clarkson, S. Fishel. *Biol.Reprod.*, 40, 183, (1989).
[236] E. de Lamirande and C. Gagnon. *Free Radic.Biol.Med.*, 14, 255, (1993).
[237] A. Zini, E. de Lamirande and C. Gagnon. *J.Androl.*, 16, 424, (1996).
[238] R.J. Aitken and S.D: Roman. *Oxid.Med.Cel.Long.* 1, 15, (2008).
[239] T.T.Turner and J.J. Lysiak. *J. Androl.*, 29, 488, (2008).

[240] R.J. Aitken and G.N. De Iuliis. *Reprod.Biomed.Online*, 14, 727, (2007).
[241] R.J. Aitken and M.A. Baker. *Mol.Cell Endocrinol.*, 250, 66, (2006).
[242]R.J. Aitken. *Reprod.Fertil. Dev.*, 16, 655, (2004).
[243] D.B. Hales, J.A. Allen, T. Shankara, P. Janus, S. Buck, T. Diemer and K.H. Hales. *Ann.NYAcad.Sci.*, 1061, 120, (2005).
[244] C.K. Naughton, A.K. Nangia and A. Agarwal. *Hum.Reprod.Update*, 7, 473, (2001).
[245] S.C. Sikka. *Curr.Med.Chem.*, 8, 851, (2001).
[246]A. Agarwal, S.Gupta and S. Sikka. *Curr.Opin.Obstet.Gynecol.*, 18, 325, (2006).
[247] W.A. Pryor, K.N. Houk, C.S. Foote, J.M. Fukuto, L.J. Ignarro, G.L. Squadrito and K.J.A. Davies. *Am.J.Physiol.Regul.Integr.Comp.Physiol.*, 291, R491,(2006). [248] C. Szabo, H. Ischiropoulus and R. Radi. *Nat.Rev.*, 6, 662, (2007). [249] V. Peltola, E. Mantyla, I. Huhtaniemi, and M. Ahotupa. *J Androl ,* 15, 353, (1994). [250] P.G. Quinn and A.H. Payne. *J.Biol.Chem.*, 259, 4130, (1984). [251] H. Chen, J. Liu, L. Luo, M.U. Baig, J.M. Kim and B.R. Zirkin. *Exp.Gerontol.*, 40, 728, (2005).
[252] D.D. Mruk, B. Silvestrini, M. Mo, C.Y. Cheng. *Contraception,* 65, 305, (2002).
[253] E. Cadenas. *Mol.AspectsMed.*, 25, 17, (2004).
[254] M. Maiorino, V. Bosello, F. Ursini, C. Foresta, A. Garolla, M. Scapin, H. Sztajer and L. Flohe. *Biol.Reprod.*, 68, 1134, (2003).
[255] T. Ischi, S. Matsuki, Y. Iuchi, F. Okada, S. Toyosaki, Y. Tomita, Y. Ikeda and Y. Fujii. *FreeRad.Res.*, 39, 695, (2005).
[256] V.R. Narra, R.W. Howell, K.S.R. Sastry and D.V. Rao. *J.Nucl.Med.*, 34, 637, (1993).
[257] R. Kutlubay, E.O. Oguz, B. Can, M.C. Guven, Z. Sinik, O.L. Tuncay and E. Vieamen. *Int.J.Toxicol.*, 26, 297, (2007).
[258] S. Uguralp, U. Usta and B. Mizrak. *Eur.J.Pediatr.Surg.*, 15, 333, (2005).
[259] M. Gavazza and A. Catala. *Int.J.Biochem.Cell Biol.*, 35, 359, (2003).
[260] J. B. Kerr, K. L. Loveland, M. K. O'Bryan, and D. M. de Kretser. *Cytology of the Testis and Intrinsic Contro*. Neil JD. Knobil and Neill's Physiology of Reproduction. Jimmy D. Neill, Ed, Elsevier, (2006), pp827-947.
[261] A. Zini and P. Schlegel. *J.Urol.*, 158, 659, (1997).
[262] F. Bauché, M.H. Fouchard and B.J. Jégou. *FEBS Let.*, 394, 392, (1994).
[263] A. Zini and P. Schlegel. *J.Androl.*, 17, 473, (1996).
[264] R.M. Vigueras-Villaseñor, D. Molina-Ortiz, G. Reyes-Torres, D. Santamaría del Angel, N.A. Moreno-Mendoza, M.E. García Cruz, O. Cuevas-Alpuche and J.C. Rojas-Castañeda. *Acta Histochem.*, 111, 127, (2009).
[265] S.B. Guimaraes, A.A. Aragao, J.M. Santos, S. Kimura Ode, P.H. Barbosa and P.R. Vasconcelos. *Acta Cir Bras*, 22, 30, (2007).
[266] A. Agarwal, S. Prabakaran and S.S. Allamaneni. *Reprod.Biomed.Online*, 12, 630, (2006).
[267] A. Zamoner, K.P. Barreto, D.W. Filho, F. Sell, V.M. Woehl, F.C. Guma, F.R. Silva and R. Pessoa-Pureur. *Mol. Cell Endocrinol.*, 267, 116, (2007).
[268] B.S.Muralidhara. *Reprod. Toxicol.*, 23, 578, (2007).
[269] M.M. Reddy, S.V. Mahipal, J. Subhashini, M.C. Reddy, K.R. Roy, G.V. Reddy, P.R. Reddy and P. *Reddanna. Reprod.Toxicol.*, 22, 493, (2006).
[270] I. Manna, K. Jana, P.K. Samanta. *Acta.Physiol.Scand.*, 178, 33, (2003).
[271] I. Manna, K. Jana, P.K. Samanta. *J. Appl. Physiol.*, 29, 172, (2004).
[272] G.B. Chainy, S. Samantaray, L. Samanta. *Andrologia,* 29, 343, (1997).

[273] S.P. Chaki, M.M. Misro, D.K. Gautam, M. Kaushik, D. Ghosh and G.B. Chainy. *Apoptosis,* 11, 1427, (2006).

[274] M.L. Conte da Frota, E. Gomes da Silva, G.A. Behr, M. Roberto de Oliveira, F. Dal-Pizzol, F. Klamt and J.C. Moreira. *Mol.Cell Biochem.*, 285, 173, (2006).

[275] H. Ozyurt, H. Pekmez, B.S. Parlaktas, I. Kus, B. Ozyur and M. Sarsilmaz. *Asian J.Androl.*, 8, 189, (2006).

[276] R. Nordmann, C. Ribiere and H. Rouach. *Alcohol Alcohol*, 25,231, (1990).

[277] A. Zafir and N. Banu. *Indian J.Biochem.Biophys.*, 46, 53, (2009).

[278] S.P. Chaki, M.M. Misro, D. Ghosh, D.K. Gautam and M. Srinivas. *Apoptosis*. 10, 395, (2005).

[279] B.R. Zirkin and H. Chen. *Biol.Reprod.*, 63, 977, (2000).

[280] T.T. Turner, H.J. Bang, J.J. Lysiak. *Urology.*, 65, 390, (2005).

[281] I. Hanukoglu. *Drug Metab Rev.*, 38, 171, (2006).

[282] L. Luo, H. Chen, M.A. Trush, M.D. Show, M.D. Anway and B.R. Zirkin. *J Androl.*, 27, 240, (2006).

[283] D.K. Gautam, M.M. Misro, S.P. Chaki and N. Sehgal. *Apoptosis*, 11, 39, (2006).

[284] M. Ikeda, H. Kodama, J. Fukuda, Y. Shimizu, M. Murata, J. Kumagai and T. Tanaka. *Biol.Reprod.*, 61, 393, (1999).

[285] C. Paul, S. Teng and P.T.K. Saunders. *Biol.Reprod.*, 80, 913, (2009).

[286] E. Kasahara, E.F. Sato, M. Miyoshi, R. Konaka, K. Hiramoto, J. Sasaki, M. Tokuda, Y. Nakano and M. Inoue. *Biochem. J.*, 365, 849, (2002).

[287] N. Aydilek, M. Aksakal and A. Z. Karaklıçık. *Andrologia*, 36, 277, (2004).

[288] S. P. Chaki, D. Ghosh and M.M. Misro. *Int.J.Androl.*, 26, 319, (2003).

[289] S. Dhanabalan and P.P. Mathur. *Exp.Toxicol.Pathol.*, 61, 415, (2009).

[290] A. Maheshwari, M.M. Misro, A. Aggarwal, R.K. Sharma and D. Nandan D. *FEBS J.*, 276, 870, (2009).

[291] A. Agarwal, R.A. Saleh and M.A. Bedaiwy. *Fert.Steril.* 79, 829, (2003).

[292] H. Sies. *Eur.J.Biochem.*, 215, 213, (1993).

[293] M. Jedlinska-Krakowska, G, Bomba, K. Jakubowski, T. Rotkiewicz, B. Jana and A. Penkowski. J.*Reprod.Dev.*, 52, 203, (2006).

[294] A. Agarwal, M.M.Misro, A. Maheshwari, N. Sehgal and D. Nandan. *Mol.Reprod.Dev.*, 77, 900, (2010).

[295] P. Das and M. Chowdhury. *Mol. Cell Biochem.* 198, 151, (1999).

[296] D. Ghosh, U.B. Das, M. Mallick and J. Debnath. *Drug.Chem.Toxicol.* 25: 281- 292. (2002).

[297] F. Gerold and J.R. Combs. *Vitamin E.* In F. Gerold and J.R. Combs (Eds.) The Vitamins: Fundamental Aspects in Nutrition and Health, (1992).pp. 223-249. New York, Academic Press.

[298] H. Wefers and H. Sies. *Eur.J.Biochem.*, 174, 353, (1988).

[299] G.R. Buettner. *Arch.Biochem.Biophys.*, 300, 525, (1993).

[300] W. Gorczyca, F. Traganos, H. Jesionowska and Z. Darzynkiewicz. *Exp.Cell Res.*, 207, 202, (1993).

[301] J.G. Sun, A. Jurisicova and R.F. Casper. *Biol.Reprod.*, 56, 602, (1997).

[302] D.S. Irvine, J.P. Twigg, E.L. Gordon, N. Fulton, P.A. Milne and R.J. Aitken. *J.Androl.*, 21, 33, (2000).

[302] G.J. Osterhuis, A.B. Mulder, E. Kalsbeek-Batenburg, C.B. Lambalk, J. Schoemaker and I. Vermes. *Fertil.Steril.*, 74, 245, (2000).
[304] X. Wang, R.K. Sharma, S.C. Sikka, A.J. Thomas, T. Falcone and A. Agarwal. *Fertil. Steril.*, 80,531, (2003).
[305] A. Agarwal, I. Ikemoto and K.R. Loughlin. *J.Urol.*, 152, 107, (1994). J.S. Armstrong, M. Rajasekaran, W. Chamulitrat, P. Gatti, W.J. Hellstrom and [306] S.C. Sikka. *Free Radic.Biol.Med.*, 26, 869, (1999).
[307] J. Lee, J.H. Richburg, S.C. Younkin and K. Boekelheide. *Endocrinology*, 138, 2081, (1997).
[308] T. Suda, T. Takahashi, P. Golstein and S. Nagata. *Cell*, 75, 1169, (1993).
[309] D. Sakkas, E. Mariethoz, G. Manicardi, D. Bizzaro, P. Bianchi and U. Bianchi. *Rev.Reprod.*, 4, 31, (1999).
[310] E.M. Hull, R.L. Meisel and B.D. Sachs. *Male Sexual Behavior*. D.W. Pfaff, A.P. Arnold, A.M. Etgen, S.E. Fahrbach, R.T. Rubin (eds). Hormones, Brain and Behavior. San Diego: Elsevier Science, (2002), pp3-137.
[311] E.B. Keverne. *Sexual and aggressive behavior in social groups of talapoin monkeys*. R. Porter, J. Whelan (eds.). Sex, hormones and behavior. Ciba Found. Symp. 63. (1979). pp.271–286.
[312] S. Yotsuyanagi, T. Mizuno, Y. Nagasaka and M. Namiki. *J.Sex. Med.*, 3, 612, (2006).
[313] K. Sugiura, H. Yoshimura and M. Yokoyama. *Psychopharmacology*, 133, 249, (1997).
[314] S. Retana-Márquez, E.D. Salazar and J. Velazquez-Moctezuma *J. Psychoneuroendocrinology*, 21, 39, (1996).
[315] P.S. D'Aquila, P. Brain and P. Willner. *Physiol.Behav.*, 56, 861, (1994).
[316] J. Grønli, R. Murison, E. Fiske, B. Bjorvatn, E. Sørensen, C.M Portas and R. Ursin. *Physiol.Behav.*, 84, 571, (2005).
[317] Y. Sato, N. Suzuki, H. Horita, H. Wada, A. Shibuya, H. Adachi, T. Tsukamoto, Y. Kumamoto and M. Yamamoto. *J.Androl.*, 17, 83, (1996).
[318] W. Hawley, E. Grissom, L. Keskitalo, T. Hastings and G. Dohanich. *Physiol Behav.*, 102, 181, (2011).
[319] D.J. Cosgrove, Z. Gordon, J.E. Bernie, S. Hami, D. Montoya, M.B. Stein, M. Monga. *Urology*, 5, 881, (2002).
[320] E.J. Letourneau, P.A. Schewe and B.C. Frueh. *J.Trauma Stress*, 10, 125, (1997).
[321] A. Kendurkar and B. Kaur. *Prim.Care Companion J.Clin.Psychiatry*, 10, 299, (2008).
[322] G. Corona, V. Ricca, E. Bandini, E. Mannucci, L. Petrone, A. Fisher, F. Lotti, G. Balercia, C. Faravelli, G. Forti and M. Maggi. J.Sex Med., 5, 458, (2008).
[323] V. Anticević and D. Britvić. *Croat.Med.J.*, 49, 499, (2008).
[324] G. Frajese, R. Lazzari, A. Magnani, C. Moretti, V. Sforza and D. Nerozzi. J. *Steroid Biochem.Molec.Biol.*, 37, 411, (1990).
[325] E.M. Hull, R.I. Wood and K.E. McKenna. *Neurobiology of male sexual behavior*. Neil JD. Knobil and Neill's Physiology of Reproduction. Jimmy D. Neill, Ed, Elsevier, (2006), pp1729-1824.
[326] F.L. Moore and L.J. Miller. *Horm.Behav.*, 18, 400, (1984).
[327] R.R. Tokarz. *Horm.Behav.*, 21, 358, (1987).
[328] J. Wingfield. Horm.Behav., 19, 174, (1985).
[329] R. Sapolsky, L.C. Krey and B.S. McEwen. *Endocr.Rev.*,7, 622, (1986).

[330] D.R. Colborn, D.L. Thompson, J.J. Capehart and K.L. White, K.L. *J.Anim.Sci.*, 69, 2556, (1991).
[331] S. Retana-Márquez, H. Bonilla-Jaime and J. Velázquez-Moctezuma. *Physiol.Behav.*, 63, 367, (1998).
[332] B. Leuner, E.R. Glasper and E. Gould. *PLoS ONE*, 5, 1, (2010).
[333] M.D. Spritzer, A.Weinberg, V. Viau, L.A.M. Galea. *Behav.Brain Res.*, 200, 106, (2009).
[334] J.G. Pfaus. *J.Sex Med.*, 6, 1506, (2009).
[335] W.A. Dornan and C.W. Malsbury. Neurosci.Biobehav.Rev., 13, 1, (1989).
[336] J. Pfaus J and B. Gorzalka. "Reexamining the role of endogenous opioids in sexual behavior". 66th Annual Meeting of theWestern Psychological Association. Seattle,WA; 1986.
[337] D.J.S. Sirinathsinghji DJS. *Brain Res.*, 407, 185, (1987).
[338] E. Keen-Rhinehart, V. Michopoulos, D.J. Toufexis, E.I. Martin, H. Nair, K.J. Ressler, M. Davis, M.J. Owens, C.B. Nemeroff and M.E. Wilson. *Mol.Psychiatry.*, 14, 37, (2009).
[339] Y. Miwa, K. Nagase, N. Oyama N, H. Akino, O. Yokoyama. *J.Sex.Med.*, 8, 688, (2011)
[340] M.J. Owens and C.B. Nemeroff. The neurobiology of corticotropin-releasing factor: implications for affective disorders. A.F. Schatberg, C.B. Nemeroff (Eds). *The Hypothalamic–Pituitary–Adrenal Axis: Physiology, Pathophysiology and Psychiatric Implications* (1988). pp 1–35. Raven Press, New York
[341] G.A. Olson, R.D. Olson and A.J. Kastin. Peptides, 15, 1513, (1994).
[342] R. Feldman, J. Meyer and L. Quenzer L. *Principles of Neuropsychopharmacology.* (1997). Saunderland, Massachusetts: Sinauer Associates Inc. Publishers; pp. 49–548.
[343] M.J. Millan, R. Przewlocki, M. Jerlics, C. Gramsch, V. Holt and A. Herz. *Brain Res.*, 208, 325, (1981).
[344] R.S. Sathe, B.R. Komisaruk, A.K. Ladas and S.V. Godbole. *Arch.Med.Res.*, 32, 221, (2001).
[345] E.A. Young. *Neuroendocrinology*, 52, 405, (1990).
[346] A.L. Vaccarino, A.J. Kastin. *Peptides*, 21, 1975, (2000).
[347] A.T. Lim and J.W. Funder. *Neuroendocrinology*, 36, 225, (1983).
[348] A. Argiolas. Neuropeptides and sexual behaviour. *Neurosci.Biobehav.Rev.*, 23, 1127, (1999).
[349] L. Matuszewich and W.A. Dornan. *Psychopharmacology*, 106,391, (1992).
[350] W.R. Van Furth, M.G. Van Emst and J.M. Van Ree. *Behav.Neurosci.*, 109, 123, (1995).
[351] J.G. Pfaus, B.J. Everitt. *The psychopharmacology of sexual behavior*. F.E. Bloom and D.J. Kupfer, eds. Psychopharmacology: the Fourth Generation in Progress. New York: Raven Press; (1995). pp. 742–58.
[352] M.R. Melis, S. Succu and A. Argiolas. *Brain Res.Bull.*, 44, 689, (1997).
[353] M.R. Melis, S. Succu, U. Iannucci and A. Argiolas A. *Naunyn-Schmiedeberg's Arch.Pharmacol.*, 355, 595, (1997).
[354] A.M. Huges, B.J. Everitt and J. Herbert. *Psychopharmacology*, 102, 243, (1990).
[355] W.R. Van Furth, G. Woltering, J.M. Van Ree. *Brain Res.Rev.*, 21, 162, (1995).
[356] A.M. Hughes, B.J. Everitt and J. Herbert. *Neuroscience*, 27, 689, (1989).

[357] G. Drolet, E.C. Dumont, I. Gosselin, R. Kinkead, S. Laforest, J.F. Trotier. *Prog.NeruoPsychopharmacol.Biol.Psychiatry*, 25, 729, (2001).

[358] H. Shang, M.M. Torregrossa, E.M. Jutkiewicz, Y.G. Shi, K.C. Rice, J.H. Woods, S.J. Watson and M.C. Ko. *Eur.J.Neurosci.*, 23, 984, (2006).

[359] D.L. Maney, R.D. Richardson and J.C. Wingfield. *Horm. Behav.*, 32, 11, (1997).

[360] G.E. Bentley, J.P. Jensen, G.J. Kaur, D.W. Wacker, K. Tsutsui and J.C. Wingfield. *Horm. Behav.*, 49, 550, 2006.

[361] L.J. Kriegsfeld, E.M. Gibson, W.P. Williams III, S. Zhao, A.O. Mason, G.E. Bentley and K. Tsutsui. *J. Neuroendocrinol.*, 22, 692, (2010).

[362] A.K. Dubey and T.M. Plant. *Biol Reprod*, 33,423, (1985).

[363] S.A. Lerman, G.K. Miller, K. Bohlman, V. Albaladejo, J.F. Léonard, V. Devas and R.L. Clark. *Reprod Toxicol*, 11, 799, (1997).

[364] N.R. Vulliemoz, E. Xiao, L. Xia-Zhang, J. Rivier and M. Ferin. *Endocrinology*, 149, 869, (2008).

[365] S.L. Berga. *Endocrinology*, 149, 867, (2008).

[366] J.C. Wingfield and R.M. Sapolsky. *J Neuroendocrinol*, 15, 711, (2003).

[367] D.M. Champagne. *Hum.Reprod.*, 21, 1651, (2006).

[368] S. Einarsson, Y. Brandt, H. Rodriguez-Martinez and A. Madej. *Theriogenology*, 70, 1197, (2008).

In: Testosterone
Editor: Konstantin Chichinadze

ISBN 978-1-62100-492-9

Chapter VI

Genetic Variants of Liver-localized *SRD5A1* and *AKR1C4* Genes Associated with Circulating Sex Steroid Levels

ChenDi Liao[1*], Jieying Jiang[1,*], Nelson L. S. Tang[1,2,†], Timothy C. Y. Kwok[3], Xingyan Wang[1], Claes Ohlsson[4], Anna L. Eriksson[5], Liesbeth Vandenput[5], Frank W. K. Chan[6], Anthony Kwok[7], Eric Orwoll[8], Jean Woo[9], Ping Chung Leung[7]

[1]Department of Chemical Pathology, The Chinese University of Hong Kong, Hong Kong SAR, China

[2]Laboratory of Genetics of disease susceptibility, Li Ka Shing Institute of Health Sciences, Hong Kong SAR, China

[3]Department of Community and Family Medicine, Faculty of Medicine, The Chinese University of Hong Kong, Hong Kong SAR, China

[4]Center for Bone Research at the Sahlgrenska Academy, Institute of Medicine, Gothenburg University, SE-413 45 Gothenburg, Sweden

[5] Center for Bone Research at the Sahlgrenska Academy, Departments of Internal Medicine and Geriatrics, Gothenburg University, Gothenburg, Sweden

[6]School of Public Health and Primary care, The Chinese University of Hong Kong, Hong Kong SAR, China

[7]Jockey Club Centre for Osteoporosis Care and Control, Faculty of Medicine, The Chinese University of Hong Kong, Hong Kong SAR, China

[8]Oregon Health & Science University, Portland, Oregon, USA

[9]Department of Medicine and Therapeutics, Faculty of Medicine, The Chinese University of Hong Kong, Hong Kong SAR, China

---

[*] These authors contributed equally.

[†] Address correspondence to: Nelson L.S. Tang, MD, PhD, FRCPA. Department of Chemical Pathology, Faculty of Medicine, The Chinese University of Hong Kong, Prince of Wales Hospital, Shatin, New Territories, Hong Kong SAR, China. Phone: +852 26322320; Fax: +852 26365090; E-mail: nelsontang@cuhk.edu.hk.

ABSTRACT

Stead-state sex steroid concentrations in the circulations show significant inter-individual variations within and across populations. Such variations are also associated with predisposition to various diseases. Genetic polymorphisms in genes encoding enzymes in the biosynthesis and metabolism pathways of sex hormones are likely to account for such inter-individual variations. In this study of over 1400 Chinese men, single nucleotide polyporphisms (SNPs) of candidate genes involved in sex steroid metabolic pathway were investigated for their association with blood androgens concentrations. We found that blood androgen concentrations correlated with SNPs in *SRD5A1* and *AKR1C4* genes. The genotype of rs11738248 in *SRD5A1* was significantly associated with circulating dihydrotestosterone(DHT) to testosterone (T) ratio while the C-T-T haplotype on *SRD5A1* could be a predictor for low DHT level. As for AKR1C4, it was found that the genotype rs17134607 was associated with androsterone level in a linear regression model. In addition, it was also observed that the G-A haplotype could be a risk haplotype for high androsterone level. This chapter is the first to reveal the potential association between circulating androgen levels and the genetic variations in *SRD5A1* and *AKR1C4* in a large cohort of healthy general population. Future studies may examine their underlying functional genetic elements that affected the sex steroid level in blood and their potential association with diseases.

INTRODUCTION

Sex steroids play important roles in human development [1]. Serum levels of various sex steroids have been associated with various clinical diseases such as prostate cancer and liver cancer [2-4]. Therefore, it is important to understand the mechanism contributing to the variation in circulating level of sex steroid among individuals and across ethnic groups which behaves as a complex trait. Twin studies have shown that inter-individual variations in circulating sex steroid concentrations could be attributed largely to genetic effects [5, 6]. In addition, there have been studies showing strong familial correlations [7-9]. However, there is limited understanding about the exact underlying determinants (in term of genetic and their variants) of circulating sex steroid level itself.

Many enzymes are involved in the biosynthesis and metabolism pathways of sex steroids. Genetic variations in these genes may alter the functional property of its encoded enzyme, such as its activity, and thus affect the steady-state sex steroid level in the circulation. Testosterone (T) is the most prominent sex steroid in men, and is transformed into its more potent metabolite, dihydrotestosterone (DHT), by 5α-reductases [10]. Two distinct genes encode for two isoenzymes have been described for 5α-reductase. They are steroid 5α-reductase type I and II (SRD5A1/2), encoded by two separate genes *SRD5A1* and *SRD5A2*, located on chromosome 5p15.5 [11] and 2p23 [12, 13] respectively. While *SRD5A2* gene has been studied more thoroughly, where it is repeatedly shown to be associated with circulating concentration of testosterone and its downstream metabolite androstane-3α, 17β-diol-glucuronide (*3α-diolG*) among different ethnic groups [14-17]. Studies of the effects of *SRD5A1* genetic variation on serum sex steroid level were very limited. Only two studies have reported an association between *SRD5A1* gene and serum DHT/T ratio, an indicator of the enzymatic activity of 5α-reductase [18, 19]. However, both studies were performed within a small group (N<60) and one with patient samples only (type 2 diabetes) [18]. Thus, the reliability and the ability to generalize the results to healthy population may be uncertain

The main difference between the two isoenzymes resides in their expression in tissue, whereas SRD5A1 is mostly expressed in liver and skin, SRD5A2 is predominantly located in the male reproductive tissues [13]. After SRD5A1 reduces T to DHT in the liver, it is further metabolized by 3α-hydroxysteroid dehydrogenase type I (AKR1C4) into less potent metabolite, 3α-androstanediol (3α-diol). In addition, AKR1C4 also has a 17β-hydroxysteroid dehydrogenase activity, which readily oxidizes 3α-diol to another metabolite androsterone [20, 21]. AKR1C4 is a liver-specific enzyme encoded by the *AKR1C4* gene from chromosome 10p14-15 [22], and genetic effect of *AKR1C4* gene has not been investigated before.

Here, we propose to study the association of these two genes involved in the sex steroid metabolic pathway of the liver with sex steroid levels in the circulation. By genotyping tagSNPs that represented the *SRD5A1* and *AKR1C4* gene in a large homogenous cohort of Chinese male population, we analyzed their associations with testosterone and its metabolites, to search for genetic predictors of circulating sex steroid levels.

METHOD

Study Population

The study population consisted of a healthy cohort of community Chinese men, which included 2000 men of 65 years old and above, recruited from community centers for the elderly and housing estates in Hong Kong. Participants were invited to the School of Public Health of the Chinese University of Hong Kong to have their body height and weight measured, as well as to collect their demographic profile and information regarding their lifestyle through a questionnaire. Peripheral blood samples were also collected from the participants in the morning (before 11AM) after an overnight fast. Serum was saved after centrifugation of clotted blood on the same day and an EDTA blood tube was saved to DNA extraction, both were stored at –80°C until assay. Ultimately, only 1402 individuals with sufficient sample volume were available for measurements of sex steroid concentration. The study was approved by the Clinical Research Ethics Committee of the Chinese University of Hong Kong, and all participants gave written informed consent.

The method for serum sex steroid measurement has been described previously [7]. The serum sex steroid levels were quantitated using a gas chromatographic-negative chemical ionization-mass spectrometry (GC/NCI-MS) at the Laboratory of Molecular Endocrinology and Oncology, Laval University, Quebec, Canada. The assay properties were as follows: serum sex hormone binding globulin (SHBG), limit of detection 0.2nmol/l, intra-assay CV 5.6%, inter-assay CV:6.5%; testosterone, limit of detection 0.05ng/ml, intra-assay CV 2.9%, inter-assay CV 3.4%; DHT, limit of detection 0.01μg/L, intra-assay CV3.1%, inter-assay CV4.1%) [23].

Genotyping of TagSNPs

Commercial DNA extraction kit (GE Healthcare, USA) was used to extract genomic DNA from the peripheral blood samples. Genomic DNA was extracted from peripheral blood samples using commercial extraction kit according to manufacture's instruction. The extracted DNA samples were stored at -80°C before genotyping.

From the International HapMap Phase project (release #21a/phase II, Mar08), we obtained all SNPs located within the *SRD5A1* and *AKR1C4* gene and its surrounding 5kb region (both upstream and downstream) in the Han Chinese Beijing (CHB) population. Using a spectral decomposition algorithm [24-26] covering all SNPs with minor allele frequencies of at least 5% in Asians, factors accounting for the polymorphisms in each gene were identified: three for *SRD5A1* and two were found for *AKR1C4* (Table 1). These factors corresponded to the SNPs representing the overall genetic variation in the genic region including coding and non-coding sequences of the two genes. The 3 tagSNPs of *SRD5A1* identified were rs248807, rs11738248 and rs824811, while the 2 tagSNPs of *AKR1C4* were rs1334473 and rs17134607, together covering 90% of variance in both genes.

Table 1. Gene SNP factor component analysis and resulting tagSNPs

Gene	Component in spectral decomposition	% of variance	Cumulative %	Representative SNP in the component
SRD5A1	1	45.15	45.15	rs248807
	2	35.86	81.01	rs11738248
	3	8.41	*89.48*	rs824811
AKR1C4	1	73.50	73.50	rs1334473
	2	16.33	*90.00*	rs17134607

We performed melting temperature-shift allele-specific genotyping method in a single-tube PCR to genotype the tagSNPs, which was described previously [8, 17, 27]. In brief, two allele-specific primers containing a different length of 5'GC sequence and one complementary primer <20bp downstream from the SNP were designed for each SNP. The varying length of GC tail would generate a 3–4°C difference in melting temperature between the allele-specific PCR products, enabling genotype identification by its distinct melting profile. Primer sequences of the tagSNPs and the PCR conditions are presented in Table 2. Biomek® 2000 robotic system (Beckman Coulter) was used to set up the PCRs. The PCR amplification conditions and melting curve analysis method described previously was used [8, 17], and we obtained the tagSNP genotype information by monitoring analysis on the LightCycler® 480 real-time PCR system (Roche Applied Science).

Statistics

Deviation from the Hardy-Weinberg Equilibrium (HWE) was examined for the tagSNPs genotype distribution using the χ^2test. Using the ANOVA univariate analysis, differences in serum sex steroid concentrations among the three genotypes of each tagSNP was assessed after adjusting for age and body mass index (BMI). Multivariate linear regression was used to evaluate the associations of the SNPs with sex steroid levels in a model that included age, BMI, smoking habits, drinking habits and SHBG as covariates. All single-point statistical analyses were performed using SPSS 11.5 (SPSS Inc., Chicago, IL). The study population was also divided into three equal sub-groups according to their serum sex steroids level to examine for association between sex steroid levels and the gene haplotyes. Haploview 4.1 [28] was used to infer *SRD5A1* and *AKR1C4* haplotypes using an accelerated expectation maximization algorithm, and the haplotypic frequencies of subjects with sex steroid levels within the higher tertile are compared with those within the lower tertile. Using the Haploview implemented permutation test, another measure of significance corrected for multiple testing bias was also obtained for the association results. Analysis results were considered significant at a 2-tailed *P*-value of <0.05 for all tests.

Table 2. Allele-specific primer sequence for genotyping the tagSNPs of *SRD5A1* and *AKR1C4* gene

tagSNPs	Primer type	Primer Sequence
SRD5A1		
rs248807	Allele C	5'-gcgggcagggcggcCAGTCTTTGTCGGCTCTGGG-3'
	Allele A	5'-gattaccgCAGTCTTTGTCGGCTCTGGT-3'
	Common	5'-CAACTGAGCCATATCAGTAACATCCAT-3'
rs11738248	Allele C	5'-gcgggcagggcggcTGGGCTTATGAGCAAACTGC-3'
	Allele T	5'-gattaccgTGGGCTTATGAGCAAACTGT-3'
	Common	5'-AGAGGAAGCGGCTCCTTGGGATG-3'
rs824811	Allele C	5'-gcgggcagggcggcAACGTCAGTGTTATCTCATTTGTTTC-3'
	Allele T	5'-gattaccgAACGTCAGTGTTATCTCATTTGTTTT-3'
	Common	5'-TGAAGAAGTGAGTAATGGCTCATTTCTC-3'
AKR1C4		
rs1334473	Allele C	5'-gcgggcagggcggcTGGTTTGAAGTTTAGCCTAAAGCTC-3'
	Allele T	5'-gattaccgTGGTTTGAAGTTTAGCCTAAAGCTT-3'
	Common	5'-CAGAAACAGGACGAGACTGAGTTCAGG-3'
rs17134607	Allele G	5'-gcgggcagggcggcCAGACAACTTTTTGAAAAGTTGGG-3'
	Allele A	5'-gattaccgCAGACAACTTTTTGAAAAGTTGGA-3'
	Common	5'-TCTCAAAGTGCTTTGGCCAGTAGC-3'

Results

The basic demographic and serum sex steroid data of the study participants are summarized in Table 3. The final study cohort consisted of 1402 Chinese men with available sex steroid levels and DNA for genotyping. The mean age of the study cohort was 72.5 ± 5.0, while the mean BMI was 23.4 ± 3.1 kg/m^2. Overall, 64.0% were smokers (smoked >5 packs of cigarette) and 72.5% were alcoholic drinkers (drank >12 alcoholic drinks). The mean serum sex steroid levels are summarized in Table 3 as mean ± SD.

Table 3. Characteristics of study participants

Variables	Subjects (N=1402)
Age(yr)	72.5 ± 5.0
Body Mass Index(BMI)	23.4 ± 3.1
Smokers	897 (64.0%)
Alcohol drinkers	1016 (72.5%)
Serum sex steroids	
Testosterone (μg/L)	5.47 ± 1.99
DHT (μg/L)	0.47 ± 0.22
SHBG (nmol/L)	51.2 ± 20.4
Androsterone (μg/L)	0.22 ± 0.082

Data are presented as means±SD for continuous variables, and frequency (percentage) for categorical variables.

Table 4. Genotype and allele frequencies of the tagSNPs

SNPs	Position	Type	Ancestral allele	Genotype	Frequency (%)	Frequency in CHB
SDR5A1						
rs248807	Chr. 5	Intron 1	C	CC (1)	825 (60.7%)	55.6%
(N=1359)	6,696,374			CA (2)	454 (33.4%)	40.0%
				AA (3)	80 (5.9%)	4.4%
				HWE	$P = 0.56$	
rs11738248	Chr. 5	Intron 3	C	CC (1)	835 (71.8%)	75.6%
(N=1163)	6,710,494			CT (2)	301 (25.9%)	22.2%
				TT (3)	27 (2.3%)	2.2%
				HWE	$P = 0.12$	
rs824811	Chr. 5	Intron 4	T	CC (1)	15 (1.3%)	1.0%
(N=1161)	6,718,781			CT (2)	225 (19.4%)	32.5%
				TT (3)	921 (79.3%)	67.4%
				HWE	$P = 0.51$	
AKR1C4						
rs1334473	Chr.10	Intron 7	C	CC (1)	641 (55.7%)	62.8%
(N=1150)	5,245,689			CT (2)	436 (37.9%)	30.2%
				TT (3)	73 (6.3%)	7.0%
				HWE	$P = 0.92$	
rs17134607	Chr.10	3' near	G	GG (1)	916 (78.2%)	68.9%
(N=1172)	5,251,910	gene		AG (2)	239 (20.4%)	30.1%
				AA (3)	17 (1.4%)	1.0%
				HWE	$P = 0.98$	

Table 5. Univariate association between tagSNP genotypes and serum sex steroid levels

***SRD5A1* SNP**	**Genotype**	**T (μg/L)**	**DHT (μg/L)**	**DHT/T**	**SHBG (nmol/L)**
rs248807	CC (60.7%)	5.45 ± 2.01	0.47 ± 0.22	0.087 ± 0.027	51.04 ± 20.47
(N=1359)	CA (33.4%)	5.49 ± 2.02	0.49 ± 0.23	0.088 ± 0.025	50.87 ± 20.21
	AA (5.9%)	5.66 ± 2.09	0.48 ± 0.21	0.088 ± 0.027	54.84 ± 18.52
	***P*-value**	0.95	0.50	0.51	0.25
rs11738248	CC (71.8%)	5.48 ± 2.01	0.48 ± 0.22	0.088 ± 0.27	50.20 ± 19.45
(N=1163)	CT (25.9%)	5.49 ± 1.92	0.46 ± 0.22	0.082 ± 0.25	49.70 ± 20.31
	TT (2.3%)	5.25 ± 2.61	0.45 ± 0.28	0.086 ± 0.31	49.78 ± 25.00
	***P*-value**	0.99	0.43	**0.036**	0.93
rs824811	CC (1.3%)	5.99 ± 2.22	0.59 ± 0.23	0.099 ± 0.025	49.41 ± 18.49
(N=1161)	CT (19.4%)	5.49 ± 2.06	0.47 ± 0.21	0.087 ± 0.026	49.67 ± 19.77
	TT (79.3%)	5.46 ± 1.98	0.47 ± 0.22	0.087 ± 0.027	50.06 ± 19.49
	***P*-value**	0.25	**0.027**	0.12	0.96
***AKR1C4* SNP**	**Genotype**	**Adt (μg/L)**			**SHBG (nmol/L)**
rs1334473	CC (55.7%)	0.22 ± 0.08	-	-	49.20 ± 18.61
(N=1150)	CT (37.9%)	0.22 ± 0.09	-	-	51.21 ± 21.36
	TT (6.3%)	0.22 ± 0.09	-	-	47.63 ± 18.99
	***P*-value**	0.69	-	-	0.16
rs17134607	GG (78.2%)	0.21 ± 0.08	-	-	49.98 ± 19.88
(N=1172)	AG (20.4%)	0.23 ± 0.08	-	-	49.97 ± 19.88
	AA (1.4%)	0.27 ± 0.14	-	-	49.08 ± 14.13
	***P*-value**	**0.003**	-	-	0.98

T=testosterone, DHT=dihydrotestosterone, Adt=androsterone, SHBG=sex hormone binding globulin. Values are given as mean ± SD. P-values are obtained from ANOVA analysis of age- and BMI-adjusted sex steroid standardized residual value.

Single SNP Analysis

The genotype frequencies for the 3 tagSNPs of *SRD5A1* and 2 tagSNPs of *AKR1C4* are shown in Table 4. Genotype frequency distribution of all tested SNPs followed the HWE (P>0.05).

Table 5 showed the univariate analysis of association between the tested SNPs and various age- and BMI-adjusted serum sex steroid levels. For the three *SRD5A1* SNPs, the DHT concentration was significantly different among the three genotypes of rs824811 (P = 0.027), with the CC genotypes associated with the highest level; whereas DHT/T ratio was found to be significantly different in rs11738248 (P = 0.036), with CC genotype being the highest. While for *AKR1C4* gene, the three genotypes of rs17134607 showed significantly different androsterone level after adjustment for age and BMI (P = 0.003).

The observed associations were further analyzed in multivariate linear regression models with age, BMI, smoking and drinking status and SHBG as covariates (Table 6). The SNP rs11738248 of *SRD5A1* remained significantly associated to DHT/T ratio (P = 0.03), however, SNP rs824811 only showed a trend towards association with DHT after the adjustment for confounding factors (P = 0.094). As for SNP rs17134607 of *AKR1C4*, the association with androsterone level remained significantly in the multivariate analysis (P = 0.002).

Haplotype Analysis

Results for haplotypes analysis of *SRD5A1* and *AKR1C4* gene are shown in Table 7. The three SNPs on the *SRD5A1* gene composed four *SRD5A1* haplotypes, with C-C-T haplotype being the most common, accounting for about 50% of all haplotypes in the population samples. The haplotype C-T-T, which represented around 16% of population haplotypes, appeared to be a risk haplotype for individuals with low serum DHT levels and DHT/T ratio (nominal chi-square test, P = 0.012 and 0.039, respectively). After 10,000 permutation test that corrected for multiple testing bias, the association between C-T-T haplotype and serum DHT level remained significant at P = 0.045. However, no associations were found for any haplotypes and serum testosterone levels.

Among the three possible haplotypes composed by the two SNPs of *AKR1C4*, G-G haplotype was the most prevalent, comprised of more than 60% of population haplotypes. The haplotype G-A accounted for about 11% in the population, and was found to be associated with high serum androsterone level (P = 0.019). The ssociation remained marginally significant at P = 0.049, after permutation analysis adjusting for multiple testing.

Discussion

The variation in circulating sex steroid levels concentrations between individuals have been attributed to genetic and environmental (life-style factors) effects. Male twin studies revealed that familial factors accounted for 50% or more of the variations in plasma sex steroid levels [29], while a heritability estimate of >85% was observed for the production rate of T and DHT [30]. Therefore, we investigated the underlying genetic factors that may have affected the production and circulating levels of sex steroid level among genes involved in the sex steroid metabolic pathways.

Table 6. Association of *SRD5A1* and *AKR1C4* SNPs with sex steroid levels in linear regression models including demographic, life style factors and SHBG as covariates

SNPs	Sex steroid	$\beta \pm S.E.$	*P*
SRD5A1			
rs11738248	DHT/T	-0.003 ± 0.002	**0.030**
rs824811	DHT	-0.019 ± 0.011	0.094
AKR1C4			
rs17134607	Androsterone	0.016 ± 0.005	**0.002**

Table 7. Association between *SRD5A1* and *AKR1C4* haplotypes in the high vs. low tertile groups of serum sex steroid levels

Haplotype	High tertile frequency	Low tertile frequency	Overall frequency	*P*-value	*P*-value after 10,000 permutations
SRD5A1 Haplotype (rs248807-rs11738248-rs824811)					
DHT	(N=934)	(N=934)			
C-C-T	0.494	0.506	0.500	0.627	0.999
A-C-T	0.249	0.221	0.235	0.185	0.508
C-T-T	0.132	0.179	0.156	**0.012**	**0.045**
C-C-C	0.123	0.094	0.108	0.062	0.212
T					
C-C-T	0.486	0.519	0.502	0.187	-
A-C-T	0.254	0.228	0.241	0.226	-
C-T-T	0.140	0.151	0.145	0.548	-
C-C-C	0.120	0.101	0.111	0.223	-
DHT/T					
C-C-T	0.510	0.527	0.519	0.520	0.977
A-C-T	0.235	0.209	0.222	0.217	0.571
C-T-T	0.138	0.176	0.158	**0.039**	0.141
C-C-C	0.114	0.087	0.100	0.073	0.248
AKR1C4 Haplotype (rs1334473-rs17134607)					
Adt	(N=772)	(N=784)			
G-G	0.614	0.637	0.626	0.344	0.605
A-G	0.254	0.268	0.261	0.520	0.796
G-A	0.132	0.094	0.113	**0.019**	**0.049**

SRD5A1 haplotypes are composed of three SNPs, rs248807-rs11738248-rs824811, and *AKR1C4* haplotypes are composed of two SNPs, rs1334473 and rs17134607, both in specified order. N equals to numbers of chromosomes within each tertile group. Haploview 4.1 was used to infer haplotypes using an accelerated expectation maximization algorithm.

This is the first report in a large cohort of a healthy general population, regarding the association between circulating sex steroid level and the *SRD5A1* and *ARK1C4* gene. Although there were prior reports about sex steroid levels and the *SRD5A1* gene, their studies restricted to small samples of patients with disorder [18, 19]. Nevertheless, our results showed consistency with previous findings that the genetic variations of the *SRD5A1* gene were associated with DHT/T ratio [18, 19]. The T-allele of the intronic SNP rs11738248 was significantly associated with lower serum DHT/T ratio ($\beta = -0.003$, $P = 0.030$), and the C-T-T haplotype (containing the T-allele) was associated with both lower serum DHT level and DHT/T ratio. While for the *AKR1C4* gene, no previous report studied the relationship between its genetic variations and sex steroid levels. In our study, the A-allele of SNP rs17134607 was significantly associated with higher androsterone level ($\beta = 0.016$, $P = 0.002$). The *AKR1C4* haplotype analysis further supported this observation, where the G-A haplotype appeared to be a risk haplotype for higher androsterone level.

Although none of our studied SNPs are exonic SNPs and have no known influence on the amino acid structure of the encoding enzyme, it is possible that other functional regulatory elements or alleles are in linkage disequilibrium with these SNPs or their haploblocks. It is also possible that these SNP or haplotype variants exert more subtle regulatory effects on the expression of the *SRD5A1* and *AKR1C4* genes. Nonetheless, both may result in altered the 5α-reducatse and the 3α-hydroxysteroid dehydrogenase activity, and thus causing variation in circulating sex steroid level.

Since both of these genes are predominantly expressed in the liver, it is plausible that the effects of their genetic variations on the sex steroid level may also be related to liver diseases. Studies have consistently demonstrated that the serum testosterone or DHT levels were significantly lowered in patients with liver disease such as cirrhosis and hepatocellular carcinoma [3, 31, 32]. As we've shown here that genetic variations within *SRD5A1* and *AKR1C4* were significantly associated with serum sex steroid level, it may be interesting to further examine whether these same genetic variations may be risk factors for other diseases, which have been associated with blood androgen levels, such as prostate cancer.

Conclusion

In summary, our study of a large homogeneous cohort of Chinese general population revealed that genetic variants of *SRD5A1* and *AKR1C4* gene could affect circulating level of sex steroids among healthy individuals, including DHT, DHT/T ration and androsterone. Further studies on the androgen metabolism will help to determine the underlying functional genetic factors that affected the circulating sex steroid level and their possible association with various diseases.

Acknowledgment

This study was supported partly by a Hong Kong RGC grant (CUHK 4439/05m), the Swedish Research Council, the Swedish Foundation for Strategic Research, Avtal omLäkarutbildning och Forskning/Läkarutbildningsavtalet research grant in Gothenburg, the Lundberg Foundation, the Torsten and Ragnar Söderberg's Foundation and the Novo Nordisk

REFERENCES

[1] B. B. Yeap, *Nat Clin Pract Endocrinol Metab* 5, 113 (2009).

[2] A. W. Hsing, J. K. Reichardt and F. Z. Stanczyk, *Prostate* 52, 213 (2002).

[3] H. Kuper, C. Mantzoros, P. Lagiou, A. Tzonou, R. Tamimi, L. Mucci, V. Benetou, E. Spanos, S. O. Stuver and D. Trichopoulos, *Oncology* 60, 355 (2001).

[4] G. Severi, H. A. Morris, R. J. MacInnis, D. R. English, W. Tilley, J. L. Hopper, P. Boyle and G. G. Giles, *Cancer Epidemiol Biomarkers Prev* 15, 86 (2006).

[5] E. A. Kuijper, C. B. Lambalk, D. I. Boomsma, S. van der Sluis, M. A. Blankenstein, E. J. de Geus and D. Posthuma, *Hum Reprod* 22, 2153 (2007).

[6] H. Z. Ring, C. N. Lessov, T. Reed, R. Marcus, L. Holloway, G. E. Swan and D. Carmelli, *J Clin Endocrinol Metab* 90, 3653 (2005).

[7] A. L. Eriksson, M. Lorentzon, L. Vandenput, F. Labrie, M. Lindersson, A. C. Syvanen, E. S. Orwoll, S. R. Cummings, J. M. Zmuda, O. Ljunggren, M. K. Karlsson, D. Mellstrom and C. Ohlsson, *J Clin Endocrinol Metab* 94, 1033 (2009).

[8] J. Jiang, N. L. Tang, C. Ohlsson, A. L. Eriksson, L. Vandenput, F. W. Chan, J. K. Ching, A. Kwok, E. Orwoll, T. C. Kwok, J. Woo and P. C. Leung, *Clin Chim Acta* 411, 53 (2009).

[9] M. W. Yu, S. W. Cheng, M. W. Lin, S. Y. Yang, Y. F. Liaw, H. C. Chang, T. J. Hsiao, S. M. Lin, S. D. Lee, P. J. Chen, C. J. Liu and C. J. Chen, *J Natl Cancer Inst* 92, 2023 (2000).

[10] D. W. Russell and J. D. Wilson, *Annu Rev Biochem* 63, 25 (1994).

[11] E. P. Jenkins, C. L. Hsieh, A. Milatovich, K. Normington, D. M. Berman, U. Francke and D. W. Russell, *Genomics* 11, 1102 (1991).

[12] L. W. Chu, J. K. Reichardt and A. W. Hsing, *Curr Opin Endocrinol Diabetes Obes* 15, 261 (2008).

[13] A. E. Thigpen, R. I. Silver, J. M. Guileyardo, M. L. Casey, J. D. McConnell and D. W. Russell, *J Clin Invest* 92, 903 (1993).

[14] J. Ahn, F. R. Schumacher, S. I. Berndt, R. Pfeiffer, D. Albanes, G. L. Andriole, E. Ardanaz, H. Boeing, B. Bueno-de-Mesquita, S. J. Chanock, F. Clavel-Chapelon, W. R. Diver, H. S. Feigelson, J. M. Gaziano, E. Giovannucci, C. A. Haiman, B. E. Henderson, R. N. Hoover, L. N. Kolonel, P. Kraft, J. Ma, L. Le Marchand, K. Overvad, D. Palli, P. Stattin, M. Stampfer, D. O. Stram, G. Thomas, M. J. Thun, R. C. Travis, D. Trichopoulos, J. Virtamo, S. J. Weinstein, M. Yeager, R. Kaaks, D. J. Hunter and R. B. Hayes, *Hum Mol Genet* 18, 3749 (2009).

[15] N. E. Allen, M. S. Forrest and T. J. Key, *Cancer Epidemiol Biomarkers Prev* 10, 185 (2001).

[16] V. M. Hayes, G. Severi, E. J. Padilla, H. A. Morris, W. D. Tilley, M. C. Southey, D. R. English, R. L. Sutherland, J. L. Hopper, P. Boyle and G. G. Giles, *Int J Cancer* 120, 776 (2007).

[17] J. Jiang, N. L. Tang, C. Ohlsson, A. L. Eriksson, L. Vandenput, C. Liao, X. Wang, F. W. Chan, A. Kwok, E. Orwoll, T. C. Kwok, J. Woo and P. C. Leung, *Clin Chem* 56, 1742 (2010).

[18] J. A. Ellis, S. Panagiotopoulos, A. Akdeniz, G. Jerums and S. B. Harrap, *J Hum Genet* 50, 534 (2005).

[19] A. Tria, O. Hiort and G. H. Sinnecker, *Horm Res* 61, 180 (2004).

[20] T. M. Penning, M. E. Burczynski, J. M. Jez, C. F. Hung, H. K. Lin, H. Ma, M. Moore, N. Palackal and K. Ratnam, *Biochem J* 351, 67 (2000).

[21] T. M. Penning, Y. Jin, S. Steckelbroeck, T. Lanisnik Rizner and M. Lewis, *Mol Cell Endocrinol* 215, 63 (2004).

[22] M. Khanna, K. N. Qin, R. W. Wang and K. C. Cheng, *J Biol Chem* 270, 20162 (1995).

[23] L. Vandenput, F. Labrie, D. Mellstrom, C. Swanson, T. Knutsson, R. Peeker, O. Ljunggren, E. Orwoll, A. L. Eriksson, J. E. Damber and C. Ohlsson, *J Bone Miner Res* 22, 220 (2007).

[24] B. D. Horne and N. J. Camp, *Genet Epidemiol* 26, 11 (2004).

[25] Z. Lin and R. B. Altman, *Am J Hum Genet* 75, 850 (2004).

[26] Z. Meng, D. V. Zaykin, C. F. Xu, M. Wagner and M. G. Ehm, *Am J Hum Genet* 73, 115 (2003).

[27] J. Wang, K. Chuang, M. Ahluwalia, S. Patel, N. Umblas, D. Mirel, R. Higuchi and S. Germer, *Biotechniques* 39, 885 (2005).

[28] J. C. Barrett, B. Fry, J. Maller and M. J. Daly, *Bioinformatics* 21, 263 (2005).

[29] A. W. Meikle, D. T. Bishop, J. D. Stringham and D. W. West, *Metabolism* 35, 1090 (1986).

[30] A. W. Meikle, J. D. Stringham, D. T. Bishop and D. W. West, *J Clin Endocrinol Metab* 67, 104 (1988).

[31] J. Guechot, N. Peigney, F. Ballet, M. Vaubourdolle, J. Giboudeau and R. Poupon, *Cancer* 62, 760 (1988).

[32] P. B. Luppa, M. Thaler, E. Schulte-Frohlinde, A. Schreiegg, U. Huber and J. Metzger, *Clin Chem Lab Med* 44, 967 (2006).

In: Testosterone
Editor: Konstantin Chichinadze

ISBN 978-1-62100-492-9

Chapter VII

Non-Gonadotropin Regulation of Testosterone Biosynthesis

***Ho Lin*[1], *Kai-Lee Wang*[2], *Paulus S. Wang*[2,*] *and Shyi-Wu Wang*[3,*]**
[1]Department of Life Sciences, National Chung Hsing University, Taichung, Taiwan
[2]Department of Physiology, School of Medicine, National Yang-Ming University, Taipei, Taiwan
[3]Department of Physiology, Collage of Medicine, Chang-Gung University, Taoyuan, Taiwan, Republic of China

Abstract

Testosterone, a potent androgen, is mainly synthesized in the testicular Leydig cells. It is well known that biosynthesis and the secretion of testosterone are stimulated by gonadotropin, especially the luteinizing hormone (LH) released from the anterior pituitary gland resulting from the activation of the hypothalamus-pituitary-testis (H-P-T) axis. A significant negative feedback regulation between testosterone and LH had been well established. In addition to gonadotropin, some factors may regulate testosterone production by acting, either directly or indirectly, on the Leydig cells. For example, thyroxine (T_4) and prolactin enhance testosterone production by acting directly at the testicular interstitial cells (TIC) or Leydig cells. However, some cardiac glycosides, e.g. digoxin and digitoxin, as well as the cardiotonic steroid isolated from Chausu, such as bufalin, may inhibit testosterone production *via* attenuation of the activities of adenylyl cyclase and cytochrome P450scc, and cause a decrease of testicular accumulation of adenosine 3', 5'-cyclic monophosphate (cAMP). Not only the cardiotonic steroids, some other Chinese herbs, such as evodiamine, *S*-petasin and the extracts of adlay hull can also decrease testosterone production *via* the inhibition of cAMP production, 17β-hydroxysteroid dehydrogenase (17β-HSD) enzyme activity in Leydig cells and gonadotropin-releasing hormone (GnRH)-induced LH secretion. Meanwhile, testosterone production can be altered by some abusive drug (e.g. amphetamine) and environmental pollutants (e.g. nonylphenol, polybrominated diphenol ethers). We have previously

[*] These two authors have equal contributions to this work.

demonstrated that testosterone production can be increased by a gonadotropin-independent mechanism through a direct action of lactate on Leydig cells. We have also found out that hypoxia increases cell proliferation and testosterone production in Leydig cells *via* an increase of the production of vascular endothelial growth factor (VEGF). These results indicate that many factors, including Chinese herb medicine, toxicants, environmental pollutants and lactate, as well as VEGF, may alter the biosynthesis of testosterone *via* a gonadotropin-independent mechanism, such as the changes of the activities of cAMP pathway, intracellular calcium and steroidogenic enzymes. The changes of testosterone production, either synthesis or secretion, might be associated with the alterations of metabolisms and carcinogenesis in the reproduction organs, e.g. prostate gland.

1. EFFECTS OF CHINESE HERBAL MEDICINE

1.1. Introduction

Testosterone is critical to physiological activities of men and the male animals. The interference of testosterone production may finally cause infertility. There are so many internal or external factors may affect testosterone production. In this section, the authors focus on the evidence showing the effects of external natural compounds derived from Chinese herbs on testosterone production. The compounds include cardiac glycosides, evodiamine, *S*-petasin, adlay, cinnamon, and catechins. Some compounds which inhibit testosterone production might be useful in androgen-related diseases, such as prostate cancer. For other compounds which stimulate testosterone production may be applied in androgen deficiency syndrome. Nevertheless, the application of those medicine or food products which contain these compounds should still be attentive.

Chinese herbal medicine has been believed containing many therapeutic applications against diseases [128]. In this section, evidence was collected to introduce both inhibitory and stimulatory effects of some Chinese herb-derived compounds on testosterone production. Hope these descriptions will lead readers to a greater understanding about the potentials of Chinese herbs.

1.1.1. Cardiac Glycosides

1.1.1.1. Bufalin

Bufalin is a steroid compound isolated from Chansu, a galenical preparation of the dried white venom of Chinese *Bufo bufo gargarizans* [50, 94]. Several lines of evidences indicate that bufalin enables to block vasodilation, increase vasoconstriction, vascular resistance and blood pressure *via* inhibiting Na^+, K^+-ATPase [3, 30, 92]. These findings suggest that bufalin belongs to an endogenous digitalis-like factor. The effects of bufalin on regulation of testosterone production are interesting to investigate. Wang *et al.* used male rats as an animal model to determine the effects of bufalin on the regulation of testosterone production *in vivo* and *in vitro* [129]. Their results indicate that a single intravenous injection of bufalin decreases both basal and human chorionic gonadotropin (hCG)-stimulated levels of plasma testosterone. Administration of bufalin *in vitro* results in an inhibition of both basal and hCG-stimulated release of testosterone. Bufalin significantly diminishes adenosine 3’, 5’-cyclic monophosphate (cyclic AMP, cAMP) accumulation in rat testes. However, the basal levels of plasma and medium luteinizing hormone (LH) are not altered by bufalin administration. The LH response to gonadotropin-releasing hormone (GnRH) is diminished by bufalin both *in vivo* and *in vitro*. These results show the effects and possible mechanisms of bufalin on testosterone production by rat model.

1.1.1.2. Chansu

Chansu, similar as bufalin, is also prepared from dried white venom of Chinese *Bufo bufo gargarizans* and is one of the major components of Kyushin, a traditional Chinese medicine. Kyushin is reported to have a cardiotonic effect due to the action of bufadienolides such as bufalin and cinobufagin [50]. According to the above results indicating the bufalin effects, it is reasonable to speculate that Chansu may possess hypogonadal effects in male rats. The same group (Wang *et al.*) took similar strategy to identify the effects of the methanol extract of Chansu on hypothalamic-pituitary-testicular (H-P-T) function in male rats [132]. At first, they extracted crude Chansu by methanol and purified by a Sep-Pak C18 column. They showed no activity of bufalin, cinobufagin, estradiol, or digoxin in purified methanol extract was detected. A single intravenous injection of Chansu results in a decrease of the basal and hCG-induced levels of plasma testosterone and the GnRH-induced level of plasma LH. Administration of Chansu *in vitro* decreases basal and hCG-stimulated testosterone production, as well as spontaneous and forskolin- or 3-isobutyl-l-methylxanthine (IBMX)-induced accumulation of cAMP in rat testicular interstitial cells. Although LH release by rat anterior pituitary glands is diminished, GnRH release by the rat mediobasal hypothalamus is enhanced by administration of Chansu *in vitro*. These results suggest that the bufalin-free extracts of Chansu inhibit testosterone secretion and also provide the mechanism how Chansu proceeds its functions.

1.1.1.3. Digoxin

Digoxin is a cardiac glycoside derived from the flowering plant *Digitalis lanata* (foxglove). It has been well known about the effects on treating congestive heart failure. The direct positive inotropic actions of digoxin are similar as bufalin which has been attributed to inhibition of Na^+-K^+-ATPase. The primary sexual problems reported in male patients suffering from cardiovascular disease are the decrease of sexual desire and excitement phase [88]. Studies of patients receiving long-term digoxin therapy have detected changes in plasma testosterone and LH [88, 114]. In order to understand the correlation between sexual problem and digoxin, Lin *et al.* performed *in vivo* and *in vitro* experiments to examine inhibitory effects of digoxin on testosterone secretion and to determine possible underlying mechanisms [70]. Indeed, they found intravenous injection of digoxin decreases the basal and hCG-stimulated plasma testosterone concentrations in adult male rats. Digoxin also decreases the basal and hCG-stimulated release of testosterone from rat testicular interstitial cells. The basal and hCG-stimulated production of cyclic AMP and the stimulatory effects of forskolin and 8-Br-cyclic AMP on testosterone production are all inhibited by digoxin treatment. Their data also indicate that digoxin enables to inactivate the cytochrome P450 side chain cleavage enzyme (cytochrome P450scc) without influencing the activity of other steroidogenic enzymes. These results suggest that digoxin, just like bufalin and Chansu, has the ability to inhibit testosterone production and they further provide the targets, adenylyl cyclase and cytochrome P450scc, can be attacked by digoxin. The authors used purified rat Leydig cells and have similar findings as above ones (Lin's unpublished data). Furthermore, they found that the expression of steroidogenic acute regulatory protein (StAR) is decreased by digoxin. Estrogen production in Leydig cells is not affected by digoxin, which suggests that digoxin effects are nothing to do with aromatase activity. Finally, ouabain, another compound of digitalis, has no effects on testosterone production suggesting that digoxin effects are specific and Na^+-K^+ ATPase-independent.

1.1.1.4. Digitoxin

Digitoxin is highly hydrophobic and completely absorbed from the gastrointestinal tract and possesses a longer half-life [62]. Overdose of digitoxin could produce digitalis intoxication which results in some symptoms: anorexia, nausea, and vomiting, and noncardiac symptoms-gastrointestinal complaint [42, 111]. Wang *et al.* has reported that intravenous injection of digitoxin decreases hCG-stimulated, but not basal, plasma testosterone levels [131]. Administration of digitoxin *in vitro* results in an inhibition of both basal and hCG- as well as 8-Br-cAMP-stimulated release of testosterone. In addition, digitoxin diminished hCG-stimulated cAMP accumulation in rat testicular interstitial cells and inhibited the activity of cytochrome P450scc but failed to affect the activities of other steroidogenic enzymes. Their efforts contribute not only the acute inhibitory effect of digitoxin on the testosterone production but also provide the mechanism how digitalis acts. On the other hand, adrenal gland is also an important source of steroids in the animal. The same group first identifies that digoxin and digitoxin inhibit not only testosterone production but also corticosterone production in rat adrenal cortical cells through Na^+-K^+ ATPase-independent pathway [133]. This implies that digitalis might possibly affect androgen production in adrenals. This issue is still interesting to further investigate.

1.1.2. Evodiamine

Evodiamine is isolated from the dry unripened fruit of *Evodia rutaecarpa Bentham* (a Chinese medicine named Wu-chu-yu). It was also found to affect vasotension, anoxia, and the body temperature [20, 124, 137]. Although evodiamine indeed has many biological effects, its effects on the endocrine system are not clear. Lin *et al.* have first demonstrated that evodiamine was effective to reduce both basal and hCG-stimulated testosterone secretion in rat testicular interstitial cells [69]. The stimulatory effect of forskolin on testosterone release is prevented by administration of evodiamine. Evodiamine also decreases 8-Br-cAMP- and androstenedione-stimulated testosterone secretion. These results suggest that evodiamine reduces testosterone secretion via a specific mechanism involving reduced activity of cAMP-related pathways and 17β-hydroxysteroid dehydrogenase.

1.1.3. S-Petasin

S-petasin, a kind of sesquiterpene ester, is the anti-inflammatory and analgesic component of the butterbur (*Petasites hybridus*) [72]. The clinical benefit of *S*-petasin is the spasmolytic activity [9]. Lin *et al.* identify the effects of *S*-petasin on the secretion of testosterone *in vivo* and *in vitro* [68]. They found that single intravenous injection of *S*-petasin decreases basal plasma testosterone concentration in adult male rats. In the culture medium of rat testicular interstitial cells, *S*-petasin is effective to reduce the basal and hCG-stimulated release of testosterone. *S*-petasin also diminishes forskolin- or androstenedione-stimulated testosterone secretion. These results suggest that *S*-petasin may specifically inhibit the activities of adenylyl cyclase and 17-ketosteroid reductase and causes the reduction of testosterone production.

1.1.4. Adlay

Coix lachryma-jobi L. var. *ma-yuen* Stapf. (a Chinese medicinal plant named Yi-yi-lan) that is commonly known as adlay (Job's tears) is an annual crop. It is widely cultivated in Taiwan, Japan, and China and is considered a health food supplement. From ancient times, adlay has been used in Asian countries for the treatment of rheumatism, warts, neuralgia, and disorders of the female endocrine system [Li, Pen-t's sao kang mu (Systematic Pharmacopoeia), China, 1596]. Hsia *et al.* are interesting in understanding whether adlay can affect testosterone secretion [52]. They used the methanol extracts of adlay hull (AHM) to treat rat Leydig cells and the results suggest that AHM decreases testosterone release *via* the inhibition of either PKA and PKC pathways or 17β-hydroxysteroid dehydrogenase activity. In addition, they found GnRH-induced LH secretion by anterior pituitary tissues is also inhibited by adlay treatment.

1.1.5. Cinnamon

Cinnamon bark has been used to treat menstrual pain and infertility. While several pharmacological studies have suggested anti-inflammatory properties [65, 117], the mechanisms by which the herb exerts its various activities have not been well understood. Iwaoka *et al.* used cinnamaldehyde (a major component of cinnamon) to treat human adrenal cells, H295R, and analyzed the testosterone concentration in culture medium by a highly sensitive LC-electrospray ionization-tandem mass spectrometry [56]. They found that testosterone and dehydroepiandrosterone concentrations are decreased in the presence of cinnamaldehyde. Oppositely, exposure of cinnamaldehyde increases progesterone release but the releases of cortisol or estradiol are not affected by cinnamaldehyde. This is an interesting case indicating that a herbal compound, such as cinnamaldehyde, may contain selectivity to affect steroid production in human endocrine cells.

1.1.6. Cathechin

Catechins have been reported to have many pharmacological properties such as the effects of anti-oxidative, anti-inflammatory, anticarcinogenic, anti-ultraviolet, and reduction of blood pressure as well as glucose and cholesterol levels [5, 85, 90, 106, 138]. Yu *et al.* used different catechin-related components (include catechin, epicatechin, epigallocatechin gallate) to test their effects on rat testosterone production [141]. The data show that catechins increase plasma testosterone *in vivo* in male rats. *In vitro*, low-dose concentrations of catechins increase GnRH-stimulated LH release by anterior pituitary gland and hCG-stimulated testosterone release. The authors conclude that the stimulatory effects of catechins might be due to increasing the action of cAMP, but not P450scc, steroidogenesis acute regulatory protein or the activity of intracellular calcium in Leydig cells. Interestingly, one of the catechins, called epicatechin, specifically increases the testosterone secretion *via* the activation of 17β-hydroxysteroid dehydrogenase. This is a seldom example in Chinese herb which contains stimulatory effects on androgen production and arecoline is another example which is discussed elsewhere in this section.

2. Effects of Environmental Xenosteroids

2.1. Environmental Agent

More than 7×10^6 chemicals have been created and there are currently more than 80,000 chemicals registered with Environmental Protection Agency (EPA). Some of the artificial chemicals have adverse effects on endocrine system in wild life, experimental animals or humans. These chemicals could release into the environment and are so called endocrine disrupting chemicals (EDCs) such as alkylphenol, flame retardants or pesticide. The sources and levels of exposure to EDCs are diverse and very widely around the world [28, 51]. In the past five years, we have also focused on the effects of several EDCs on reproductive functions, especially the hypothalamus- pituitary-testis (H-P-T) axis.

2.2. Nonylphenol (NP)

Nonylphenol (NP) is one of the stable metabolites from nonylphenol polyethoxylate (NPE), a non-ionic surfactant widely used as component of detergents [15, 39]. The chemical structure of NP is similar to estradiol and has been reported to have xenoestrogenic effects by binding to estrogen receptor (ER) [10, 113]. NP has the potential to interfere with female reproduction as well as development.

The NP effects on testicular function were also investigated in rats. In our previous studies [135, 136], we found that NP has different effects on testosterone release both *in vivo* and *in vitro*. In an *in vitro* study, NP could stimulate basal whereas abolished hCG-evoked testosterone release in rat Leydig cells. The stimulatory effect of NP on testosterone release is, at least in part, through elevating the activity of P450scc and stimulating protein activation of steroidogenic acute regulatory protein (StAR). Whereas the same concentration of NP abolished hCG-evoked testosterone release, at least in part, through inhibiting the activity of 17β-hydroxysteroid dehydrogenases type 3 (17βHSD3) [135]. Moreover, our *in vivo* study has also demonstrated that plasma testosterone level is elevated after oral gavage of NP (100 μg/kg/day) for 7 days. However, the plasma testosterone level is reduced by 50 percent after oral administration of the same concentration of NP for 30 days. In contrast, a lower dose of NP (10 μg/kg/day) administration did not have any effect on the Leydig cell function [136]. These effects may associate with enhancement of NP on intracellular Ca^{2+} level (unpublished data).

2.3. Polybrominated Diphenyl Ethers (PBDEs)

Polybrominated diphenyl ethers (PBDEs), a class of flame retardants, have been used since 1960s [107]. PBDEs are wildly used in a variety of housewares and electronic equipment, such as textiles, carpets, ceiling, air conditioning, electronic cables, computers, television set, and vehicles. The chemical structures of PBDEs are similar to thyroid hormones. PBDEs affect thyroid hormones hormeostasis [107] by binding to thyroxine carrier proteins [45] and its receptors [61]. PBDEs have been shown to alter thyroid hormone homeostasis, maturation of nervous system, as well as male or female reproductive system.

In our recent studies, the effects of PBDEs on testosterone release both *in vivo* and *in vitro* have been investigated. Because lower-brominated diphenyl ethers are the dominant ones observed in organisms, we used PBDE-710, one of the PBDEs mixture composed by 85% of tetra- and penta-BDEs, to mimic the internal conditions. PBDE-710 stimulated testosterone release from rat Leydig cells. PBDE-710 also enhanced cAMP production as well as activity of cytochrome P450, family 11, subfamily A, polypeptide 1 (CYP11A1) which is also known as cholesterol side-chain cleavage cytochrome P450 (P450scc). PBDE-710 also increased plasma testosterone levels after intravenous injection for 1 h in the presence of hCG (unpublished data).

2.4. Maneb

Pesticide effects on reproduction system has also been investigated in recent years [12, 37]. Disruption of endocrine function as well as induction of cytotoxicity in Sertoli cell, Leydig cell or spermatozoa has been reported. A positive correlation between poorer sperm concentration and motility and pesticides concentration has been found in Americans [115, 116]. Maneb, one of the most frequently used pesticides, was found to alter sperm quality after daily administration for 5 weeks [80].

Recently, we found decreased plasma testosterone level after daily intraperitoneal injection of maneb (4 mg/kg) for more than 14 days. This inhibitory effect can be reversed by hCG treatment. In contrast, administration of maneb for 6, 7 or 9 days did not alter plasma testosterone levels and Leydig cell function. Testosterone release is not altered in Leydig cells after 1 h treatment with maneb [120]. These results implied that maneb could alter Leydig cell function only after long term exposure.

3. Effects of Drugs and Metabolites

3.1. Propylthiouracil (PTU)

Propylthiouracil (PTU) is a thionamide drug with anti-thyroid effects. The principal action of PTU is to inhibit the synthesis of thyroid hormones and the deiodination of thyroxine (T_4) to its active form, triiodothyronine (T_3) in the peripheral tissues [140]. Clinical studies have shown that PTU treatment in hyperthyroid patients results in leucopenia [22], jaundice, hepatocellular dysfunction, hepatitis [26], and hepatomegaly [67, 57].

Besides the toxic effects on liver and immune systems, PTU has been found to have side effects on steroidogenesis in adrenal cortex [74], testis [16-19] and ovary [14]. It has been shown that PTU treatment in rats decreases the basal and adrenocorticotropin (ACTH)-stimulated secretion of corticosterone in vivo and in vitro through its inhibition on the activity of 11β-hydroxylase and production of monophosphate cAMP in rat zona fasciculata-reticularis (ZFR) cells [74] Since co-treatment of T_4 with PTU in rats may reduce the levels of plasma thyroid stimulating hormone (TSH) and increase the levels of plasma T_4 but only partially reverse the levels of plasma corticosterone and does not change the *in vitro* production of corticosterone and cAMP in ZFR cells, it is suggested that PTU may act directly on the ZFR cells to inhibit the production of corticosterone [74].

The acute and direct effects of PTU on testosterone secretion in primates and rodents have been examined [16-18]. In male monkeys infused intravenously with PTU for 30 min, PTU decreases plasma testosterone but not plasma T_4 and LH [16]. Administration of PTU *in vitro* results in a dose-dependent inhibition of basal and hCG- , as well as forskolin-stimulated testosterone release by monkey and rat testicular interstitial cells [16, 17]. It has also been found that PTU acts directly on rat Leydig cells to diminish testosterone production by inhibiting P450scc function and the expression of StAR [18].

Not only testosterone production but also progesterone production is inhibited by the administration of PTU. The *in vitro* results have demonstrated that PTU decreases the progesterone production by granulosa cells *via* a thyroid-independent mechanism involving the inhibition of post-cAMP pathway, and the activities of intracellular calcium, steroidogenic enzyme and StAR protein functions [14].

Overall, these studies indicate that PTU may inhibit the production of testosterone from testis and that of progesterone from ovary *via* an acute and direct effect on the steroidogenic cells in reproductive tissues.

3.2. Arecoline

Arecoline (1, 2, 5, 6-tetrahydrol-1-methyl-3-pyridinecarboxylic acid methyl ester) is the most abundant plant alkaloid extracted from betel nuts (*Areca Catechu* L.) [33]. Epidemiological studies have reported a high correlation between betel nut-chewing habit and oral cancer [55, 63, 119], carcinogenicity [55, 101, 108], immunotoxicity [105], and teratogenicity [109] in animals. Besides to the above dysfunctions, arecoline has been shown to affect the endocrine systems including the increase of the levels of plasma epinephrine ACTH [97], and plasma T_3 concentrations [93]. The effects of arecoline on reproductive functions were also explored. Arecoline treatment causes suppression of pineal activity but stimulates testicular function [104]. Administration of arecoline increases not only the basal and hCG-induced levels of testosterone but also the production of testosterone *in vitro* in response to hCG, forskolin, 8-Br-cAMP and androstenedione from rat Leydig cells [130]. Furthermore, the testosterone production induced by arecoline can be attenuated by the blockers (e.g. nifedipine, nimodipine, and tetrandrine) of L-type intracellular calcium channels. Western blot indicates that arecoline increases StAR protein expression in rat Leydig cells compared with vehicle [130]. Therefore, it is suggested that arecoline increases testosterone production by acting directly on Leydig cells *via* mechamisms involving an activation of L-type calcium channels, including the activity of 17β-hydroxysteroid dehydrogenase and enhancing the expression of StAR.

3.3. Amphetamine

It has been well known that amphetamine is a dopamine agonist which increases dopamine release [24, 29, 60]. Sudden abstinence in human beings who abuse amphetamine chronically might precipitate an organic mood disorder that mimics many syndromes of depression [122]. It has been shown that amphetamine exposure and withdrawal in rats modifies the responses of the hypothalamic-pituitary-adrenal (H-P-A) axis and regional brain catecholamine levels, then influence the hypothalamic-pituitary- gonad axis [84]. After incubation of rat testicular interstitial cells with amphetamine, the production of testosterone, either basal or challagnd by hCH, 3β-HSD, P450c17, or 17-KSR, was attenuated, but generation of cAMP is increased [121]. The association between the increase of cAMP generation and the decrease of testosterone production need further study.

3.4. Hydrogen Peroxide (H_2O_2)

Hydrogen peroxide (H_2O_2) is one of reactive oxygen species (ROS) which can be produced continuously in normal cellular metabolism and in the steroidogenic pathway [95]. It has been well known that H_2O_2 plays a key role in regulating the biosynthesis of thyroid hormones [91]. Meanwhile, H_2O_2 inhibits activation of adenylyl cyclase caused by receptor-bound gonadotropin and inhibits the basal and evoked production of progesterone in both granulosa and luteal cells [6, 7, 31, 79].

In the male reproductive system, H_2O_2 has been shown to decrease sperm motility and viability [78]. In Leydig cells, steroidogenic cytochrome P450 enzymes produce ROS as the by-product during their catalytic sections [98, 99]. Tsai *et al.* [123] have examined the effects of H_2O_2 on testosterone release from rat Leydig cells and demonstrated that H_2O_2 acts on rat Leydig cells to attenuate the basal and hCG-induced testosterone release, abolish forskolin- or 8-Br-cAMP- evoked testosterone release. H_2O_2 also inhibits pregenolone production in the presence of trilostane (an inhibitor of 3β-hydroxysteroid dehydrogenase) therefore diminishes the activity of P450scc in Leydig cells. These results suggest that H_2O_2 acts directly on rat Leydig cells to diminish testosterone production by inhibiting P450scc activity and StAR protein expression.

4. Adaptation to Exercise and Hypoxia

4.1. Exercise and Lactate

Exercise or physical activity can be considered as a kind of stress for human body. This kind of stress, exercise, is known to be a powerful stimulus for endocrine system [44]. However, the hormonal response seems to be related to the exercise intensity, volume, and time duration [73]. Studies showed that elevated [13, 41, 48, 53, 64, 86, 102, 118, 126], unchanged [49, 76], decreased [8, 25, 38, 40, 81, 89, 127], decreased but not significant [134] plasma testosterone concentrations were found immediately after exercise for different time intervals. Also, increased testosterone from muscle has been observed after a single bout of exercise in rats [1].

Lactate is the product of glucose after glycolysis [96]. It is well known that plasma lactate can be stimulated by exercise [100]. The action of lactate on the target cells is through a pH-dependent monocarboxylate transporter (MCT) system [58, 59]. Among these MCT family, MCT1 has been identified on the membrane of Leydig cells [87]. Also, testicular Sertoli cells are able to produce lactate *in vitro* [36]. Mero has demonstrated that that change of plasma testosterone in positively correlated with lactate production in exercise [35, 83]. After swimming and lactate administration, increased plasma testosterone has been observed [75]. Rats were subjected to swim training routine (10 min in length 2 times per day) for 1 wk. The water immersion rats were used as controls. Increased plasma lactate in testicular vein and trunk were found in swimming rats compared to water immersion rats. Plasma LH (secreted from anterior pituitary gland) and testosterone were increased after swimming. Meanwhile, lactate stimulates GnRH (secreted from hypothalamus), LH, and testosterone released *in vitro*. Moreover, testicular cAMP increased after lactate stimulation *in vitro*. Lin *et al.* showed that lactate at the physiological level (10 mM) stimulates testosterone production in rat Leydig cells through a mechanism involving the increased activities of adenylyl cyclase, cytochrome P450scc, and L-type Ca^{2+} channel [71]. These studies indicate that the mechanism exerted by lactate on testosterone production may either through the hypothalamus- pituitary-testis axis or through the direct stimulation on steroidogenesis in Leydig cells.

4.2. Hypoxia and Vascular Endothelial Growth Factor (VEGF)

Hypoxia is defined as the inadequate oxygen supply to the tissues or cells [34, 43, 47]. In mouse TM3 Leydig cell lines, the basal VEGF release and the response of VEGF production to hCG are increased [54]. In addition, the proliferation of TM3 cells were stimulated by hypoxia (5%) after 16 h. Moreover, hCG or VEGF augmented the proliferation of TM3 cells, which was abolished by VEGF antibody. Meanwhile, increased testosterone release was observed in Leydig cells treated with different doses of VEGF. Enhanced phosphorylated extracellular signal-regulated kinase (p-ERK) expression was observed in Leydig cells treated with VEGF. Therefore, the cell proliferation and the secretion of testosterone in Leydig cells can be stimulated by hypoxia *via* an enhanced VEGF production [54]. Hypoxia-inducible factors (HIFs) are called the "master regulators" for the adaptation of the cell to hypoxia [77]. HIF-1α has been found to be constitutively expressed in murine testis [82]. Also, HIF-1α enhanced the 3β-hydroxysteroid dehydrogenase type 1 (Hsd3b1), which is the enzyme for conversion of pregnenolone to progesterone and to testosterone in testis [77]. Moreover, birth hypoxia stimulated plasma testosterone in human may act through augmented ACTH secretion, not LH [11]. In contrast, testosterone in man induces HIF-1α and its downstream angiogenesis through hypoxia and epidermal growth factor receptor (EGFR) signaling [103]. Therefore, hypoxia could induce testosterone secretion from Leydig cells through the enhanced VEGF protein expression, augmented LH secretion, and HIF-1α-induced Hsd3b1 protein.

In contrast to hypoxia-induced testosterone secretion from Leydig cells, Farias *et al.* found chronic hypobaric hypoxia, significantly decreased plasma LH after 5 days exposure, inhibited plasma testosterone in rat after 30 days exposure [32]. Meanwhile, Coste *et al.*

showed no significant change in plasma testosterone in human after diurnal exposure to mild hypobaric hypoxia (up to 12,000 ft) [23]. Dehydroepiandrosterone (DHEA), another kind of androgens synthesized from cholesterol in gonad and adrenal gland, reduced HIF-1α accumulation and may be related to the reduction of hypoxia in pulmonary arterial hypertension [27].

4.3. Ischemia by Testicular Torsion

Although testicular torsion occurs in all age group, it often occurs either at puberty or soon after birth. Torsion can lead to testicular damage, ischemia, hemorrhagic infarction, testicular necrosis, and finally infertility [110, 112]. In contrast, the majority of animal studies showed that testicular torsion often occurs in adult animals [46]. It is well established that testicular torsion-detorsion has been identified as an ischemia/reperfusion (IR) model of testicular damage.

Loss of spermatogenesis, reduction of serum testosterone, and decreased testicular venous plasma testosterone have been found in rats after unilateral spermatic cord torsion [21, 46, 125]. Also, low plasma LH has been observed in the torsion rats [21]. Moreover, torsion causes impaired testosterone secretion from the cultured rat testicular interstitial cells [21] and the reduced testosterone response to hCG stimulation in boys [66]. In contrast to the reduced testosterone after torsion, reserved steroidogenesis can be found in patients [2] or rats [4] after torsion. Cho *et al.* have found that the testosterone levels of the testicular interstitial fluid in ipsilateral testes were significantly enhanced after 2 h torsion, but suppressed in the contralateral testes [21]. This increased testosterone in ipsilateral testes caused by torsion may lead to cell apoptosis through the decreased serum- and glucocorticoid-inducible kinase-1(SGK1), phosphoinositide-dependent protein kinase-1 (PDK1), and forkhead box O3 (FOXO3a) phosphorylation [21]. However, heme oxygenase -1 induced by torsion might provide a protection for testes suffering torsion-detorsion injury [139].

5. Conclusion

Although the major control of testosterone production in Leydig cells is gonadotropin, especially the LH, from the anterior pituitary gland, many factors, including Chinese herb medicine, toxicants, clinical drugs, abused drugs, and some metabolites, might regulate the biosynthesis and secretion of testosterone. In many cases, these non-gonadotropin modulators may act directly on the Leydig cells to regulate the biosynthesis of testosterone *via* mechanisms involving the alterations of steroidogenesis, activities of steroidogenic enzymes, cAMP generation, cAMP functions and/or intracellular calcium levels. In the near future, it should be interesting to study the regulation of non-gonadotropin modulators on the expressions of LH receptor, at either transcription or translation levels.

We hope that the information in this chapter will be helpful for the future studies not only in the side effects of toxicants and drugs, but also in the study of male reproduction, e.g. anti-cancer effects on the prostate cancer in human beings.

Acknowledgments

We are grateful to Miss Yi-Ting Chen and Miss Wan-Yun Chen for their assistance in the preparation of this article.

References

[1] Aizawa, K; Iemitsu, M; Otsuki, T; Maeda, S; Miyauchi, T; and Mesaki, N. Sex differences in steroidogenesis in skeletal muscle following a single bout of exercise in rats. *J. Appl. Physiol.* 2008; 104: 67-74.

[2] Arap, MA; Vicentini, FC; Cocuzza, M; Hallak, J; Athayde, K; Lucon, AM; Arap, S; and Srougi, M. Late hormonal levels, semen parameters, and presence of antisperm antibodies in patients treated for testicular torsion. *J. Androl.* 2007; 28:528-532.

[3] Bagrov, AY; Roukoyatkina, NI; Fedorova, OV; Pinaev, AG; Ukhanova, MV. Digitalis-like and vasoconstrictor effects of endogenous digoxin-like factor(s) from the venom of Bufo marinus toad. *Eur. J. Pharmacol.*1993; 234:165-172.

[4] Baker, LA; and Turner, TT. Leydig cell function after experimental testicular torsion despite loss of spermatogenesis. *J. Androl.* 1995; 16:12-17.

[5] Basu, A; Lucas, EA. Mechanisms and effects of green tea on cardiovascular health. *Nutr. Rev.* 2007;65:361-375.

[6] Behrman, HR; Aten, RF. Evidence that hydrogen peroxide blocks hormone-sensitive cholesterol transport into mitochondria of rat luteal cells. *Endocrinology* 1991; 128:2958-2966.

[7] Behrman, HR; Preston, SL. Luteolytic actions of peroxide in rat ovarian cells. *Endocrinology* 1989; 124:2895-2900.

[8] Berg, U; Enqvist, JK; Mattsson, CM; Carlsson-Skwirut, C; Sundberg, CJ; Ekblom, B; and Bang, P. Lack of sex differences in the IGF-IGFBP response to ultra endurance exercise. *Scand. J. Med. Sci. Sports.* 2008; 18: 706-714.

[9] Bickel, D; Roder, T; Bestmann, HJ; Brune, K. Identification and characterization of inhibitors of peptido-leukotriene-synthesis from Petasites hybridus. *Planta Med.* 1994; 60:318-322.

[10] Blom, A; Ekman, E; Johannisson, A; Norrgren, L; Pesonen, M. Effects of xenoestrogenic environmental pollutants on the proliferation of a human breast cancer cell line (MCF-7). *Arch. Environ. Contam. Toxicol.* 1998; 34:306-310.

[11] Boksa, P; and Zhang, Y. Global birth hypoxia increases the neonatal testosterone surge in the rat. *Neuroendocrinology* 2008; 88:266-275.

[12] Bretveld, R; Brouwers, M; Ebisch, I; Roeleveld, N. Influence of pesticides on male fertility. *Scand. J. Work Environ. Health.* 2007; 33:13-28

[13] Buresh, R; Berg, K; and French, J. The effect of resistive exercise rest interval on hormonal response, strength, and hypertrophy with training. *J. Strength. Cond. Res.* 2009; 23:62-71.

[14] Chen, JJ; Wang, SW; Chein, EJ; Wang, PS. Direct effect of propylthiouracil on progesterone release in rat granulosa cells. *Brit. J. Pharmacol.* 2003; 139:1564-1570.

[15] Cheng, CY; Wu, CY; Wang, CH; Ding, WH. Determination and distribution characteristics of degradation products of nonylphenol polyethoxylates in the rivers of Taiwan. *Chemosphere* 2006; 65:2275-2281.

[16] Chiao, YC; Chao, HL; Huang, SW; Wang, PS. Direct effects of propylthiouracil on testosterone production in monkeys. Chinese J. Physiol. 2000a; 43:55-59.

[17] Chiao, YC; Lin, H; Wang, SW; Wang, PS. Direct effects of propylthiouracil on testosterone secretion in rat testicular interstitial cells. Birt. J. Pharmacol. 2000b;130:1477-1482

[18] Chiao, YC; Cho, WL; Wang, PS. Inhibition of testosterone production by propylthiouracil in rat Leydig cells. *Biol. Reprod.* 2002; 67:416-422.

[19] Chiao, YC; Lee, HY; Wang, SW; Hwang, JJ; Chien, CH; Huang, SW; Lu, CC; Chen, JJ; Tsai, SC; Wang, PS. Regulation of thyroid hormones on the production of testosterone in rats. *J. Cell. Biochem.* 1999; 73:554-562.

[20] Chiou, WF; Chou, CJ; Shum, AY; Chen, CF. The vasorelaxant effect of evodiamine in rat isolated mesenteric arteries: mode of action. *Eur. J. Pharmacol.* 1992; 215:277-283.

[21] Cho, YM; Pu, HF; Huang, WJ; Ho, LT; Wang, SW; and Wang, PS. Role of serum- and glucocorticoid-inducible kinase-1 in regulating torsion-induced apoptosis in rats. *Int. J. Androl.* 2010.

[22] Cooper, DS. Antithyroid drugs. *N. Engl. J. Med.* 1984; 311:1353-1362.

[23] Coste, O; Van Beers, P; Charbuy, H; Bogdan, A; and Touitou, Y. Simulation of long-haul flights in humans: prolonged mild hypoxia does not alter the circadian time structure of plasma testosterone and gonadotrophins. *Steroids* 2006; 71:214-221.

[24] Crowley, WR; Zemlan, FP. Neurotransmitter systems: anatomy and pharmacology. *In Neuroendocrinology of Reproduction: Physiology and Behavior*. Ed. Adler, N.T. 1981, pp.71-73. New York: Plenum.

[25] Daly, W; Seegers, CA; Rubin, DA; Dobridge, JD; Hackney, AC. Relationship between stress hormones and testosterone with prolonged endurance exercise. *Eur. J. Appl. Physiol.* 2005; 93: 375-380.

[26] Deidiker, R; deMello, DE. Propylthiouracil-induced fulminant hepatitis: case report and review of the literature. *Pediatr. Pathol. Lab. Med.* 1996; 16:845-852.

[27] Dessouroux, A; Akwa, Y; Baulieu, EE. DHEA decreases HIF-1alpha accumulation under hypoxia in human pulmonary artery cells: potential role in the treatment of pulmonary arterial hypertension. *J. Steroid Biochem. Mol. Biol.* 2008; 109:81-89.

[28] Diamanti-Kandarakis, E; Bourguignon, JP; Giudice, LC; Hauser, R; Prins, GS; Soto, AM; Zoeller, RT; Gore, AC. Endocrine-disrupting chemicals: an Endocrine Society scientific statement. *Endocr. Rev.* 2009; 30:293-342.

[29] Dluzen, DE; Ramirez, VD. *In vitro* progesterone modulation of amphetamine-stimulated dopamine release from the corpus striatum of ovariectomized estrogen-treated female rats: response characteristics. *Brain Res.* 1990; 517:117-122.

[30] Eliades, D; Swindall, B; Johnston, J; Pamnani, M; Haddy, F. Hemodynamic effects of bufalin in the anesthetized dog. *Hypertension* 1989; 13:690-695.

[31] Endo, T; Aten, RF; Leykin, L; Behrman, HR. Hydrogen peroxide evokes antisteroidogenic and antigonadotropic actions in human granulose luteal cells. *J. Clin. Endocrinol. Metab.* 1993; 76:337-342.

[32] Farias, JG; Bustos-Obregon, E; Tapia, PJ; Gutierrez, E; Zepeda, A; Juantok, C; Cruz, G; Soto, G; Benites, J; Reyes, JG. Time course of endocrine changes in the hypophysis-gonad axis induced by hypobaric hypoxia in male rats. *J. Reprod.* 2008; 54:18-21.

[33] Farnsworth, ER. Betel nut--its composition, chemistry, and uses. *Sci. New Quinea* 1976; 4:85-90.

[34] Fedele, AO; Whitelaw, ML; Peet, DJ. Regulation of gene expression by the hypoxia-inducible factors. *Mol. Interv.* 2002; 2:229-243.

[35] Fellmann, N; Beaune, B; Coudert, J. Blood lactate after maximal and supramaximal exercise in 10- to 12-year-old Bolivian boys. Effects of altitude and socioeconomic status. *Int. J. Sports Med.* 1994; 15 Suppl 2: S90-S95.

[36] Foucault, P; Carreau, S; Kuczynski, W; Guillaumin, JM; Bardos, P; and Drosdowsky, MA. Human Sertoli cells *in vitro*. Lactate, estradiol-17 beta and transferrin production. *J. Androl.* 1992; 13:361-367.

[37] Fry, DM. Reproductive effects in birds exposed to pesticides and industrial chemicals. *Environ. Health Perspect.* 1995; 103:165-171.

[38] Ginsburg, GS; O'Toole, Rimm, E; Douglas, PS; Rifai, N. Gender differences in exercise-induced changes in sex hormone levels and lipid peroxidation in athletes participating in the Hawaii Ironman triathlon. Ginsburg-gender and exercise-induced lipid peroxidation. *Clin. Chim. Acta* 2001; 305:131-139.

[39] Gong, Y; Han, XD. Effect of nonylphenol on steroidogenesis of rat Leydig cells. *J. Environ. Sci. Health.* B 2006; 41:705-715.

[40] Gonzalezjurado, JA; Teresa, C; Molina, E; de la Pradas, F; Guisado B, R; J Naranjo O, J. Effects of the consumption of Phlebodium Decumanum on plasma cortisol and testosterone levels in subjects participating in an exercise program. *Rev. Med. Chil.* 2009; 137: 497-503.

[41] Goto, K; Takahashi, K; Yamamoto, M; Takamatsu, K. Hormone and recovery responses to resistance exercise with slow movement. *J. Physiol. Sci.* 2008; 58:7-14.

[42] Greenblatt, DJ; Smith, TW. Digitalis. Clinical implications of new facts about an old drug. *Postgrad. Med.*1976; 59:134-139.

[43] Haase, VH. Hypoxia-inducible factors in the kidney. *Am. J. Physiol. Renal. Physiol.* 2006; 291:F271-F281.

[44] Hackney, AC. Stress and the neuroendocrine system: the role of exercise as a stressor and modifier of stress. *Expert. Rev. Endocrinol. Metab.* 2006; 1: 783-792.

[45] Hamers, T; Kamstra, JH; Sonneveld, E; Murk, AJ; Kester, MH; Andersson, PL; Legler, J; Brouwer, A. *In vitro* profiling of the endocrine-disrupting potency of brominated flame retardants. *Toxicol. Sci.* 2006; 92:157-173.

[46] Heindel, RM; Pakyz, RE; Cosentino, MJ. Spermatic cord torsion. Contralateral testicular degeneration at various ages in the rat. *J. Androl.* 1990; 11:506-513.

[47] Höckel, M; Vaupel, P. Tumor hypoxia: Definitions and current clinical, biologic, and molecular aspects. *J. Natl. Cancer Inst.* 2001; 93:266-276.

[48] Hoffman, JR; Im, J; Rundell, KW; Kang, J; Nioka, S; Spiering, BA; Kime, R; Chance, B; Speiring, BA. Effect of muscle oxygenation during resistance exercise on anabolic hormone response. *Med. Sci. Sports Exerc.* 2003; 35: 1929-1934.

[49] Hoffman, JR; Ratamess, NA; Kang, J; Rashti, SL; Kelly, N; Gonzalez, AM; Stec, M; Anderson, A; Bailey, BL; Yamamoto, LM; Hom, LL; Kupchak, BR; Faigenbaum, AD;

Maresh, CM. Examination of the efficacy of acute L-alanyl-L-glutamine ingestion during hydration stress in endurance exercise. *J. Int. Soc. Sports Nutr.* 2010; 7:8-19.

[50] Hong, Z; Chan, K; Yeung, HW. Simultaneous determination of bufadienolides in the traditional Chinese medicine preparation, liu-shen-wan, by liquid chromatography. *J. Pharm. Pharmacol.* 1992; 44:1023-1026.

[51] Hotchkiss, AK; Rider, CV; Blystone, CR; Wilson, VS; Hartig, PC; Ankley, GT; Foster, PM; Gray, CL; Gray, LE. Fifteen years after "Wingspread"--environmental endocrine disrupters and human and wildlife health: where we are today and where we need to go. *Toxicol. Sci.* 2008; 105:235-259.

[52] Hsia, SM; Tseng, YW; Wang, SW; Kuo, YH; Huang, DW; Wang, PS; Chiang, W. Effect of adlay (Coix lachryma-jobi L. var. ma-yuen Stapf.) hull extracts on testosterone release from rat Leydig cells. *Phytother. Res.* 2009; 23:687-695.

[53] Hulmi, JJ; Ahtiainen, JP; Selanne, H; Volek, JS; Hakkinen, K; Kovanen, V; Mero, AA. Androgen receptors and testosterone in men-effects of protein ingestion, resistance exercise and fiber type. *J. Steroid Biochem. Mol. Biol.* 2008; 110:130-137.

[54] Hwang, GS; Wang, SW; Tseng, WM; Yu, CH; Wang, PS. Effect of hypoxia on the release of vascular endothelial growth factor and testosterone in mouse TM3 Leydig cells. *Am. J. Physiol. Endocrinol. Metab.* 2007; 292: E1763-E1769.

[55] IARC. *Betel-quid and Areca Nut Chewing. Monographs on the Evaluation of the Carcinogenic Risk of Chemicals to Humans.* Lyon, France: IARC Scientific Publications, 1985, pp. 141-202.

[56] Iwaoka, Y; Hashimoto, R; Koizumi, H; Yu, J; Okabe, T. Selective stimulation by cinnamaldehyde of progesterone secretion in human adrenal cells. *Life Sci.* 2010;86:894-898.

[57] Jonas, MM; Eidson, MS. Propylthiouracil hepatotoxicity: two pediatric cases and review of the literature. *J. Pediatr. Gastroenterol. Nutr.* 1988; 7: 776-779.

[58] Juel, C. Lactate-proton cotransport in skeletal muscle. Physiol. Rev. 1997; 77:321-358.

[59] Juel, C; Halestrap, AP. Lactate transport in skeletal muscle - role and regulation of the monocarboxylate transporter. *J. Physiol.* 1999; 517: 633-642.

[60] Keiser, HR. Pheochromocytoma and other diseases of the sympathetic nervous system. In *Principles and Practice of Endocrinology and Metabolism*. ed. Beccker, K.L. 1990, pp. 676-679. Philadelphia: J. B. Lippincott Company.

[61] Kitamura, S; Kato, T; Iida, M; Jinno, N; Suzuki, T; Ohta, S; Fujimoto, N; Hanada, H; Kashiwagi, K; Kashiwagi, A. Anti-thyroid hormonal activity of tetrabromobisphenol A, a flame retardant, and related compounds: Affinity to the mammalian thyroid hormone receptor, and effect on tadpole metamorphosis. *Life Sci.* 2005; 76:1589-1601.

[62] Kley, HK; Abendroth, H; Hehrmann, R; Muller, A; Keck, E; Schneitler, H; Elsasser, H; Kruskemper, HL. [No effect of digitalis on sex and adrenal hormones in healthy subjects and in patients with congestive heart failure]. *Klin. Wochenschr.*1984; 62:65-73.

[63] Ko, YC; Huang, YL; Lee, CH; Chen, MJ; Lin, LM; Tsai, CC. Betel quid chewing, cigarette smoking and alcohol consumption related to oral cancer in Taiwan. *J. Oral. Pathol. Med.* 1995; 24:450-453.

[64] Kraemer, RR; Acevedo, EO; Synovitz, LB; Hebert, EP; Gimpel, T; Castracane, VD. Leptin and steroid hormone responses to exercise in adolescent female runners over a 7-week season. *Eur. J. Appl. Physiol.* 2001; 86:85-91.

[65] Kreydiyyeh, SI; Usta, J; Copti, R. Effect of cinnamon, clove and some of their constituents on the Na(+)-K(+)-ATPase activity and alanine absorption in the rat jejunum. *Food Chem. Toxicol.* 2000;38:755-762.

[66] Kubini, K; Zachmann, M; Albers, N; Hiort, O; Bettendorf, M; Wölfle, J; Bidlingmaier, F; and Klingmüller, D. Basal inhibin B and the testosterone response to human chorionic gonadotropin correlate in prepubertal boys. *J. Clin. Endocrinol. Metab.* 2000; 85:134-138.

[67] Levy, M. Propylthiouracil hepatotoxicity. A review and case presentation. *Clin. Pediatr.* 1993; 32:25-29.

[68] Lin, H; Chien, CH; Lin, YL; Chen, CF; Wang, PS. Inhibition of testosterone secretion by *S*-petasin in rat testicular interstitial cells. *Chinese J. Physiol.* 2000;43: 99-103.

[69] Lin, H; Tsai, SC; Chen, JJ; Chiao, YC; Wang, SW; Wang, GJ; Chen, CF;Wang, PS. Effects of evodiamine on the secretion of testosterone in rat testicular interstitial cells. *Metabolism* 1999; 48:1532-1535.

[70] Lin, H; Wang, SW; Tsai, SC; Chen, JJ; Chiao, YC; Lu, CC; Huang, WJ; Wang, GJ; Chen, CF; Wang, PS. Inhibitory effect of digoxin on testosterone secretion through mechanisms involving decreases of cyclic AMP production and cytochrome P450scc activity in rat testicular interstitial cells. *Brit. J. Pharmacol.*1998; 125:1635-1640.

[71] Lin, H; Wang, SW; Wang, RF; Wang, PS. Stimulatory effect of lactate on testosterone production by rat Leydig cells. *J. Cell. Biochem.* 2001; 83: 147-154.

[72] Lin, YL; Mei, CH, Huang, SL, Kuo, YH. Four new sesquiterpenes from Petasites formosanus. *J. Nat. Prod.* 1998; 61:887-890.

[73] Liu, TC; Kuo, CH; Wang, PS. Exercise and testosterone. Adapt. Med. 2009; 1:26-31.

[74] Lo, MJ; Wang, SW; Kau, MM; Chen, JJ; Chen, YH; Fang, VS; Ho, LT; Wang, PS. Pharmacological effects of PTU on corticosterone secretion in male rats. *J. Invest. Med.* 1998; 46:444-452.

[75] Lu, SS; Lau, CP; Tung, YF; Huang, SW; Chen, YH; Shih, HC; Tsai, SC; Lu, CC; Wang, SW; Chen, JJ; Chien, EJ; Chien, CH; Wang, PS. Lactate and the effects of exercise on testosterone secretion: evidence for the involvement of a cAMP-mediated mechanism. *Med. Sci. Sports Exerc.* 1997; 29: 1048-1054.

[76] Lucía, A; Chicharro, JL; Pérez, M; Serratosa, L; Bandrés, F; and Legido, JC. Reproductive function in male endurance athletes: sperm analysis and hormonal profile. *J. Appl. Physiol.* 1996; 81:2627-2636.

[77] Lysiak, JJ; Kirby, JL; Tremblay, JJ; Woodson, RI; Reardon, MA; Palmer, LA; Turner, TT. Hypoxia-inducible factor-1□ is constitutively expressed in murine Leydig cells and regulates 3β-hydroxysteroid dehydrogenase type 1 promoter activity. *J. Androl.* 2009; 30:146-156.

[78] MacLeod, J. The role of oxygen in the metabolism and motility of human spermatozoa. *Am. J. Physiol.* 1943; 138:512-518.

[79] Margolin, Y; Aten, RF; Behrman, HR. Antigonadotropic and antisteroidogenic actions of peroxide in rat granulose cells. *Endocrinology* 1990; 127:245-250.

[80] Mallem, L; Boulakoud, MS; Franck, M. Hypothyroidism after medium exposure to the fungicide maneb in the rabbit *Cuniculus lepus*. *Commun. Agric. Appl. Biol. Sci.* 2006; 71:91-99.

[81] Manna, I; Jana, K; Samanta, PK. Effect of intensive exercise-induced testicular gametogenic and steroidogenic disorders in mature male Wistar strain rats: a correlative approach to oxidative stress. *Acta Physiol. Scand.* 2003; 178:33-40.

[82] Marti, HH; Katschinski, DM; Wagner, KF; Schäffer, L; Stier, B; Wenger, RH. Isoform-specific expression of hypoxia-inducible factor-1□ during the late stages of mouse spermiogenesis. *Mol. Endocrinol.* 2002; 16:234-243.

[83] Mero, A. Blood lactate production and recovery from anaerobic exercise in trained and untrained boys. *Eur. J. Appl. Physiol. Occup. Physiol.* 1988; 57: 660-666.

[84] Moberg, GP. Influence of the adrenal axis upon the gonads. In *Oxford Reviews of Reproductive Biology*. ed. Clarke, J.R. 1981, pp.456-496. New York: Raven Press.

[85] Mukhtar, H; Ahmad, N. Green tea in chemoprevention of cancer. *Toxicol. Sci.* 1999;52:111-117.

[86] Murray, FT; Cameron, DF; Vogel, RB; Thomas, RG; Wyss, HU; Zauner, CE. The pituitary-testicular axis at rest and during moderate exercise in males with diabetes mellitus and normal sexual function. *J. Androl.* 1988; 9:197-206.

[87] Nakai, M; Chen, L; Nowak, RA. Tissue distribution of Basigin and monocarboxylate transporter 1 in the adult male mouse: a study using the wild-type and Basigin gene knockout mice. *Anat. Rec. Part A* 2006; 288A:527-535.

[88] Neri, A; Zukerman, Z; Aygen, M; Lidor, Y; Kaufman, H. The effect of long-term administration of digoxin on plasma androgens and sexual dysfunction. *J. Sex. Marital. Ther.* 1987; 13:58-63.

[89] Nindl, BC; Kraemer, WJ; Deaver, DR; Peters, JL; Marx, JO; Heckman, JT; Loomis, GA. LH secretion and testosterone concentrations are blunted after resistance exercise in men. *J. Appl. Physiol.* 2001; 91:1251-1258.

[90] Nomura, M; Kaji, A; He, Z; Ma, WY; Miyamoto, K; Yang, CS; Dong, Z. Inhibitory mechanisms of tea polyphenols on the ultraviolet B-activated phosphatidylinositol 3-kinase-dependent pathway. *J. Biol. Chem.* 2001; 276:46624-46631.

[91] Nunez, J; Pommier, J. Formation of thyroid hormones. *Vitam. Horm.* 1982; 39:175-229.

[92] Pamnani, MB; Chen, S; Yuan, C M; Haddy, FJ. Chronic blood pressure effects of bufalin, a sodium-potassium ATPase inhibitor, in rats. *Hypertension* 1994; 23:I106-I109.

[93] Panda, S; Kar, A. Dual role of betel leaf extract on thyroid function in male mice. *Pharmacol. Res.* 1998; 38:493-496.

[94] Panesar, NS. Bufalin radioimmunoassays: in search of the endogenous digitalis-like substance. *J. Immunoassay* 1994; 15:371-391.

[95] Peltola, V; Huhtaniemi, I; Metsa-Ketela, T; Ahotupa, M. Induction of lipid peroxidation during steroidogenesis in the rat testis. *Endocrinology* 137:105-112.

[96] Philp, A; Macdonald, AL; Watt, PW. Lactate - a signal coordinating cell and systemic function. *J. Exp. Biol.* 2005; 208:4561-4575.

[97] Polinsky, RJ; Brown, RT; Curras, MT; Baser, SM; Baucom, CE; Hooper, DR; Marini, AM. Central and peripheral effects of arecoline in patients with autonomic failure. *J. Neurol. Neurosurg. Psychiatry.* 1991; 54:807-812.

[98] Quinn, PG; Payne, AH. Oxygen-mediated damage of microsomal cytochrome P-450 enzymes in cultured Leydig cells. Role in steroidogenic desensitization. *J. Biol. Chem.* 1984; 259:4130-4135.

[99] Quinn, PG; Payne, AH. Steroid product-induced, oxygen-mediated damage of microsomal cytochrome P-450 enzymes in Leydig cell cultures. Relationship to desensitization. *J. Biol. Chem.* 1985; 260:2092-2099.

[100] Quistorff, B; Secher, NH; Van Lieshout, JJ. Lactate fuels the human brain during exercise. *FASEB J.* 2008; 22:3443-3449.

[101] Rao, AR; Das, P. Evaluation of the carcinogenicity of different preparations of areca nut in mice. *Int. J. Cancer.* 1989; 43:728-732.

[102] Ratamess, NA; Kraemer, WJ; Volek, JS; Maresh, CM; Vanheest, JL; Sharman, MJ; Rubin, MR; French, DN; Vescovi, JD; Silvestre, R; Hatfield, DL; Fleck, SJ; Deschenes, MR. Androgen receptor content following heavy resistance exercise in men. *J. Steroid Biochem. Mol. Biol.* 2005; 93:35-42.

[103] Rudolfsson, SH; Bergh, A. Testosterone-stimulated growth of the rat prostate may be driven by tissue hypoxia and hypoxia-inducible factor-1α *J. Endocrinol.* 2008; 196:11-19.

[104] Saha, I; Chatterji, U; Chaudhuri-Sengupta, S; Nag, TC; Nag, D; Banerjee S; Maiti ,BR. Ultrastructural and hormonal changes in the pineal-testicular axis following arecoline administration in rats. *J. Exp. Zool.* 2007; 307A:187-198.

[105] Selvan, RS; Selvakumaran, M; Rao, AR. Influence of arecoline on immune system. II. Suppression of thymus-dependent immune responses and parameter of non-specific resistance after short-term exposure. *Immunopharmacol. Immunotoxicol.* 1991;13:281-309.

[106] Shapiro, H; Lev, S; Cohen, J; Singer, P. Polyphenols in the prevention and treatment of sepsis syndromes: rationale and pre-clinical evidence. *Nutrition* 2009;25:981-997.

[107] Siddiqi, MA; Laessig, RH; Reed, KD. Polybrominated diphenyl ethers (PBDEs): new pollutants-old diseases. *Clin. Med. Res.* 2003; 1:281-290.

[108] Singh, A; Rao, AR. Effect of arecanut on the black mustard (*Brassica niger, L.*)-modulated detoxication enzymes and sulfhydryl content in the liver of mice. *Cancer Lett.* 1993; 72:45-51.

[109] Sinha, A; Rao, AR. Embryotoxicity of betel nuts in mice. *Toxicology* 1985; 37:315-326.

[110] Smith, GI. Cellular changes from graded testicular ischemia. *J. Urol.* 1955; 73:355-362.

[111] Smith, TW. Digitalis. Mechanisms of action and clinical use. *N. Engl. J. Med.* 1988; 318:358-365.

[112] Somani BK, Watson G, and Townell, N. Testicular torsion. *Brit. Med. J.* 2010; 341:c3213.

[113] Soto, AM; Justicia, H; Wray, JW; Sonnenschein, C. p-Nonyl-phenol: an estrogenic xenobiotic released from "modified" polystyrene. *Environ. Health Perspect.* 1991; 92:167-173.

[114] Stoffer, SS; Hynes, KM; Jiang, NS; Ryan, RJ. Digoxin and abnormal serum hormone levels. *J. Am. Med. Assoc.* 1973; 225:1643-1644.

[115] Swan, SH. Semen quality in fertile US men in relation to geographical area and pesticide exposure. *Int. J. Androl.* 2006; 29:62-68.

[116] Swan, SH; Kruse, RL; Liu, F; Barr, DB; Drobnis, EZ; Redmon, JB; Wang, C; Brazil, C; Overstreet, JW. Semen quality in relation to biomarkers of pesticide exposure. *Environ. Health Perspect.* 2003; 111:1478-1484.

[117] Tanaka, S; Yoon, YH; Fukui, H; Tabata, M; Akira, T; Okano, K; Iwai, M; Iga, Y; Yokoyama, K. Antiulcerogenic compounds isolated from Chinese cinnamon. *Planta Med.*1989; 55:245-248.

[118] Thomas, NE; Leyshon, A; Hughes, MG; Davies, B; Graham, M; Baker, JS. The effect of anaerobic exercise on salivary cortisol, testosterone and immunoglobulin (A) in boys aged 15-16 years. *Eur. J. Appl. Physiol.* 2009; 107:455-461.

[119] Thomas, S; Kearsley, J. Betel quid and oral cancer: a review. *Eur. J. Cancer. B. Oral. Oncol.* 1993; 29:251-255.

[120] Tsague-Manfo, FP; Chao, WF; Fewou-Moundipa, P; Pugeat, M; Wang, PS. Effects of maneb on testosterone release in male rats. *Drug Chem. Toxicol.* 2011; 34:120-128.

[121] Tsai, SC; Chen, JJ; Chiao, YC; Lu, CC; Lin, H; Yeh, JY; Lo, MJ; Kau, MM; Wang, SW; Wang, PS. The role of cyclic AMP production, calcium channel activation and enzyme activities in the inhibition of testosterone secretion by amphetamine. *Brit. J. Pharmacol.* 1997; 122:949-955.

[122] Tsai, SC; Chiao, YC; Lu, CC; Doong, ML; Chen, YH; Shih, HC; Liaw, C; Wang, SW; Wang, PS. Inhibition by amphetamine of testosterone secretion through a mechanism involving an increase of cyclic AMP production in rat testes. *Brit. J. Pharmacol.* 1996; 118:984-988.

[123] Tsai, SC; Lin, CS; Wang, PS. Antisteroidogenic actions of hydrogen peroxide on rat Leydig cells. *J. Cell. Biochem.* 2003; 90:1276-1286.

[124] Tsai, TH; Lee, TF; Chen, CF; Wang, LC. Thermoregulatory effects of alkaloids isolated from Wu-chu-yu in afebrile and febrile rats. *Pharmacol. Biochem. Behav.* 1995; 50:293-298.

[125] Turner, TT; Bang, HJ; Lysiak, JJ. Experimental testicular torsion: reperfusion blood flow and subsequent testicular venous plasma testosterone concentrations. *Urology* 2005; 65:390-394.

[126] Volek, JS; William J. Kraemer, WJ; Jill A. Bush, JA; Thomas Incledon, T; Mark Boetes, M. Testosterone and cortisol in relationship to dietary nutrients and resistance exercise. *J. Appl. Physiol.* 1997; 82:49-54.

[127] Wade, CE; Stanford, KI; Stein, TP; Greenleaf, JE. Intensive exercise training suppresses testosterone during bed rest. *J. Appl. Physiol.* 2005; 99:59-63.

[128] Wang, J; van der Heijden, R; Spruit, S ; Hankermeier, T; Chan, K; van der Greef, J; Xu, G; Wang, M. Quality and safety of Chinese herbal medicines guided by a systems biology perspective. *J. Ethnopharmacol.* 2009; 126:31-41.

[129] Wang, SW; Chiao, YC; Tsai, SC; Lu, CC; Chen, JJ; Shih, HC; Chen, YH; Lin, H; Hwu, CM; Wang, PS. Inhibition of bufalin on pituitary and testicular function in rats. *J. Pharmacol. Exp. Ther.* 1997; 283:528-532.

[130] Wang, SW; Hwang, GS; Chen, TJ; Wang, PS. Effects of arecoline on testosterone release in rats. *Am. J. Physiol. (Endocrinol. Metab.)* 2008; 295:E497-E504.

[131] Wang, SW; Lin, H; Hwang, JJ; Wang, PS. Inhibition of testosterone secretion by digitoxin in rat testicular interstitial cells. *J. Cell. Biochem.* 1999; 74:74-80.

[132] Wang, SW; Lin, H; Tsai, SC; Hwu, CM; Chiao, YC; Lu, CC; Chen, JJ; Wang, GJ; Chou, CJ; Lin, LC; Chen, CF; Wang, PS. Effects of methanol extract of Chansu on hypothalamic-pituitary-testis function in rats. *Metabolism* 1998; 47:1211-1216.

[133] Wang, SW; Pu, HF; Kan, SF; Tseng, CI; Lo, MJ; Wang, PS. Inhibitory effects of digoxin and digitoxin on corticosterone production in rat zona fasciculata-reticularis cells. *Brit. J. Pharmacol.* 2004; 142:1123-1130.

[134] Woody, CJ; Weber, SL; Laubach, HE; Ingram-Willey, V; Amini-Alashti, P; Sturbaum, BA. The effects of chronic exercise on metabolic and reproductive functions in male rats. *Life Sci.* 1998; 62:327-332.

[135] Wu, JJ; Wang, KL; Hsai, SM; Mao, IF; Chen, ML; Wang PS. Effects of oral nonylphenol on testosterone production in rat Leydig cells. *Adapt. Med.* 2010a; 2:47-52.

[136] Wu, JJ; Wang, KL; Wang, SW; Hwang, GS; Mao, IF; Chen, ML; Wang PS. Differential effects of nonylphenol on testosterone secretion in rat Leydig cells. *Toxicology* 2010b; 268:1-7.

[137] Yamahara, J; Yamada, T; Kitani, T; Naitoh, Y; Fujimura, H. Antianoxic action of evodiamine, an alkaloid in Evodia rutaecarpa fruit. *J. Ethnopharmacol.* 1989; 27:185-192.

[138] Yang, CS; Wang, X; Lu, G; Picinich, SC. Cancer prevention by tea: animal studies, molecular mechanisms and human relevance. *Nat. Rev. Cancer.* 2009; 9:429-439.

[139] Yang, S; Shih, HJ; Chow, YC; Tsai, PS; Wang, TY; Wang, PS; and Huang, CJ. The protective role of heme oxygenase-1 induction on testicular tissues after testicular torsion and detorsion. *J. Urol.* 2007; 177:1928-1933.

[140] Yang, Y; Gordon, CJ. Regulated hypothermia in the hypothyroid rat induced by administration of propylthiouracil. *Am. J. Physiol.* 1997; 272:1390-1395.

[141] Yu, PL; Pu, HF; Chen, SY; Wang, SW; Wang, PS. Effects of catechin, epicatechin and epigallocatechin gallate on testosterone production in rat leydig cells. *J. Cell. Biochem.* 2010; 110:333-342.

In: Testosterone
Editor: Konstantin Chichinadze

ISBN 978-1-62100-492-9

Chapter VIII

Development of Novel Proton-Affinitive Derivatives for Simultaneous Analysis of Testosterone and Dihydrotestosterone in Human Serum and Prostate Tissue by LC-ESI-MS/MS

Kouwa Yamashita*
Faculty of Pharmaceutical Sciences, Tohoku Pharmaceutical University
Aoba-ku, Sendai, Miyagi, Japan

Abstract

High performance liquid chromatography-tandem mass spectrometry (HPLC-MS/MS) is a powerful method for microanalysis of compounds in biological matrices. In this review, we introduce the recent development of HPLC-MS/MS analysis for the quantification of testosterone (T) and dihydrotestosterone (DHT). By adding an effective proton-affinitive tag to T and DHT, T and DHT were determined simultaneously with limits of quantification LOQs) of 1 pg/0.2 ml serum, and T and DHT with LOQs of 0.5 pg and 1 pg/3 mg prostate tissue, respectively. In addition, sufficient specificity of this method was achieved by selected reaction monitoring (SRM).

Keywords: Picolinyl derivatization; Testosterone; Dihydrotestosterone; High performance liquid chromatography-tandem mass spectrometry; Electrospray ionization

* Tel. +81-22-727-0138; Fax +81-22-727-0137; E-mail: kyama@tohoku-pharm.ac.jp.

1. Introduction

Testosterone (T) is metabolized to dihydrotestosterone (DHT) by 5α-reductase, which exists in the prostate, testis, brain and skin. As DHT showed 3-10 times stronger biological activities as male hormone than those of T, and DHT can play important hormonal roles in the prostate, skin and brain [1-3]. The blood level of DHT is approximately 10-20% of T level, and the production of DHT is inhibited by 5α-reductase inhibitors [4]. Therefore, the blood level of DHT might be an important biomedical index for evaluating clinical inhibitory potential of such inhibitors in the treatment of prostatic hypertrophy.

The DHT level in prostate tissue of patients with benign prostatic hyperplasia (BPH) is higher than that of patients with prostate cancer (PCa) [5]. Recent bioanalytical data have shown decreased 5α-reductase activity in prostatic carcinoma (PCa) when compared to BPH [6]. Negative correlation between the degree of malignancy in PCa and prostate DHT levels was also reported [7]. Therefore, the measurement of serum and prostate DHT levels in addition to T may be clinically useful for obtaining the supportive data in the discriminative diagnosis of these diseases.

Past four decades, radio-immunoassay (RIA) and enzyme-immunoassay (EIA) have been considered to be state-of-the-art methods in measurement of steroid hormones in biological specimen with their simplicity and high sensitivity for clinical diagnosis. In the case of T and DHT, the concentrations of these compounds have also routinely been measured by these immunochemical methods. However the direct measurement of T and DHT by immunoassay has been fraught with accuracy and imprecision problems originated from the inherent cross-reactivity of antisera used in the assay [8]. In order to eliminate the effect of cross-reactivity, it was necessary to separate T and DHT from one another in serum and prostate tissue prior to measurement by immunoassay [5, 9, 10].

Mass spectrometry coupled with gas chromatography (GC-MS) has been accepted to quantify T and DHT in serum and prostate tissue. However, the previous GC-MS procedures have the following limitations: a large amount of serum or tissue is normally required one analysis; much time is required for sample preparation and analysis; and the specificity and sensitivity are insufficient in low levels [11-13]. However, during last decade, high performance liquid chromatography-tandem mass spectrometry (HPLC-MS/MS) has also come to be employed conveniently for steroid analyses [14-19] because this method does not always require deconjugation and derivatization processes prior to analysis.

In this review, we introduce the recent development in HPLC-MS/MS method for the quantification of T and DHT in biological samples. An effective deriavtzation steps, thorough chromatographic separation and selected reaction monitoring (SRM) by MS/MS have achieved excellent sensitivity and specificity for this method. These methods have become a central approach for the simultaneous quantification of T and DHT in small amounts of biological samples.

2. DERIVATIZATION TO ENHANCE DETECTION SENSITIVITY OF TESTOSTERONE AND RELATED COMPOUNDS IN HPLC-MS/MS

Advances in ionization techniques have greatly contributed to the development of HPLC-MS assay of steroid hormones. At first, electron ionization was applied to HPLC-MS with particle beam interface. By this ionization, T and DHT were analyzed at LOQ of 0.17 ng as an injected amount due to a low efficiency of ionization [20]. Atmospheric pressure chemical ionization (APCI) was found to be attractive for measurement of serum testosterone because of low matrix effect. In HPLC-APCI-MS/MS, large volume of serum sample (1 ml) was necessary to analyze testosterone [19, 21]. To gain much higher sensitivity and reduce serum sample volume, researcher have developed some derivatization testosterone was converted to oxime derivative or acetyl derivative. Niwa et al have demonstrated the use of ethyloxime-acetyl derivative as proton-affinitive tag to detect plasma testosterone concentrations as low as 0.2 ng/ml in a 0.05 ml rat plasma [22].

Use of an electrospray ionization (ESI) as an interface of HPLC provided the ability to ionize samples wide range of polarity and molecular weight, however it had previously been considered that ESI was not suitable for the analysis of neutral and steroids, especially sterols with high sensitivity [23, 24]. In reports utilizing HPLC-ESI-MS/MS of steroids, T in serum was analyzed with limit of quantification of 86 pg/ml [14] or 100 pg/ml [25] without derivatization of intact molecule. Of course, these methods have sufficient sensitivity and accuracy for analyzing tetstosterone in samples of adult males, but are not sufficient for measuring testosterone in samples from women and children [26]. In addition, it was generally proposed that the presence of interfering peaks co-existing in biological matrices and co-eluting with analyte of interest resulted in causing ionization suppression to reduce detection sensitivity [27, 28].

In order to improve these limitations, steroid molecules have been derivataized to exhibit more polar chemical properties. Proposed derivatives were listed in Figure 1. Among these derivatives, N-methylpyridinium (NMP) ether [29, 30], 2-hydradino-N- methylpyridine-hydrazone (HMP)[25, 31], 4-(4-dimethyl-1-piperadinium)-3-nitro- carbamate (MAPZ) [32] and Girard-P [33] derivatives were permanently charged derivatives. Testosterone was analyzed with LOD of 1.5-pg using the NMP derivative [25], and sensitivity was improved approximately 13 times. It was reported that dihydrotestosterone was also analyzed with this derivative with LOQ of 5 pg/ml serum [29]. HMP and Girard-P were developed as derivatizing reagents for carbonyl functional group of androgens, and the detection sensitivity of the HMP derivatives for T and DHT were 0.3 pg/on column and 0.5 pg/on column, and sensitivity were improved by approximately 70 and 1600 times, respectively [25]. The derivative obtained for T with Girard-P reagent exhibited LOD of 3 pg/on column, and sensitivity was enhanced by 7 times. However, the formation of geometric *syn*- and *anti*-isomers originated from imine-moiety seemed to be inevitable and resulted in reducing the detection sensitivity [25]. It is also known that the HMP derivatization is not suitable for steroids that have two carbonyl groups, such as androst-4-ene-3, 17-dione and progesterone, because of the production of a number of ions as $[M-H]^-$ and $[M]^{2+}$ without the formation of a single charged positive ion [25].

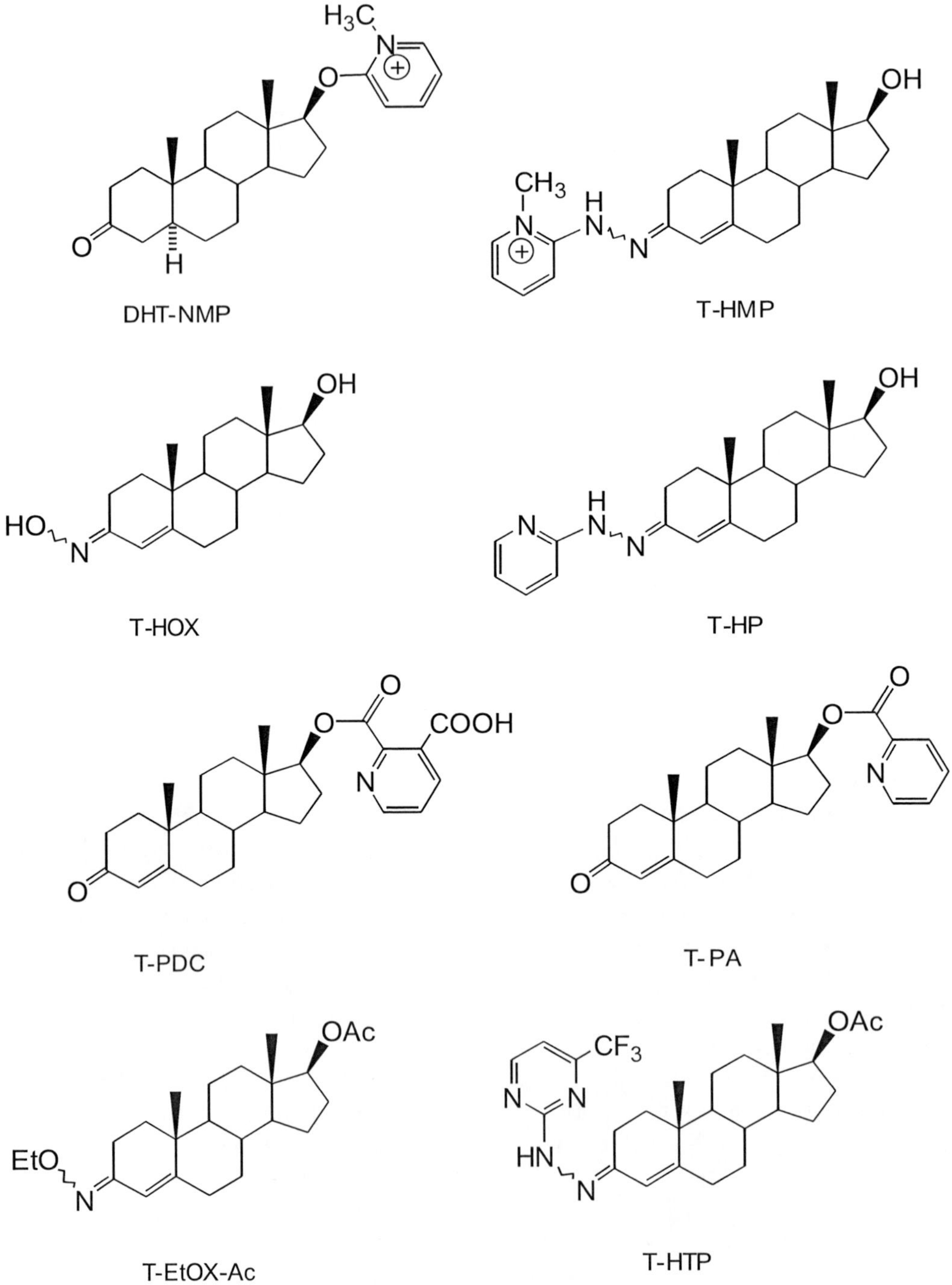

Figure 1. Proposed derivatives of testosterone and dihydrotestosterone for HPLC-MS.

On the other hand, pyridine-2, 3-dicarboxylic acid (PDC) [34], picolinic acid (PA)[35-39], hydroxylamine (HOX)[40], 2-hydrazinopyridine (HP)[41] and 2-hydrazino-4-trifluoromethylpyrimidine (HTP)[42] were used for the derivatization of testosterone. These are all proton-affinitive derivatives. Of these derivatives, PDC and PA derivatives were used for hydoxyl group of testosterone molecule. In the preparation of PDC derivatives, PDC anhydride was used as a reagent, and the derivatives were obtained as a mixture of 2-carboxylate and 3-craboxylate of testosterone. The HOX and HTP derivatization were also introduced to the carbonyl group of testosterone, and the formation of geometric *syn-* and *anti-*isomers originated from imine-moiety seemed to be inevitable and resulted in reducing the sensitivity in a similar manner as shown in the case of HMP and Girard-P derivatives. The detection limits of testosterone were 0.12 pg/on column and 0.7 pg/on column as their HOX [40] and HP derivatives [41], respectively. The HP derivatives of androstenedione and progesterone showed improvement in detection sensitivity when compared to those permanently charged HMP derivatives of them. The LOQ of PDC ester of T was 200 pg/ml [34] and the LOQ of PA of T exhibited higher LOQ of 1 pg/0.2 ml serum and 0.5 pg/3 mg prostate tissue [44], respectively. Recently, the HTP derivative of T was reported and the LOQ for T was 0.1 ng/ml serum [42].

3. CHARACTERIZATION OF THE PICOLINYL (PA) DERIVATIVES OF T AND DHT [43, 44]

We have successfully introduced a picolinyl moiety as proton-affinitive tag into the hydroxyl group of various kinds of steroids, including T and related androgens. The initial efforts were directed to the synthesis of derivatives and compare the behaviors of various kinds of pyridine carboxylate derivatives, nicotinate, isonicotonate, 2-methoxynicotinate, 6-methylpicolinate, of hydroxysteroids. We have also demonstrated that the picolinyl ester derivatization is a simple and versatile method for sensitive and specific quantification using positive HPLC-ESI-MS/MS in a micro-scale.

In microdetermination, extraction of T and DHT from serum was performed as mentioned below prior to derivatization. Human serum (0.2 ml) was mixed with internal standard to make volume of 1 ml with purified water. Diethyl ether was added to the diluted serum sample, and the mixture was shaken for 10 min. The aqueous phase was frozen and the organic layer was separated and then evaporated to dryness at 40°C under N_2 stream. The residue was dissolved in the reagent mixture, and the resulting mixture was allowed to stand at room temperature for 30 min.

As shown in Figure 2, the reagent mixture, consisting 2-methyl-6-nitrobenzoic anhydride, 4-dimethylaminopyridine, picolinic acid (or other pyridine-carboxylates), triethylamine and tetrahydrofuran was added to the authentic samples or purified extracts obtained from serum and prostate samples. Picolinoyl chloride in pyridine solution was also useful for derivatization. Excess reagents were then removed by solid phase extraction using Oasis-HLB cartridges and the picolinyl derivatives of T and DHT, as well as other steroids, were eluted with 80% MeCN-H_2O.

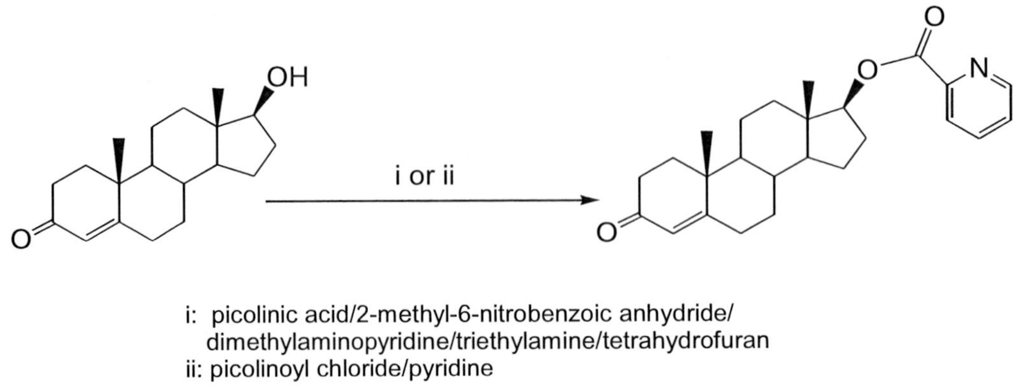

Figure 2. Proton-affinitive derivatization of testosterone with picolinic acid.

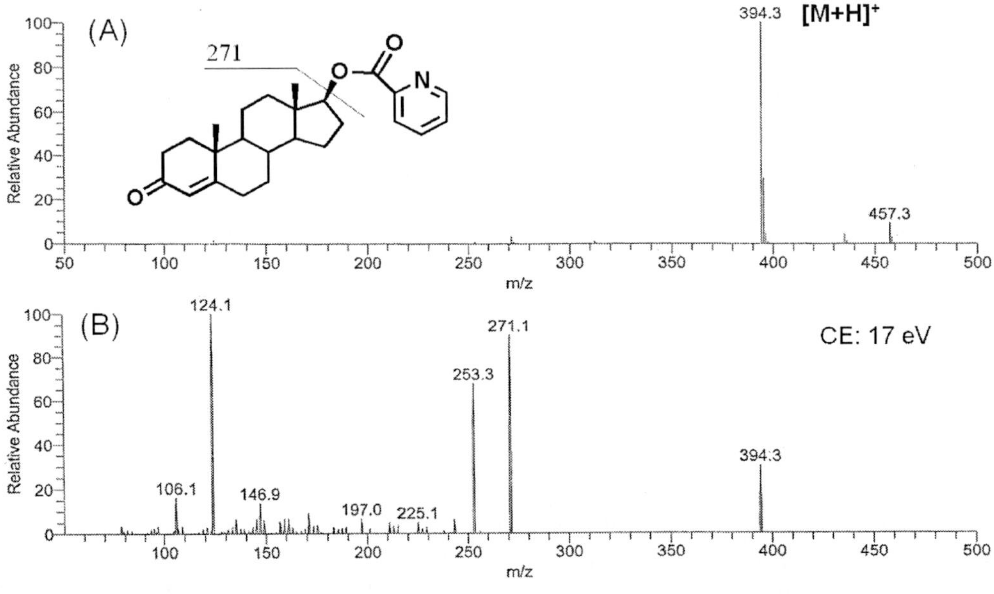

Figure 3. Typical ESI-mass spectrum and its product ion spectrum of the picolinyl derivative of testosterone.

Among these derivatives, the picolinyl derivatives showed the best HPLC-ESI-MS/MS behaviors and approximately 100-fold higher detection response by SRM compared with underivatized molecule.

Absolute recovery rates of T and DHT during the process of extraction, derivatization and purification from serum and prostate tissue were more than 80%. The extraction of T and DHT from prostate tissue was achieved with the highest recovery rate than other solvents such as methanol, acetone and acetonitrile.

In positive ESI-mass spectrometry, the picolinyl derivatives of T and DHT showed protonated molecule at *m/z* 394 and *m/z* 396 as base peaks. Collision of these protonated molecule of the picolinyl derivative resulted in the formation of characteristic product ions of *m/z* 271 and 253 for T and *m/z* 273 and 255 for DHT, respectively. These product ions were assigned for the elimination of picolinyl moiety from the protonated molecule and subsequent elimination of H_2O and used as SRM transitions. Positive ESI-mass spectrum and the representative product ion spectrum of the picolinyl derivative of T were shown in Figure 3.

The picolinyl derivatization has been successfully applied to the determination of estrogens [36], corticosteroids [37, 38], aldosterone [45] and sterols [24, 39].

Table 1. Intra- and inter-assay accuracy and precision for T and DHT in serum and prostate tissue

Matrices	T				DHT			
	Added (pg)	Found[b,c] (pg)	Accuracy[d] (%)	Precision (%)	Added (pg)	Found[b,c] (pg)	Accuracy[d] (%)	Precision (%)
Human serum[a] (0.2 mL)								
Intra assay	0	0.04 ± 0.08	-	-	0	0.02 ± 0.04	-	-
	1	1.15 ± 0.05	115.2	4.7	1	1.10 ± 0.17	110.2	15.3
	10	11.24 ± 0.39	112.4	3.5	10	10.56 ± 0.58	105.6	5.5
	1000	985.86 ± 52.65	98.6	5.3	1000	996.90 ± 19.29	99.7	1.9
Inter assay	0	0.17 ± 0.26	-	-	0	0.10 ± 0.12	-	-
	1	0.96 ± 0.12	96.0	12.9	1	1.01 ± 0.15	100.7	15.0
	10	10.93 ± 0.40	109.3	3.7	10	10.49 ± 0.65	104.9	6.2
	1000	1028.17 ± 24.02	102.8	2.6	1000	965.62 ± 30.69	96.6	3.2
Human Prostate (3 mg)								
Intra assay	0	0.28 ± 0.06	-	-	0	4.60 ± 0.24	-	-
	0.5	0.52 ± 0.06	104.4	11.4	1	1.02 ± 0.17	102.2	17.1
	5	5.04 ± 0.15	100.8	3.0	5	5.31 ± 0.13	106.3	2.6
	10	10.27 ± 0.15	100.3	1.5	10	10.73 ± 0.15	107.3	1.5
Inter assay	0	0.10 ± 0.09	-	-	0	4.73 ± 0.29	-	-
	0.5	0.51 ± 0.07	101.5	13.2	1	1.03 ± 0.13	103.3	12.5
	5	4.81 ± 0.16	96.1	3.2	5	4.81 ± 0.30	96.2	5.9
	10	9.72 ± 0.41	97.2	4.1	10	9.62 ± 0.52	96.2	5.2

[a] Charcoal-treated serum.

[b] Data were espressed as mean +/-S.D. of five experiments (intra-assay) and three experiments (inter-assay, 3 days).

[c] Results are expressed after subtraction of the mean endogenous serum or prostate concentration.

[d] Data were calculated after subtraction of the mean endogenous concentration of each case.

4. Evaluation of Assay Performance Utilizing PA Derivatization

Calibration graphs were constructed for T and DHT by means of T-d3 and DHT-d3 as internal standards. The calibration graph for T and DHT standard spiked in purified water or charcoal-treated human serum, at 6 concentration levels (0.5–1000 pg/tube) showed good linearity with correlation coefficients (r) of more than 0.999 and the similar slopes in both matrices. The signal intensities corresponding to the retention times for both internal standards in SRM obtained for serum (0.2 ml) and prostate tissue (15 mg) samples were measured with or without internal standards (T-d_3, DHT-d_3, each 100 pg) in the presence of T and DHT (10 pg for serum and 100 pg for prostate tissue) Neither serum nor prostate sample showed little interference (0.05% and 0.03% against T-d_3 and DHT-d_3-signals: 100 pg each in serum and 0.9% and 0.34% against T-d_3 and DHT-d_3-singal: 100 pg each in prostate tissue). This result verified that the interfering peaks overlapped to retention times of both internal standards were negligible in HPLC-ESI-MS/MS.

When the limit of quantification (LOQ) was defined as the lowest concentration of the spiked analyte measured in serum and prostate tissue with accepted accuracy (bias:< 20%) and precision (< 20%), and signal-to-noise ratio of at least 5, the LOQs of T and DHT in serum were 1 pg/0.2 ml. The LOQs of T and DHT in prostate tissue were 0.5 and 1 pg/3 mg. respectively.

The results of intra-assay and inter-assay accuracy and precision of T and DHT were shown in Table 1. Accuracy and precision of T and DHT in serum were calculated for three different concentrations of low, medium and high QC samples. Accuracies for both intra- and inter-assay procedures in serum and prostate tissue were in the range of 96-115.2% and 96.1-104.4%, respectively. Precisions for both intra- and inter-assay procedures were also 2.6-12.9% and 1.5-13.2%, respectively.

5. Application for Simultaneous Determination of T and DHT in Human Serum and Prostate Tissue

Typical SRM chromatograms of the picolinyl derivatives of T and DHT in the extract obtained from prostate tissue homogenates are shown in Figure 4. Signal corresponding to the picolinyl derivative of dehydroepiandrosterone (DHEA) was observed in the same SRM chromatogram with the same transition for T. As shown in this Figure 4, T and DHT in human prostate tissue were simultaneously determined by SRM with excellent signal-to-noise ratio after conversion to their picolinyl derivatives with injected amount of sub-picograms.

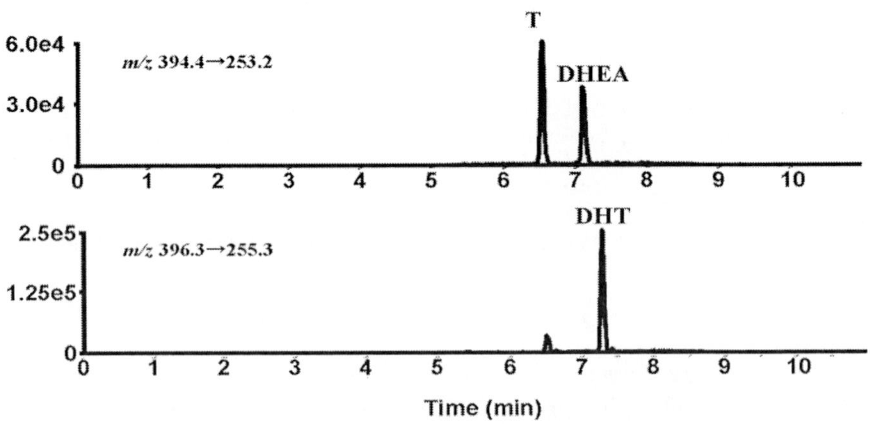

Figure 4. Typical selected reaction monitoring of the picolinyl derivatives of androgens extracted from human prostate tissue (T: 1 pg, DHT: 2 pg as injected amounts) in a positive mode using protonated molecules as precursor ions.API-5000 LC-MS, column; Cadenza CDC18 (150 mm x 3 mm i.d., 3 μm), mobile phase; HCOOH-H_2O (1 : 99, v/v, solvent B), MeCN-MeOH (50 : 50, v/v, solvent C), C/B = 60/40 to 90/10 for 0-5.0 min, 90/10 for 5.0-7.0 min, 100/0 for 7.0-9.0 min, 100/10 to 60/40 for 9.0-11.0 min, temperature; 40°C.

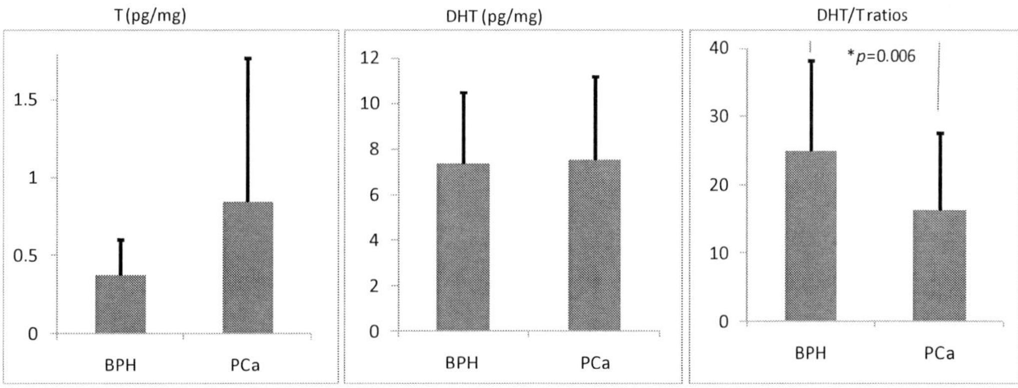

Figure 5. Prostatic T and DHT levels, and DHT/T ratios in benign prostate hyperplasia (BPH) and prostate cancer (PCa) patients. Results are expressed as the mean ± SD.

The developed method was applied to the simultaneous determination of T and DHT levels in human serum and prostate tissues. The serum levels of T and DHT in healthy males and females with respect to age were analyzed using this method and the results are shown in Table 2. As shown in Table 2, T and DHT levels gradually decreased with age in females but decrease was not significant in males. Both T and DHT levels were higher in males than in females, and DHT/T ratios were higher in females than in males.

The levels of T and DHT in prostate samples obtained from the patients with BPH (n=30) or PCa (n=37) *via* needle biopsy were shown in Figure 6. The prostate levels of DHT were similar in PCa and BPH. On the other hand, the prostate levels of T in BPH accounted for 5% of DHT, and 11% in PCa patients. Significant DHT/T ratio between BPH (24.7±13.3, n=30) and PCa (16.4±11.3, n=37) was observed (p=0.0006, Student's *t*-test) .

Table 2. Gender differences in serum T and DHT levels, and DHT/T ratios

Male					Female				
Age	n	T[a]	DHT[a]	DHT/T	Age	n	T[a]	DHT[a]	DHT/T
-20	8	6.14±1.65	0.51±0.18	0.08±0.02	21-30	7	0.31±0.091	0.072±0.035	0.23±0.084
21-30	10	5.61±0.94	0.50±0.10	0.09±0.02	31-50	4	0.18±0.088	0.058±0.014	0.43±0.36
31-40	8	4.40±1.60	0.42±0.10	0.10±0.04	51-65	3	0.13±0.072	0.028±0.017	0.23±0.15
41-50	6	4.04±0.94	0.35±0.08	0.09±0.02					
51-60	9	4.47±1.77	0.48±0.15	0.11±0.03					
61-70	8	5.07±2.03	0.58±0.29	0.12±0.07					
71-	11	3.69±1.78	0.53±0.32	0.15±0.05					

Results are expressed as the mean+/-S.D.
[a] ng/mL.

6. Perspectives

HPLC-MS/MS does not require derivatization step before the analysis of steroids, which is advantageous for high-throughput assay. However, the addition of the derivatization step has markedly improved the detection sensitivity of neutral steroids such as T and related androgens. Synthesized T was further metabolized to biologically active DHT and other hydroxylated metabolites with various kinds of enzymes. Since many T metabolites have the same molecular weight and similar structures, a thorough chromatographic separation is essential to maintain the selectivity even if the latest model of mass spectrometer is operated in a high-resolution mode.

The recent development of steroid biochemistry has demonstrated that T metabolites are promising probes for the evaluation of enzyme activity of T metabolism. Therefore, not only sensitive and specific quantification of targeted T and DHT but also metabolomic analysis of whole T metabolic profiles will become an important methodology for androgen biochemistry and its clinical application.

References

[1] Bruchovsky, N. and Wilson, J. (1999). Discovery of the role of dihydrotestosterone in androgen action. *Steroids, 64*, 753-759.

[2] Torres, J. M. and Ortega, E. (2006). Steroid 5α-reductase isoenzymes in the adult female rat brain: central role of dihydrotestosterone. *J. Mol. Endcrinol. 36*, 239-245.

[3] Grah, M. (2003). Male Japanese quails with female brains do not show male sexual behaviors. *Pro. Nat. Acad. Sci.*, 100, 7859-7864.

[4] Bartsch, G., Rittmaster, R. S., Klocker, M. (2000). Dihydrotestosterone and the concept of 5α-reductase inhibition in human benign prostate hyperplasia. *Eur. Urol.*, 37, 367-380.

[5] Ghanadian, R., Pauh, C. M. (1981). Relationships between oestradiol-17β, testosterone, dihydrotestosterone and 5α-androstane-3α,17β-diol in human benign hypertrophy and carcinoma of prostate. *J. Endocrinol.*, 88, 255-262.

[6] Montogomery, R. B., Mostaghel, E. A., Vessella, R., Hess, D. L., Kalhorn, T. F., Higano, C. S. (2008). Maintenance of intratumoral androgens in metastatic prostate cancer: a mechanism of castration resistant tumor growth. *Cancer Res.*, 68, 4447-4454.

[7] Nishiyama, T., Ikarashi, T., Hashimoro, Y., Suzuki, K., Takahashi, K. (2006. Association between the dihydrotestosterone levels in the prostate and prostate cancer aggressiveness using the Gleason score. *J. Urol.*, 176, 1387-1391.

[8] Taibe, J., Benattar, C., Birr, A.S., Lindenbaum, A. (2002). Limitation of steroid determination by direct immunoassay. *Clin Chem.*, 48, 583-585.

[9] Krieg, M., Nass, R., Tunn, S. (1993). Effect of aging on endogenous level of 5a-dihydrotestosterone, testosterone, estradiol and estrone in epithekium and stroma of normal and hyperplastic human prostate. *J. Clin. Endocrinol Metab.*, 77, 375-381.

[10] Shibata, Y., Ito, K., Suzuki, K., Nakano, K., Fukabori, Y., Suzuki, R, Kawabe, Y., Honma, S., Yamanaka, H. (2000). Changes in the endocrine environment of human prostate transition zone with aging: simultaneous quantitative analysis of prostatic sex steroids and comparison with human prostatic histological composition. *Prostate*, 42, 45-55.

[11] Moneti, G., Costantini, A., Guarna, A., Salerno, R., Pazzagli, M., Natali, A. et al. (1986). Measurement of testosterone 5a-reductase metabolites in human prostatic tissues using isotope dilution mass spectrometry. *J. Steroid Biochem.*, 25, 765-772.

[12] Tieb, J., Mathian, B., Millot, B., Patriot, M-C., Mathieu, E., Queyrel, N., et al. (2003). Testosterone measured by 10 immunoassays and by isotope-dilution gas chromatography-mass spectrometry in sera from 116 men, women, and children. *Clin. Chem.*, 49, 1381-1395.

[13] Fitzgerald, R. L., Herold, D. A. (1996). Serum total testosterone: immunoassay compared with negative chemical ionization mass spectrometry. *Clin. Chem.*, 42, 749-755.

[14] Cawood, M. L., Field, H. P., Ford, C. G., Gilligwater, S., Kicman, A., Cowan, D., Barth, J. H. (2005). Testosterone measurement by isotope-dilution liquid chromatography-tandem mass spectrometry: validation of method for routine clinical practice. *Clin. Chem.*, 51, 1472-1479.

[15] Neslon, R. E., Grebe, S. K., Okane, D. J., Singh, R. J. (2004). Liquid chromatography-tandem mass spectrometry assay for simultaneous measurement of estradiol and estrone in human plasma. *Clin. Chem.*, 50, 373-384.

[16] Hauser, B., Deschner, T., Boesch, C. (2008). Development of a liquid chromatography-tandem mass spectrometry method for the determination of 23 endogenous steroids in small quantities of primate urine. *J. Chromatogr. B*, 862, 100-112.

[17] Guo, T., Taylor, R. L., Singh, R. J., Soldin, S. J. (2006). Simultaneous determination of 12 steroids by isotope dilution liwuid chromatography-photospray ionization tandem mass spectrometry. *Clin. Chim. Acta*, 372, 76-82.

[18] Mitamura, K., Nakagawa, T., Shimada, K., Namiki, M., Koh, E., Mizakami, A., Honma, S. (2002). Identification of dehydroepiandrosterone metabolites formed from human prostate homogenate using liquid chromatography-mass spectrometry and gas chromatography-mass spectrometry. *J. Chromatogr. A*, 961, 97-105.

[19] Starcevic, B., DiStefano, E., Wang, C., Catlin, D. H. (2003). Liquid chromatography–tandem mass spectrometry assay for human serum testosterone and trideuterated testosterone. *J. Chromatogr. B*, 792, 197-204.

[20] Cappielo, A., Famiglini, G., Palma, P., Siviero, A. (2005). Liquid chromatography-electron ionization mass spectrometry: fields of application and evaluation of the performance of a direct-EI interface. *Mass Spectrom. Rev.*, 24, 978-989.

[21] Wang, C., Catlin, D. H., Demers, L. M., Starcevic, B., Swerdloff, R. S. (2004). Measurement of total serum testosterone in adult men: comparison of current laboratory methods versus liquid chromatography-tandem mass spectrometry. *J. Clin. Endocrinol. Metab.*, 89, 534-544.

[22] Niwa, M., Watanabe, N., Ochiai, H., Yamashita, K. (2005). Determination of testosterone concentration in rat plasma using liquid chromatography-atmospheric pressure chemical ionization mass spectrometry combined with ethyloxime and acetyl ester derivatization. *J. Chromatogr. B*, 824, 258-266.

[23] MaDonald, J. G., Thompson, B. M., McCrum, E. C., Russell, D. W. (2007). Extraction and analysis of sterols in biological matrices by high performance liquid chromatography eletcrospray ionization mass spectrometry. *Methods Enzymol.*, 432, 145-170.

[24] Honda, A., Miyazaki, T., Ikegami, T., Iwamoto, J., Yamashita, K., Numazawa, M., Matsuzaki, Y. (2010). Highly sensitive and specific analysis of sterol profiles in biological samples by HLC-ESI-MS/MS. *J. Steroid Biochem. Mol. Biol.*, 121, 556-564.

[25] Higashi, T., Yamauchi, A., Shimada, K. (2005). 2-Hydrazino-1-methylpyridine: a highly sensitive derivatization reagent for oxosteroids in liquid chromatography-electrospray ionization-mass spectrometry. *J. Chromatogr. B*, 825, 214-222.

[26] Kushnir, M. M., Rockwood, A. L., Roberts, W. L., Pattison, E. G., Bunker, A. M., Fitzgerald, R. L., Meikle, A. W. (2006). Performance characteristics of a novel tandem mass spectrometry assay for serum testosterone. *Clin. Chem.*, 52, 120-128.

[27] Taylor, P. J. (2005). Matrix effects: the Achilles heel of quantitative high-performance liquid chromatography-electrospray-tandem mass spectrometry. *Clin. Biochem.*, 38, 328-334.

[28] Hernandéz, F., Sancho, J. V., Pozo, O. J., (2005). Critical review of the application of liquid chromatography/mass spectrometry to the determination of pesticide residues in biological samples. *Anal. Bioanal. Chem.*, 382, 934-946.

[29] Nakagawa, Y., Hashimoto, Y. (2002). Polar derivatization of 5α-dihydro- testosterone and sensitive analysis by semimicro-LC-ESI-MS. *J. Mass Sepctrom. Soc. Jpn.*, 50, 593-599.

[30] Nishiyama, T., Hashimoto, Y., Takahashi, K. (2004). The influence of androgen deprivation therapy on dihydrotestosterone levels in the prostatic tissue of patients with prostate cancer. *Clin. Cancer Res.*, 10, 7121-7126.

[31] Shibayama, Y., Higashi, T., Shimada, K., Odani, A., Mizokami, A., Konaka, H., Koh, E., Namiki, M. (2009). Simultaneous determination of salivary testosterone and dehydroepiandrosterone using LC–MS/MS: Method development and evaluation of applicability for diagnosis and medication for late-onset hypogonadism. *J. Chromatogr. B*, 877, 2615-2623.

[32] Nishio, T., Higashi, T., Funaishi, A., Tanaka, J., Shimada, K. (2007). Development and application of electrospray-active derivatization reagents for hydroxysteroids *J. Pharm. Biomed. Anal.*, 44, 786-795.

[33] Griffith, W. J., Liu, S., Alvelius, G. and Sjvöll. (2003). Derivatization for the characterization of neutral oxosteroids by electrospray and matrix-assisted laser desorption/ionization mass spectrometry. *Rapid Commun. Mass Spectrom., 17,* 924-935.

[34] Licea-Perez, H., Wang, S., Szapacs, M. E. and Yang, E. (2008). Development of a highly sensitive and selective UPLC/MS/MS method for the simultaneous determination of testosterone and 5α-dihydrotestosterone in human serum to support testosterone replacement therapy for hypogonadism. *Steroids, 73,* 601-610.

[35] Yamashita, K., Okuyama, M., Watanabe, Y., Honma, S., Kobayashi, S. and Numazawa, M. Highly sensitive determination of estrone and estradiol in human serum by liquid chromatography-electrospray ionization tandem mass spectrometry. *Steroids, 72,* 819-827.

[36] Yamashita, K., Okuyama, M., Watanabe, Y., Honma, S., Kobayashi, S. and Numazawa, M. Highly sensitive determination of estrone and estradiol in human serum by liquid chromatography-electrospray ionization tandem mass spectrometry. *Steroids, 72,* 819-827.

[37] Yamashita, K., Takahashi, M., Tsukamoto, S., Numazawa, M., Okuyama, M. and Honma, S. (2007). Use of novel derivatization for simultaneous quantification of six corticosteroids by liquid chromatography-electrospray ionization tandem mass spectrometry. *J. Chromatogr. A,* 1173, 120-128.

[38] Yamashita, K., Nakagawa, R., Okuyama, M., Honma, S., Takahashi, M. and Numazawa, M. (2008). Simultaneous determination of tetrahydrocortisol, allotetrahydrocortisol and tetrahydrocortisone in human urine by liquid chromatography-electrospray ionization mass spectrometry. *Steroids, 73,* 727-737.

[39] Honda, A., Yamashita, K., Miyazaki, H., Shirai, M., Ikegami, T., Xu, G., Numazawa, M., Hara, T. and Matsuzaki, Y. (2008). Highly sensitive analysis of sterol profiles in human serum by LC-ESI-MS/MS. *J. Lipid Res.,* 49, 2063-2073.

[40] Kalhorn, T. F., Page, S. T., Howald, W. N., Mostaghel, E. A. and Nelson, P. S. (2007). Analysis of testosterone and dihydrotestosterone from biological fluids as the oxime derivatives using high-performance liquid chromatography/tandem mass spectrometry. *Rapid Commun. Mass Spectrom.,* 21, 3200-3206.

[41] Higashi, T., Nishio, T., Hayashi, N., Shimada, K. (2007). Alternative procedure for charged derivatization to enhance detection responses of steroids in electrospray ionization-MS. *Chem. Pharm. Bull.*, 55, 662-665.

[42] Weng, Y., Xie, F., Xu, L., Zagorevski, D., Spink, D. C., Ding, X. (2010). Analysis of testosterone and dihydrotestosterone in mouse tissues by liquid chromatography-electrospray ionization-tandem mass spectrometry. *Anal. Biochem.*, 402, 121-128.

[43] Yamashita, K. Kobayashi, S., Tsukamoto, S., Numazawa, M. (2007). Synthesis of pyridine-carboxylate derivatives of hydroxysteroids for liquid chromatography-mass spectrometry. *Steroids*, 72, 50-59.

[44] Yamashita, K., Miyashiro, Y., Maekubo, H., Okuyama, M., Honma, S., Takahashi, M., Numazawa, M. (2009). Development of highly sensitive quantification method for testosterone and dihydrotestosterone in human serum and prostate tissue by liquid chromatography-electrospray ionization tandem mass spectrometry. *Sreroids*, 74, 920-926.

[45] Yamashita, K., Okuyama, M., Nakagawa, R., Honma, S., Satoh, F., Morimoto, R., Ito, S., Takahashi, M., Numazawa, M. (2009). Development of sensitive derivatization method for aldosterone in liquid chromatography-electrospray ionization tandem mass spectrometry of corticosteroids. *J. Chromatogr. A*, 1200, 114-121.

In: Testosterone
Editor: Konstantin Chichinadze

ISBN 978-1-62100-492-9

Chapter IX

Effects of Testosterone on Vascular Tone

Oguzhan Yildiz**, *Melik Seyrek
Department of Pharmacology, Gulhane School of Medicine , 06018 Ankara, Turkey

ABSTRACT

Testosterone has classically been considered to exert an unfavourable effect upon the cardiovascular system. However, numerous recent clinical and epidemiological studies have reported a controversial relationship between testosterone and lipid profiles, inflammatory responses, hypertension, and altered vascular smooth muscle reactivity with regard to cardiovascular disease. Previous animal studies have demonstrated that testosterone exhibits a vasodilatory action in vasculature of experimental animals and more recently in isolated human pulmonary artery. Accordingly, we have recently shown that testosterone relaxes isolated human spermatic vein and corpus cavernosum as well as isolated human mesenteric, internal mammary and radial arteries. Because these effects occur in seconds to minutes, we and others have suggested that this action is likely to be mediated via the interactions with receptors on the membrane (nongenomic effect) rather than by interaction with the nucleus (genomic effect). Furthermore, several studies have shown the presence of the androgen receptor on the membrane of vascular smooth muscle cells, suggesting that the proposed mechanism is likely. While this effect frequently has been observed in large arteries at micromolar concentrations, more recent studies have reported vasorelaxation of smaller resistance arteries at nanomolar (physiological) concentrations. The data from in vitro studies suggest that vasodilatory effect of testosterone is mediated via inhibition of Ca^{2+} influx into the smooth muscle cell. On the basis of the data reported to date, the exact mechanisms underlying this physiological effect of testosterone remain unclear and might involve activation of K^+ channels and antagonism of Ca^{2+} channels, are likely to be of nongenomic signaling, and might not require the endothelium. Taken as a whole, a considerable body of evidence suggests that

* Correspondence to: Oguzhan Yildiz MD PhD. Department of Pharmacology, Gulhane School of Medicine , 06018 Ankara, Turkey; Fax: +90 312 3042150 Tel: +90 312 3044766; E-mail: oyildiz@gata.edu.tr.

testosterone causes relaxation of the vasculature and it could have useful therapeutic roles in hypertension, angina, erectile dysfunction, prostatic ischemia, or other vascular dysfunctions.

INTRODUCTION

Globally, cardiovascular disease is the most common cause of mortality in the world despite aggressive control of known risk factors such as systemic hypertension, diabetes, dyslipidemia, and smoking. The life expectancy for men is significantly less than that for women and consistent observations have shown that the risk of developing coronary artery disease and hypertension is twice as much higher in men than in premenopausal women [1,2]. Hence, the possible role of sex steroids in this gender difference has stimulated current research on mechanism by which sex steroids affect heart disease and mortality. Historically, it was suggested that cardiovascular protection during the reproductive age in women was lost after menopause, and was recovered in postmenopausal women who receive estrogen replacement therapy [3]. These observations together have led to the dogmatic supposition that estrogen is beneficial and testosterone is detrimental to the cardiovascular system.

There is a plethora of evidence that estrogens may play an important cardiovascular protective role not only by means of long-term systemic effects, like those on serum lipid profile, but also by means of direct effects of vascular structure and function, such as inhibition of vascular growth and modulation of vascular tone [4,5]. However, the results from major trials concluded that postmenopausal estrogen supplementation might be associated with increased risk of cardiovascular disease rather that reducing the risk [6,7]. Estrogen administration to male survivors of myocardial infarction led excess coronary and thrombotic events [8]. In addition, initial randomized and placebo-controlled trials combining estrogen and progestin in menopausal women showed no cardiovascular benefits [6,7]. Hence, opinions on influence of hormones on cardiovascular disease have been seriously changed with more interest on identifying the role of endogenous testosterone on cardiovascular disease progression.

Testosterone is related to many aspects of cardiovascular health in men, but the controversy surrounding relationship between male hormone testosterone and cardiovascular disease still continues. Numerous clinical and epidemiological studies strongly suggest that a decline in testosterone levels predisposes men to increased risk of cardiovascular disease and mortality. Previously, Phillips et al. [9] reported that testosterone deficiency might increase cardiometabolic risk and disease. Shores et al. [10] reported that testosterone levels, which were determined twice, and survival rates decreased in male veterans over 5 years. Maggio et al. [11] noted that low level of testosterone in older men was an independent determinant of mortality in their 6-year CHIANTI study. Khaw et al. [12] studied the relationship between risk of all-cause mortality and testosterone in a nested case control study (EPIC-Norfolk) over 6–10 years with 11 606 men ranging in age between 40 and 79 years. The authors found an inverse relationship between endogenous testosterone concentrations and cardiovascular disease, as well as all-cause, related mortality. They also concluded that low testosterone levels could be a predictive marker for those men at high risk of cardiovascular disease.

Araujo et al. [13] reported that, with age adjustment, free testosterone was associated with respiratory mortality and low 5□-dihydrotestosterone and sex hormone binding globulin levels were associated with ischemic heart disease mortality. Laughlin et al. [14] followed 794 men for up to 20 years with an average of 11.8 years in the Rancho Bernardo study and they found that if men had total testosterone and bioavailable testosterone in the lowest quartile, independent of age and other cardiovascular mortality risks, they lived shorter than those with higher levels. This association was only attenuated by inflammatory cytokines such as IL-1β, IL-6, tumor necrosis factor alpha, and C-reactive protein. Additionally, a correlation between low serum testosterone and increased mortality risk was reported in male dialysis patients [15]. A weaker association was found in 1 686 men who were followed longitudinally for over 15 years in The Massachusetts Male Aging Study [13]. Several studies discuss the potential mechanisms pertaining to androgen deficiency and mortality. For example, reduced testosterone levels are associated with increased cardiovascular risk factors, such as increased fat mass [14,16-20] and subsequent cardiovascular disease, and even with death [12]. Smith et al. [21] followed more than 2 500 men for a mean of 16.5 years in the Caperhilly Study (South Wales), and they found that the cortisol/testosterone ratio had a specific relation to ischemic heart disease, which was possibly related to chronic illness, mediated through insulin resistance. In brief, endogenous testosterone concentrations are generally inversely related to cardiovascular risk factors in men, however the evidence is not conclusive regarding a generalized positive or negative effect of testosterone treatment.

Apart from sexual aspects including libido and erectile function, replacement therapy with testosterone might have beneficial vascular as well as metabolic effects. On the other hand, while some animal studies suggest that testosterone may exert deleterious effects on vascular wall by enhancing vascular tone through acute [22] or chronic mechanisms [23-25], accumulating evidence suggest that testosterone and other androgens may play an important roles in the acute regulation of vascular tone. In fact, numerous experimental studies have indicated that this rapid effect of testosterone has been observed at micromolar concentrations in a variety of large arteries (aorta, coronary and umbilical arteries) as well as small resistance arteries (mesenteric, pulmonary, prostatic and subcutenous) from several animal species (mouse, rat, rabbit, pig and dog) and human (coronary, umbilical, pulmonary, internal mammary, radial arteries in addition to human spermatic vein) [26-57] (Tables 1 and 2). Accordingly, previous clinical studies also suggested that acute intracoronary or intravenous infusion of testosterone provided rapid improvements in myocardial ischemia [58,59] and testosterone replacement therapy improved myocardial ischemia in patients with coronary artery disease, an effect presumably due to testosterone -induced coronary vasodilatation [60]. Moreover, in nonandrogen -deficient men with coronary artery disease, acute peripheral vein infusion of testosterone (2.3 mg, producing 100-fold elevation in blood testosterone concentration) increases flow-mediated dilatation (FMD, a noninvasive test for endothelial function) compared with placebo 1 h after administration, whereas a lower dose (23–46 μg, producing a 3-fold elevation) had no significant effect [61]. Another study in similar men reported that 12-wk treatment with oral testosterone undecanoate increased both FMD and nitrate-induced dilatation [62]. These reports together suggest maked vasodilating effect of testosterone, however some questions related to the mechanisms involved still arise.

Table 1. Studies suggesting that testosterone –induced vasodilatory effect is mediated by potassium channel opening action

Species	Preparation	Method	Type of potassium channel & other mechanisms	Reference
Rabbit	Coronary arteries and thoracic aorta	Isolated organ bath	K_{Ca} and/or K_V	Yue et al. (1995)
Dog	Coronary arteries	Simultaneous intravascular two-dimensional and Doppler ultrasound, in vivo	K_{ATP}	Chou et al. (1996)
Rat	Thoracic aorta	Isolated organ bath	K_{ATP}	Honda et al. (1999)
Rat	Thoracic aorta	Isolated organ bath	K_V	Ding & Stallone (2001)
Pig	Coronary arteries	Isolated organ bath and Patch-clamp studies	BK_{Ca}	Deenadayalu et al. (2001)
Rat	Mesenteric arterial bed	Isolated organ bath	BK_{Ca} and, in part NO and endothelium-dependent pathways.	Tep-areenan et al. (2002)
Rabbit	Coronary arteries	Isolated organ bath	K_V	Won et al. (2003)
Pig	Coronary arteries	Isolated organ bath and, simultaneous intravascular two-dimensional and Doppler ultrasound, in vivo	K_{ATP}	Hutchison et al (2005)
Human	Internal mammary artery	Isolated organ bath	BK_{Ca}	Yildiz et al (2005)
Human	Radial artery	Isolated organ bath	K_{ATP}	Seyrek et al (2007)
Rat	Thoracic aorta	Isolated organ bath	BK_{Ca} and, endothelium derived substance (PGI_2 etc.) induced mechanisms.	Unemoto et al. (2007)
Human	Umbilical artery	Isolated organ bath	BK_{Ca} and K_V	Cairraö et al (2008)
Human	human corporal smooth muscle	Whole-cell and cell-attached configuration patch-clamp techniques	BK_{Ca} and K_{ATP}	Han et al. (2008)
Human	Corpus cavernosum	Isolated organ bath	K_{ATP}	Yildiz et al (2009)
Human	Spermatic vein	Isolated organ bath	K_{ATP}	Seyrek et al (In press)

List of abbreviations: K_{ATP}=ATP-sensitive potassium channel; K_{Ca}=Calcium-activated potassium channel; K_v=Voltage-sensitive potassium channel; NO=nitric oxide; PGI_2= Prostacyclin.

Table 2. Studies suggesting that testosterone –induced vasodilatory effect is mediated by calcium channel antagonistic action

Species	Preparation	Method	Type of potassium channel & other mechanisms	Reference
Rat	Thoracic aorta	Isolated organ bath	VOCC/ROCC	Perusquia & Villalon (1999)
Pig	Coronary arteries	Isolated organ bath $^{45}Ca^{2+}$ influx, scintillation counter	VOCC/ROCC	Crews & Khalil (1999)
Rat	Thoracic aorta	Isolated organ bath $^{45}Ca^{2+}$ influx, scintillation counter	VOCC/ROCC	Crews & Khalil (1999)
Pig	Coronary artery smooth muscle cells	Single cell isolation and contractility study by using microscope Measurement of calcium influx by Fura-2 method	VOCC/ROCC	Murphy & Khalil (1999)
Rat	Coronary arteries	Automated wire myograph	VOCC/ROCC & some activity upon PKC	English et al. (2002)
Rat	Pulmonary arteries	Automated wire myograph	VOCC/ROCC & some activity upon PKC	Jones et al. (2002)
Rat	Aorta	Isolated organ bath	Inhibition of Ca influx modulated by endothelium-derived prostanoids & BK_{Ca} opening action	Tep-Areenan et al. (2003)
Rat	Coronary artery and thoracic aorta	Automated wire myograph Smooth muscle cell culture and flow cytometric analysis	VOCC/SOCC	Jones et al. (2004)
Human	A7r5 smooth muscle cell line and HEK 293 cells stably expressing either L- or T-type Ca^{2+} channels	Whole-cell patch-clamp technique	VOCC (L-type)	Scragg et al. (2004)

Table 2. Continued

Species	Preparation	Method	Type of potassium channel & other mechanisms	Reference
Human	Myometrium	Isolated organ bath Measurement of calcium influx by Fura-2 method	VOCC (L-type)	Perusquia et al. (2005)
Human	A7r5 smooth muscle cell line expressing L-type Ca^{2+} channels	Microfluorimetry	VOCC (L-type)	Hall et al. (2006)
Human	HEK293 cells expressing L-type Ca^{2+} channels	Whole-cell patch-clamp technique	VOCC (L-type)	Scragg et al. (2007)
Human	Umbilical artery	Isolated organ bath	VOCC	Perusquia et al. (2007)
Pig	Prostatic small arteries	Microvascular myograph	VOCC (L-type) and non-L-type Ca^{2+} channels	Navarro-Dorado (2008)
Rat	Thoracic aorta	Isolated organ bath Patch-clamp technique Measurement of calcium influx by Fura-2 method	VOCC (L-type) & cAMP production.	Montano et al. (2008)
Rabbit	Renal arteries	Isolated organ bath Western blotting	Modulation by muscular thromboxane A_2, partially mediation by endothelial prostacyclin, and blocking of extracellular Ca^{2+} entry.	Marrachelli et al. (2010)
Rat	Aorta A7r5 smooth muscle cell line expressing L-type Ca^{2+} channels	Isolated organ bath Cell Culture of Vascular Smooth Muscle Cells Whole Cell Patch clamp technique	VOCC (L-type)	Alvarez et al. (2010)

List of abbreviations: BK_{Ca}= Large conductance calcium-activated potassium channel; HEK293=Human Embryonic Kidney 293; PKC=Protein kinase C; ROCC= Receptor-operated calcium channel; SOCC=Store-operated calcium channel; VOCC=Voltage-operated calcium channel.

Mechanisms of Testosterone-Induced Vasodilation: Questions to Be Answered

Is Androgen Receptor (AR) Involved?

In the bloodstream, most of circulating testosterone is bound to serum proteins, mainly sex hormone binding protein and albumin. In target cells, testosterone can directly bind to the nuclear androgen receptor (AR), or it is converted to dihydrotestosterone, which binds in turn to the AR, that mediates the effects through modulation of transcription of the genes. These genomic effects are inhibited by transcription blockers. Certain other effects those are not mediated by transcription or protein synthesis and are referred as non-genomic effects. These effects have much faster onset and are noticed within a few minutes after intravenous infusion of androgens while the genomic effects are noticed after a gap of a few hours.

The initial experimental studies to make clear the mechanisms of testosterone-induced vasodilation focused on the degree of involvement the classical AR transcription mediated pathways [26,27,33,35,37]. In this regard, it has been shown that the vasodilating effect of testosterone is evident within minutes of testosterone application and it is maximal by approximately in 20 min, not hours. Therefore, it seems unlikely that testosterone-mediated vasodilatation would involve classical AR and genomic signalling pathway. Furthermore, additional substantial evidence is provided by findings that testosterone-induced vasodilation is not attenuated either by the covalent linkage of testosterone analogues to albumin, thus preventing endocytosis into the smooth muscle cell [33], or by pre-treatment with the AR blocker flutamide [26,27,33,35,37]. In addiditon, Ding and Stallone [33] proposed that the relative polarity of the testosterone molecule determined its own vasorelaxation efficacy. In our laboratory, we have tested the efficacy of various testosterone analogs in human internal mammary and radial arteries [44,49]. Testosterone propionate is the most polar, least lipid soluble and smallest molecular weight (MW: 344.5) among the other esterified testosterone analogs we have tested and it's the most efficacious. Thus, our data support the suggestion that testosterone-induced vasorelaxation is a non-genomic and structurally specific effect of the testosterone molecule, which is enhanced in more polar analogs that have a lower permeability to the vascular smooth muscle cell membrane [33]. In addition, blockers of transcription (e.g. actinomycin D) and translation (e.g. cycloheximide) fail to inhibit testosterone-induced vasodilation [22]. Besides, it has also been demonstrated that testosterone-mediated vasodilatation is maintained in vessels isolated from testicular feminized mice, which lack a functional AR [63]. Furthermore, other studies have shown the presence of the androgen receptor on the membrane of vascular smooth muscle cells [64,65], suggesting that the proposed non-genomic mechanism is likely.

Is Aromatization Involved?

Another important concept to be addressed is potential conversion of testosterone to estrogen, since estrogens cause acute and long-term vasodilation and testosterone and estrogens share the same biosynthetic pathway. However, this possibility has been excluded for several reasons. First, previous studies demonstrated that inhibition of aromatase activity does not prevent testosterone-mediated vasodilatation [22,26,34]. Second, estrogen receptor antagonists does not alter testosterone-induced vasodilation [27,40,48]. Moreover, non-aromatizable dihydrotestosterone triggered similar vasodilatation to testosterone [34,33,48,66]. In this regard, we used tamoxifen, an estrogen receptor antagonist and protein kinase C inhibitor, and letrozole, a non-steroidal aromatase inhibitor, to test the role of aromatisation in testosterone-induced vasodilation in human internal mammary artery. While tamoxifen inhibited testosterone- induced relaxation, letrozole had no effect, which indicated that aromatisation did not occur in human IMA, thus estrogen did not contribute on testosterone-induced relaxation. [67]. These findings together suggest that testosterone-induced vasorelaxation is not an indirect effect mediated by local conversion of testosterone to estrogen by vascular aromatase.

Is Endothelium Involved?

The vascular endothelium, a single cell layer separating blood and vascular smooth muscle, regulates vessel tone through release of vasoactive factors such as nitric oxide (NO), endothelins, and prostanoids [68]. Numerous studies have shown that high pharmacological concentrations of testosterone (10-100 μM) induce vasodilation in endothelium-denuded vessels, suggesting an endothelium-independent mechanism [26-28,30-35,37,38,66,69,70]. Accordingly, some of these studies have reported that testosterone mediated relaxation is not inhibited by indomethacin, an inhibitor of cyclo-oxygenase responsible for the synthesis of the cyclic endoperoxide from arachidonate [26-28,37]. Moreover, testosterone –induced vasodilation has been reported to be maintained in the presence of inhibitors of nitric oxide syntase (NOS) or guanylate cylase [26,28,34,37]. Previous studies also showed that testosterone had no effects on NOS activity in human and bovine aortic endothelial cells [70,71]. In contrast, other studies have demonstrated that testosterone-induced vasorelaxation from physiological to pharmacological concentrations (100 pM-10 μM) is significantly inhibited by by the removal of endothelium or treatment with NG-nitro-L-arginine methyester, in canine coronary artery [72], rat mesenteric arterial bed [35] and human pulmonary artery [73]. We have recently shown that testosterone –induced vasodilatation in human internal mammary and radial arteries is preserved in endothelial denuded vessels or in the presence of inhibitors of nitric oxide syntase or guanylate cylase [44,49]. Clearly, these data suggest the presence of an endothelium dependent mechanism at physiological concentrations of testosterone. However, vasorelaxation induced by higher pharmacological concentrations of testosterone in many in vitro studies appears to be endothelium independent. An alternative explanation may be that testosterone induced vasorelaxation, at lower physiological concentrations, may be related to neuronal NOS activation in vascular smooth muscle [74], since studies in porcine coronary and rat mesenteric arteries employed nonselective NOS inhibitor NG-nitro-L-arginine methyester and more recent studies clearly established testosterone, at lower physiological concentrations, induced formation of NO in vascular smooth muscle [34,75].

A Calcium Antagonistic or a Potassium - Channel Opening Action?

A variety of studies has demonstrated that the key mechanism underlying the vasodilatory action of testosterone is associated with the modulation of vascular smooth muscle ion channel function, particularly blockade of membrane Ca^{2+} influx via voltage-operated Ca^{2+} channels (VOCCs) and K^+ efflux involving voltage-gated, ATP-sensitive and large conductance Ca^{2+} -activated K^+ -channels (K_v, K_{ATP} and BK_{Ca} potassium channels in vascular smooth muscle, respectively) (Table 1 and 2).

A number of previous studies in isolated vessel preparations have supported the idea that testosterone and 5α-dihydrotestosterone acts as a Ca^{2+} channel antagonist, by inhibiting VOCCs [41,42,45,47,51,76,77]. In some studies, 5α-dihydrotestosterone (5α-DHT) was found to be more potent than testosterone in relaxing potassium chloride (KCl) -induced contractions. At nanomolar concentrations, testosterone was a powerful antagonist for L-type voltage-operated Ca^{2+} channels (L-VOCCs). The data showed that 5α-DHT–induced vasorelaxation might be attributed to its selective blockade on L-VOCCs, but testosteone-induced vasorelaxation involved concentration-dependent additional mechanisms involving L-VOCC antagonists at low concentrations and increasing Ca^{2+} influx and cyclic adenosine monophosphate production at high concentrations. It has previously been demonstrated that testosterone inhibits VOCCs in isolated rat pulmonary [37], and coronary arteries [36]. Similar data were reported in porcine coronary arteries in which testosterone induced vasodilation [45]. Similarly, Cairrao et al. [52] demonstrated that testosterone induced vasodilation of human umbilical arteries via a nongenomic-dependent mechanism. Moreover, the direct vasodilatory effect of testosterone on vascular smooth muscle cells has also been examined in electrophysiological experiments, which have confirmed the findings from vascular functional studies. Scragg et al. [41,47] have employed whole-cell patch clamp recordings under non-physiological and physiological conditions in human embryonic kidney-293 cells and they have shown that testosterone inhibits L-type Ca^{2+} channels. In recent study, Hall et al. [45] have employed fluorometric recordings and they have provided evidence that testosterone can block both native and recombinant L-type voltage-gated Ca^{2+} channels with IC_{50} values (the concentration that provides 50% inhibition of maximal effect) within or close to levels of circulating testosterone concentrations in A7r5 cells. VOCC inhibition by testosterone is rapid (within 2 minutes), making it unlikely to be mediated through a genomic effect. Hall et al. [45] have also observed that testosterone and nifedipine, a L-type Ca^{2+} channel blocker, share common molecular requirements for the inhibition of VOCCs and they have proposed that some of the beneficial cardiovascular effects of testosterone arise from its ability to act like a dihydropyridine antihypertensive to suppress Ca^{2+} entry and so promote vasodilation. Although VOCC function may differ in cultured cell lines, Montano et al. [51] recently confirmed concentration -dependent inhibition of VOCC by testosterone in primary cultured and freshly dissociated primary cultures. Testosterone exhibits a greater potency than nifedipine to antagonize VOCCs at physiological to supraphysiological concentrations (10 nM-1 μM). However, testosterone may act as an antagonist on VOCCs, increasing Ca^{2+} influx through VOCCs, at pharmacological concentrations (higher than 1 μM) [51]. Accordingly, vasoconstrictor effect of high concentrations of testosterone has been reported [22]. Testosterone, at pharmacological concentrations, may induce vasodilation of blood vessels via inhibition of T-type Ca^{2+} currents [41,45], receptor -operated Ca^{2+} channels [29,30,32], as well as store -operated Ca^{2+} channels [64]. In our laboratory, we have observed that testosterone at concentrations of 100 μM and higher inhibited calcium chloride – induced contractions in human IMA [44]. Consistent with our observation, it has been recently demonstrated that testosterone, at high concentrations, inhibits Ca^{2+} influx in rat aorta [38].

A number of studies have provided evidence of a modulatory role for testosterone upon potassium channel function. Chou et al. [27] have demonstrated that glibenclamide, K_{ATP} channel inhibitor, reduces vasorelaxation to testosterone in dog coronary artery. On the other hand, Honda et al. [28] have shown that tetraethylammonium, a K_{Ca} channel inhibitor, inhibited testosterone-induced vasorelaxation in aortae from spontaneously hypertensive rats. Deenadayalu et al. [34] have also demonstrated that vasorelaxation of porcine coronary artery to testosterone is inhibited by iberiotoxin, a highly selective BK_{Ca} channel inhibitor. In addition, a patch-clamp study by Deenadayalu et al. [34] has shown that testosterone opens BK_{Ca} channels in porcine coronary smooth muscle cells. Testosterone-induced opening of BK_{Ca} channels is suggested to involve intracellular messengers [33,34]. On the other hand, Ding and Stallone [33] have demonstrated that neither incubation with glibenclamide nor tetraetylammonium (TEA), a non-selective K^+ channel inhibitor, has any effect on the vasodilatory response to testosterone in rat thoracic aorta. Instead, they have shown that incubation with 4-aminopyridine (4-AP), a K_V channel inhibitor, significantly reduces vasorelaxation to testosterone, and they have therefore proposed that testosterone acts *via* K_V channel opening action. In our study, we have also observed an inhibitory effect of TEA, but not glibenclamide and 4-AP, on vasorelaxation to testosterone, suggesting that testosterone – mediated vasodilatation may occur *via* activation of BK_{Ca} channels in human internal mammary artery [44]. However in human radial artery and corpus cavernosum, glibenclamide, but no other K^+ channel inhibitors, reduced vasorelaxation to testosterone, suggesting involvement of K_{ATP} channels [47,54].

We have observed less testosterone relaxation after potassium chloride (KCl) - precontraction compared to that after prostaglandin $F_{2\alpha}$ ($PGF_{2\alpha}$) precontraction in human internal mammary artery [44]. Previously, Deenadayalu et al. [34] reported a decrease in the response to testosterone under similar conditions with our study in human internal mammary artery [44], namely a significant reduction in the efficacy of testosterone in vessels precontracted with KCl compared to $PGF_{2\alpha}$. A possible explanation of these findings may be that the potassium channel function which is compromised in conjunction with the vasodilatory efficacy of testosterone. An alternative explanation of the difference in dilatory action testosterone may be that the types of calcium channels involved may be different, and the involvement of these channels in a testosterone-relaxant mechanism is dependent on the pathways activated by the contractile agent used. Actually, $PGF_{2\alpha}$ acts primarily at the prostanoid receptors gated directly to receptor-operated calcium channels (ROCCs) [78]. This receptor stimulation also results in phosphatidylinositol 4,5 bisphosphate hydrolysis [79] with resultant generation of inositol triphospate, which triggers calcium release from the intracellular stores [80]. The high extracellular K^+ gradient generated by milimolar KCl triggers membrane depolarization with subsequent activation of VOCCs. The variance in the testosterone –induced dilatation following preconconstiction with KCl and $PGF_{2\alpha}$, could be due to a differing inhibitory efficiacy of testosterone upon ROCCs and VOCCs.

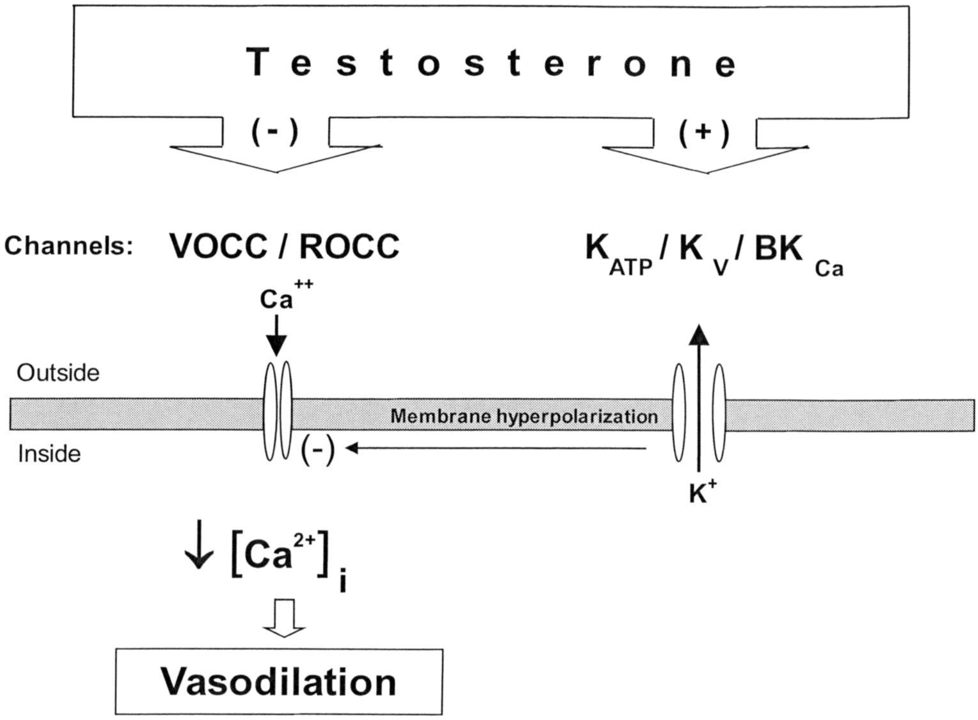

Figure 1. Proposed model for actions of testosterone. The opening of K^+ channels in the cell membrane of smooth muscle cells of blood vessels by testosterone increases K^+ efflux, which causes membrane potential hyperpolarization. This closes voltage operated calcium channels (VOCCs), decreasing Ca^{2+} entry, which leads to vasodilation. K_{ATP}: ATP-sensitive K^+ channel, BK_{Ca}: large-conductance Ca^{2+} -activated K^+ channel, K_V: a voltage-gated K^+ channel.

There is a complex-mixture of vessel-type dependent mechanisms reported about the type of the K^+ channel involved in the vasodilatory action of testosterone. Testosterone acts *via* BK_{Ca} and K_V channel opening action in rabbit, dog and pig coronary conduit arteries. However, testosterone -induced vasodilation occurs *via* K_{ATP} channel opening action in dog coronary resistance arteries [26,27,34]. Accordingly, we have recently shown that testosterone acts by way of the BK_{Ca} channel opening action in a human conduit artery, the internal mammary artery, [44]. However, testosterone -induced vasodilation occurs *via* K_{ATP} channel opening action in human radial artery similar with human corpus cavernosum [54] similar to rabbit coronary resistance arteries [26]. Actually, the radial artery shows resistance vessel characteristics because of the elastomuscular wall structure and small diameter. Therefore, we may suggest that testosterone preferentially stimulates the K_V and K_{Ca} channels in large conductance vessels, and the K_{ATP} channel in small resistance vessels. In fact, there are some differences in the vascular reactivity between large conductance and small resistance arteries. For example, it was reported that adenosine, a metabolic regulator of coronary blood flow (probably via activating K_{ATP} channels and inhibiting L-type Ca^{2+} current, had no effect on the action potential in the large coronary artery, but preferentially blocked the action potential in the small coronary artery [81]. Similarly, the coronary dilating actions of a K_{ATP} channel opening drug, levcromakalim, were heterogeneous, and it was more sensitive in small resistant coronary arteries [82]. It was also reported that the resting tone of large conductance vessels was little affected by glibenclamide [83], whereas that of small resistance vessels was affected. Therefore, the tone of the small vessels is likely to be regulated by the glibenclamide-sensitive K_{ATP} channel [84].

On the basis of the data reported to date, the exact mechanisms underlying the physiological effect of testosterone on vascular reactivity remain unclear and might involve activation of K^+ channels and antagonism of Ca^{2+} channels, are likely to be of nongenomic signaling, and might not require the endothelium. As noted above, the direct vasodilatory effect of testosterone on vascular smooth muscle cells has also been examined in electrophysiological experiments, which have confirmed the findings from vascular functional studies. As a direct evidence from patch-clamp study, Deenadayalu et al. [34] convincingly demonstrated that 200 nM testosterone-very dramatically activated BK_{Ca} channels, increasing the open probability by more 10 fold. Similarly, in rat mesenteric myocytes, 100 nM testosterone markedly activated K_v channels. In both of these studies, the selective blockade of BK_{Ca} or K_v channels markedly inhibited testosterone-induced increase in K^+ channel function [75]. On the other hand, the studies of Hall et al., Scragg et al. and Montano et al. [45,47,51] have provided electrophysiolgical evidence for a direct calcium antagonistic effect of testosterone. Indeed, either mechanism, calcium antagonistic or potassium channel opening actions, would allow vasodilation due to reduced Ca^{2+} influx through calcium channels (Figure 1).

Do Some Potential Factors Influence Testosterone Responses?

An important point of the previous in vitro studies which should be addressed is that high pharmacological concentrations of testosterone (in the micromolar levels) are required to elicit vasodilation. The physiological concentrations of testosterone are in range of 100 pM-100 nM, whereas pharmacological concentrations are higher than 100 nM. Most of the studies cited above were carried out in isolated vessel preparations; this could account for the effects of testosterone occurring only at supraphysiological concentrations (in the micromolar levels). An explanation of the discrepancy with previous studies in isolated vessels may be a consequence of access to smooth muscle ion channels, which is presumably restricted in more intact preparations lacking their natural blood supply as the lipophilic testosterone would need to cross some barriers before reaching its presumed target on smooth muscle cells. Alternatively, as a result of impaired delivery of the testosterone molecule or binding to various proteins, there may be a concentration gradient from the perfusate down to the cell membrane.

The latency for the vasodilating effect of testosterone is another point of the previous studies which should be looked up. In most of the mechanistic studies cited in this chapter, free testosterone analogues were used, and the vasodilatory action of testosterone was rapid, occuring within minutes. It has been demonstrated that the covalent linkage of testosterone analogues to a macromolecule, such as albumin, has no effect upon the timescale and magnitude of testosterone -induced vasodilatory response [33]. Since the conjugation of testosterone to albumin eliminates the permeability of testosterone to the cell membrane, and thereby, these findings again suggest a non-genomic action.

It should be noted that way of solving and delivering testosterone is of great importance. Different solvents in different concentrations have been used in various studies in humans and animals (e.g. ethanol and dimethysulphoxide). Solvents have unselective effects on ion channel activity [85], within miliseconds, which could interfere with selective actions of testosterone. However, no significant relaxant effect of final concentrations of the solvents has been reported in previous studies [26-28,33,35,37,38,60,69]. Since ethanol might induce relaxation itself we did not let the final ethanol concentration in the bath to exceed 1 % (v/v) in our studies [44,49,54,57,86-88].

Clinical Relevance of Testosterone-Induced Vasodilation

Testosterone-induced vasodilation in isolated blood vessels seem to occur at high pharmacological concentrations of testosterone (in the micromolar levels), since there are some methodological limitations related to in vitro isolated blood vessel experiments, i.e. restricted access of testosterone to smooth muscle ion channels, and concentration gradient from the perfusate down to the cell membrane due to impaired delivery of testosterone or binding to various proteins. Therefore, clinical significance and physiological relevance of this acute, non-genomic effect should be considered carefully. In previous in vitro studies, pharmacological concentrations of testosterone have been shown to cause a concentration dependent vasodilation, whereas physiological concentrations of testosterone have been reported to be effective in more recent mechanistic studies, which convincingly suggest the physiological significance of testosterone-induced vasodilation.

Testosterone-Induced Vasodilation and Coronary Artery Disease

Early studies indicating a vasodilatory effect of testosterone on isolated coronary artery [26] led further investigations into the effects of testosterone on the coronary circulation in both animals and humans. In anaesthetised animals, short term, relatively high concentrations of testosterone administration has induced vasodilation and increase in blood flow in coronary arteries, mediated at least in part by the dilator endothelium derived nitric oxide [27]. Likewise, Webb et al. [59] have reported that when physiological concentrations testosterone is instilled into the left coronary artery for short term, vasodilation ensues and coronary flow increases in men with coronary artery disease, but an endothelium-independent effect is involved. Moreover, acute administration of intravenous testosterone improves exercise tolerance and reduces angina threshold in men with coronary artery disease [58,89]. These effects were observed using supraphysiological doses, but chronic administration of low physiological replacement doses of testosterone over three months in men with chronic stable angina significantly improved exercise tolerance and angina threshold [60]. Interestingly there was no effect on angina symptoms in this and another longer-term study of testosterone treatment [60,90], however a recent study have showed that number of angina attacks and ischemic episodes reduces in men with coronary artery disease taking longer-term testosterone therapy [91]. Oral testosterone replacement in men with established coronary artery disease has a beneficial effect on baseline endothelial dysfunction [62]. In addition, epidemiological studies have shown an independent inverse relationship between endogenous testosterone concentrations and arterial stiffness, an independent predictor of coronary artery disease [92,93]. Epidemiological studies have established the inverse relationship between endogenous testosterone concentrations and extent of coronary atheroma as well [9]. Taken together, there is convincing evidence that endogenous testosterone concentrations affect risk factors for coronary artery disease and extent of coronary artery disease. In addition, testosterone has some effects directly on the blood vessel wall beyond the reproductive system of men. It would be wrong to suggest that testosterone treatment is a panacea for men with coronary artery disease, however prime candidates for benefiting from testosterone replacement therapy may be the men with coronary artery disease who are hypogonadal or have testosterone concentrations at or below the normal range [94].

Testosterone-Induced Vasodilation and Hypertension

From puberty, blood pressure is higher in men than women of a similar age [95]. Khaw et al. [2] and Fogari et al. [96] demonstrated an inverse relationship between endogenous testosterone concentrations and blood pressure independent of age and body mass index. In addition, several other clinical studies strongly demonstrated that serum testosterone levels are reduced in both hypertensive men and women [2,97-99] and testosterone replacement in hypogonadal men reduces blood pressure [100-103]. However, studies describing treatment effects of testosterone in hypertensive men are lacking. In addiditon, studies in animals suggest detrimental effects. Testosterone treatment exacerbates hypertension reduces pressure-natriuresis in male spontaneous hypertensive rats and testosterone contributed to development of hypertension and renal injury, proposed to be via up-regulation in male salt sensitive rats [104,105]. The relationship between hypertension and testosterone is complex in relationship to cardiovascular risk because multiple other risk factors are involved. As stated in introduction section of this chapter, endogenous testosterone concentrations are generally inversely related to coronary artery risk factors in men. Future studies to show whether there is a similar association between low testosterone levels and hypertension which might clarify treatment effects of testosterone in hypertensive men would be of interest.

Testosterone-Induced Vasodilation and Erectile Dysfunction

Penile erection is a vascular (hydraulic) three-step phenomenon which involves increased arterial inflow, sinusoidal smooth muscle relaxation and decreased venous drainage controlled by upper centres, as well as by peripheral regulatory mechanisms. On the basis of evidence derived from laboratory animal studies and clinical data, testosterone has a major influence on erectile function through the regulation of both the central and the peripheral steps of erection. At the peripheral level, the involved mechanisms are similar to those of the other vascular beds, and consist of a complex coordination involving adrenergic/cholinergic systems, endothelins, smooth muscle myosin phosphorilation, RhoA/Rho-kinase, as well as the recently identified sphingosine-1-phosphate signaling pathways [106]. The most important and specific pathway underlying the penile erection is nonadrenergic/ noncholinergic signaling, which, through the release of nitric oxide from the endothelium, leads to an intracellular accumulation of cyclic guanosine monophosphate, the formation and degradation of which are under testosterone control. We have recently shown that testosterone might induce relaxation in human corpus cavernosum by activation of smooth muscle K_{ATP} channels [54]. This finding suggests that testosterone, in addition to its known endothelial action, might regulate erectile function locally by its action on the smooth muscle of the human corpus cavernosum. According to meta-analysis by Isidori et al., different thresholds for sexual desire and erectile function are present in humans, the former being quite higher than the latter [107]. In humans, testosterone deficiency determines a sequence of molecular penile events leading to reduced capacity of smooth muscle and endothelial cells to relaxation as well as to increased sensitivity to contractile factors, that is, α-adrenergic agonists and deficiency of NO-induced relaxation during sexual stimulus. Serial recent studies in human have suggest that testosterone may directly control the expression and activity of phosphodiestease5 (PDE5) in human corpus cavernosum, [108,109], as it does nitric oxide synthase (NOS) [108,110,111], so that in some selected patients, that is, total-testosterone < 10 nmol/L and/or free-testosterone below 200 nmol/L, androgen supplementation may improve therapeutic efficacy to PDE5 [112]. In men with hypogonadotropic hypogonadism, the administrationof L-arginine alone did not result in an increased nitric oxide (NO) production, but the administration of L-arginine and testosterone markedly enhanced NO production in these men. Whilst some clinicians and researchers are still dubious of the influence of testosterone on penile erection, further studies are essential to understand these molecular control mechanisms as well as the influence that testosterone has on these pathways and to fully realise the roles of testosterone in erectile functions and to enhance the discovery of novel targets for drug development to treat erectile dysfunction.

Testosterone-Induced Vasodilation and Gestational Hypertension

Vasoconstriction of the umbilical cord results in growth retardation and intrauterine death of the fetus. Hence, the capability of testosterone to produce a nongenomic vasorelaxation in umbilical artery may be physiologically relevant in maintaining a sustained vasodilation in the fetoplacental circulation. Previously, we have found that testosterone has no vasodilator effect on human umbilical artery [86]. However, a more recent study has decribed relaxant effect of testosterone, 5-reduced testosterone metabolites and progestins on vascular tone of the human umbilical artery, and testosterone and its metabolites are more potent than progestins, with 5β-dihydrotestosterone being the most potent one [48]. This finding may represent another potential physiological role for the vascular effects of testosterone, which could contribute to the regulation of fetoplacental blood flow, one of the most important rate-limiting factors for normal fetal growth. Indeed, this suggestion is consistent with previous findings showing markedly increased plasma levels of dehydroepiandrosterone, androstenedione, and testosterone [113], which are produced in the maternoplacental unit [114] and have an important uterine relaxing effect throughout pregnancy [48,115]. Thus, it is reasonable to propose that a low level of testosterone and its 5-reduced metabolites, particularly 5-dihydrotestosterone, during pregnancy could partly contribute to the development of preeclamsia/eclamsia. Hence, exogenously administered vasorelaxing steroids, particularly 5-dihydrotestosterone, may be therapeutically relevant in the treatment of gestational hypertension and as well as for the endothelial dysfunction described in the maternal and fetoplacental circulation. In addition, testosterone induces similar vasorelaxation in isolated vessels from women [44,48,52,73], and the female vasculature is also acutely sensitive to androgen receptor-independent vasodilation induced by 5-dihydrotestosterone [48], which also increases its potential for use as a safe nongenomic treatment for hypertension in women.

Testosterone-Induced Vasodilation and Varicocele

In our recent study, we used human internal spermatic vein specimens from patients undergoing grade 0 and 1 varicocele operation [57,88]. We have found that direct vasodilating effect induced by testosterone occurs *via* activation of K_{ATP} channels in human internal spermatic vein [57]. We have also found that vasodilator effect of cumulative concentrations of testosterone (0.1 -300 μM) is significantly higher in patients with grade 0 and 1 than grades 2 to 3 varicocele [88]. A possible mechanism of this decrease in vasodilatory effect of testosterone in high grades may be down-regulation of androgen receptors, since testosterone concentrations are higher in internal spermatic veins than those in peripheral veins [87,116-118]. As reported in the previous studies, testosterone concentrations may increase 30 times higher than physiological concentrations in ISV of patients with varicocele and it is released into internal spermatic vein in a pulsatile fashion. These variable and high concentrations of testosterone may contribute to the pathophysiology of varicocele. The sudden increase in the prevalance of varicocele at puberty also supports the contributory role of testosterone.

Conclusion

In recent years there has been dramatic increase in research into effects of testosterone on the cardiovascular system. Several lines of evidence indicate that testosterone can exert acute vasorelaxing effects. Clearly all of the studies conducted into determining the vasodilatory mechanism of action of testosterone can be interpreted as being independent of the classical androgen receptor which mediates its effects genomically, suggesting a non-genomic action. Furthermore, it should be noted that numerous studies have shown that high pharmacological concentrations of testosterone (10-100 μM) induce vasodilation in endothelium-denuded vessels, suggesting that vasodilatory action of testosterone is independent of the endothelium. Only a few studies suggest the presence of endothelium- dependent and nitric oxide -mediated vasodilation at lower physiological concentrations of testosterone. Accumulating evidence suggests that the key mechanism behind the vasodilatory action of testosterone is through either inactivation of L type Ca^{2+} channels or activation of K_{ATP}, K_V and/or BK_{Ca} channels in vascular muscle cell membrane. Electrophysiological experiments have confirmed the findings from vascular functional studies. Deenadayalu et al. [34] convincingly demonstrated that testosterone activated BK_{Ca} channels in rat coronarty arteries by patch-clamp technique. Similarly, testosterone, as shown by patch clamp method, markedly activated K_v channels in rat mesenteric myocytes [75]. However, electrophysiolgical evidence for a direct calcium antagonistic effect of testosterone has also been reported [45,47,51]. Indeed, testosterone-induced vasodilation in isolated blood vessels in most studies occurs at pharmacological concentrations due to methodological limitations inherent to in vitro studies. However, testosterone acts at nanomolar (physiological) concentrations to inhibit L type Ca^{2+} channels or to open K^+ channels in recent electrophysiological (patch clamp) experiments [34,45,47,51,75]. These findings strongly suggest that testosterone-induced vasodilation is a physiologically relevant phenomenon. This suggestion is supported by several clinical studies that serum testosterone levels are reduced in both hypertensive men and women [2,97-99] and testosterone replacement in hypogonadal men reduces blood pressure [100-103]. Moreover, there is increasing evidence that testosterone replacement therapy significantly improves cardiovascular and metabolic functions in hypogonadal aging men [2,9,100,102,119]. In this regard, it is well known that the serum levels of testosterone components decline markedly with increasing age in otherwise normal men [120]; likewise, plasma testosterone concentrations are lower in men with cardiovascular disease [121].

The metabolism of testosterone in various target tissues yields a number of compounds with biological relevance. Apart from its aromatization, testosterone can also be converted to non aromatizable 5-reduced dihydro-metabolites which are capable of causing vascular relaxation [29,74,122]. Among non aromatizable dihidro-metabolites of testosterone, 5α-DHT exhibits only moderate vasodilator activity but potent genomic androgenic effects. In marked contrast, its isomer 5β-DHT is a higly efficacious and potent vasodilator at nanomolar to micromolar concentrations but is devoid of androgenic and estrogenic side effects. Hence, testosterone replacement therapy with vasoselective testosterone metabolites such as 5β-DHT, which exhibit little or no action on the androgen receptor, may be an emerging therapeutic option to prevent vascular dysfunction such as hypertension, erectile dysfunction, and prostatic ischemia in aging men [74].

Taken as a whole, there has been significant increase in our understanding of the role of testosterone in cardiovascular disease. Numerous reports provide evidence for the marked vasodilating effect induced by testosterone. The variance in the species and the vascular preparations used may contribute to the discrepancy between the studies in proposing a vasodilatory mechanism for testosterone. In this regard, further studies especially in different human vascular preparations and with cellular patch-clamp techniques, are essential to understand the exact mechanism of the effect testosterone and fully realize its therapeutic implications in cardiovascular diseases.

REFERENCES

[1] Messerli FH, Garavaglia GE, Schmieder RE, Sundgaard-Riise K, Nunez BD, Amodeo C. Disparate cardiovascular findings in men and women with essential hypertension. *Ann Intern Med.* 1987 Aug;107(2):158-61.

[2] Khaw KT, Barrett-Connor E. Blood pressure and endogenous testosterone in men: an inverse relationship. *J Hypertens.* 1988 Apr;6(4):329-32.

[3] Stampfer MJ, Colditz GA, Willett WC, Manson JE, Rosner B, Speizer FE, Hennekens CH. Postmenopausal estrogen therapy and cardiovascular disease. Ten-year follow-up from the nurses' health study. *N Engl J Med.* 1991 Sep 12;325(11):756-62.

[4] Simoncini T, Genazzani AR. Non-genomic actions of sex steroid hormones. *Eur J Endocrinol.* 2003 Mar;148(3):281-92. Review..

[5] Cho JJ, Cadet P, Salamon E, Mantione K, Stefano GB. The nongenomic protective effects of estrogen on the male cardiovascular system: clinical and therapeutic implications in aging men. *Med Sci Monit.* 2003 Mar;9(3):RA63-8. Review.

[6] Hulley S, Grady D, Bush T, Furberg C, Herrington D, Riggs B, Vittinghoff E. Randomized trial of estrogen plus progestin for secondary prevention of coronary heart disease in postmenopausal women. Heart and Estrogen/progestin Replacement Study (HERS) Research Group. *JAMA.* 1998 Aug 19;280(7):605-13.

[7] Rossouw JE, Anderson GL, Prentice RL, LaCroix AZ, Kooperberg C, Stefanick ML, Jackson RD, Beresford SA, Howard BV, Johnson KC, Kotchen JM, Ockene J; Writing Group for the Women's Health Initiative Investigators. Risks and benefits of estrogen plus progestin in healthy postmenopausal women: principal results From the Women's Health Initiative randomized controlled trial. *JAMA*. 2002 Jul 17;288(3):321-33.

[8] Stamler J. Prevention of atherosclerotic coronary heart disease by change of diet and mode of life. *Ther Umsch.* 1970 Mar;27(3):133-44.

[9] Phillips GB, Pinkernell BH, Jing TY. The association of hypotestosteronemia with coronary artery disease in men. *Arterioscler Thromb.* 1994 May;14(5):701-6

[10] Shores MM, Matsumoto AM, Sloan KL, Kivlahan DR. Low serum testosterone and mortality in male veterans. *Arch Intern Med.* 2006 Aug 14-28;166(15):1660-5.

[11] Maggio M, Lauretani F, Ceda GP, Bandinelli S, Ling SM, Metter EJ, Artoni A, Carassale L, Cazzato A, Ceresini G, Guralnik JM, Basaria S, Valenti G, Ferrucci L. Relationship between low levels of anabolic hormones and 6-year mortality in older men: the aging in the Chianti Area (InCHIANTI) study. *Arch Intern Med.* 2007 Nov 12;167(20):2249-54.

[12] Khaw KT, Dowsett M, Folkerd E, Bingham S, Wareham N, Luben R, Welch A, Day N. Endogenous testosterone and mortality due to all causes, cardiovascular disease, and cancer in men: European prospective investigation into cancer in Norfolk (EPIC-Norfolk) Prospective Population Study. *Circulation.* 2007 Dec 4;116(23):2694-701.

[13] Araujo AB, Kupelian V, Page ST, Handelsman DJ, Bremner WJ, McKinlay JB. Sex steroids and all-cause and cause-specific mortality in men. *Arch Intern Med.* 2007 Jun 25;167(12):1252-60.

[14] Laughlin GA, Barrett-Connor E, Bergstrom J. Low serum testosterone and mortality in older men. *J Clin Endocrinol Metab.* 2008 Jan;93(1):68-75. Epub 2007 Oct 2.

[15] Carrero JJ, Qureshi AR, Parini P, Arver S, Lindholm B, Bárány P, Heimbürger O, Stenvinkel P. Low serum testosterone increases mortality risk among male dialysis patients. *J Am Soc Nephrol.* 2009 Mar;20(3):613-20. Epub 2009 Jan 14.

[16] Basaria S, Dobs AS. Hypogonadism and androgen replacement therapy in elderly men. *Am J Med.* 2001 May;110(7):563-72. Review.

[17] Basaria S, Dobs AS. Testosterone making an entry into the cardiometabolic world. *Circulation.* 2007 Dec 4;116(23):2658-61.

[18] Basaria S. Androgen deprivation therapy, insulin resistance, and cardiovascular mortality: an inconvenient truth. *J Androl.* 2008 Sep-Oct;29(5):534-9.

[19] Montagnana M, Lippi G. Relationship between serum testosterone and cardiovascular risk profile in the general population. *Arch Intern Med.* 2008 Jun 23;168(12):1350-1

[20] Shahani S, Braga-Basaria M, Basaria S. Androgen deprivation therapy in prostate cancer and metabolic risk for atherosclerosis. *J Clin Endocrinol Metab.* 2008 Jun;93(6):2042-9.

[21] Smith GD, Ben-Shlomo Y, Beswick A, Yarnell J, Lightman S, Elwood P. Cortisol, testosterone, and coronary heart disease: prospective evidence from the Caerphilly study. *Circulation.* 2005 Jul 19;112(3):332-40.

[22] Teoh H, Quan A, Leung SW, Man RY. Differential effects of 17beta-estradiol and testosterone on the contractile responses of porcine coronary arteries. *Br J Pharmacol.* 2000 Apr;129(7):1301-8.

[23] Herman SM, Robinson JT, McCredie RJ, Adams MR, Boyer MJ, Celermajer DS. Androgen deprivation is associated with enhanced endothelium-dependent dilatation in adult men. *Arterioscler Thromb Vasc Biol.* 1997 Oct;17(10):2004-9.

[24] McCredie RJ, McCrohon JA, Turner L, Griffiths KA, Handelsman DJ, Celermajer DS. Vascular reactivity is impaired in genetic females taking high-dose androgens. *J Am Coll Cardiol.* 1998 Nov;32(5):1331-5.

[25] Schrör K, Morinelli TA, Masuda A, Matsuda K, Mathur RS, Halushka PV. Testosterone treatment enhances thromboxane A2 mimetic induced coronary artery vasoconstriction in guinea pigs. *Eur J Clin Invest.* 1994 Feb;24 Suppl 1:50-2.

[26] Yue P, Chatterjee K, Beale C, Poole-Wilson PA, Collins P. Testosterone relaxes rabbit coronary arteries and aorta. *Circulation.* 1995 Feb 15;91(4):1154-60

[27] Chou TM, Sudhir K, Hutchison SJ, Ko E, Amidon TM, Collins P, Chatterjee K. Testosterone induces dilation of canine coronary conductance and resistance arteries in vivo. *Circulation.* 1996 Nov 15;94(10):2614-9.

[28] Honda H, Unemoto T, Kogo H. Different mechanisms for testosterone-induced relaxation of aorta between normotensive and spontaneously hypertensive rats. *Hypertension.* 1999 Dec;34(6):1232-6.

[29] Perusquia M, Villalón CM. Possible role of Ca2+ channels in the vasodilating effect of 5beta-dihydrotestosterone in rat aorta. *Eur J Pharmacol.* 1999 Apr 29;371(2-3):169-78.

[30] Crews JK, Khalil RA. Antagonistic effects of 17 beta-estradiol, progesterone, and testosterone on Ca2+ entry mechanisms of coronary vasoconstriction. *Arterioscler Thromb Vasc Biol.* 1999 Apr;19(4):1034-40.

[31] Crews JK, Khalil RA. Gender-specific inhibition of Ca^{2+} entry mechanisms of arterial vasoconstriction by sex hormones. *Clin Exp Pharmacol Physiol.* 1999 Sep;26(9):707-15.

[32] Murphy JG, Khalil RA. Decreased [Ca(2+)](i) during inhibition of coronary smooth muscle contraction by 17beta-estradiol, progesterone, and testosterone. *J Pharmacol Exp Ther.* 1999 Oct;291(1):44-52..

[33] Ding AQ, Stallone JN. Testosterone-induced relaxation of rat aorta is androgen structure specific and involves K+ channel activation. *J Appl Physiol.* 2001 Dec;91(6):2742-50

[34] Deenadayalu VP, White RE, Stallone JN, Gao X, Garcia AJ. Testosterone relaxes coronary arteries by opening the large-conductance, calcium-activated potassium channel. *Am J Physiol Heart Circ Physiol.* 2001 Oct;281(4):H1720-7

[35] Tep-areenan P, Kendall DA, Randall MD. Testosterone-induced vasorelaxation in the rat mesenteric arterial bed is mediated predominantly via potassium channels. *Br J Pharmacol.* 2002 Feb;135(3):735-40.

[36] English KM, Jones RD, Jones TH, Morice AH, Channer KS. Testosterone acts as a coronary vasodilator by a calcium antagonistic action. *J Endocrinol Invest.* 2002 May;25(5):455-8.

[37] Jones RD, English KM, Pugh PJ, Morice AH, Jones TH, Channer KS. Pulmonary vasodilatory action of testosterone: evidence of a calcium antagonistic action. *J Cardiovasc Pharmacol.* 2002 Jun;39(6):814-23.

[38] Tep-areenan P, Kendall DA, Randall MD. Mechanisms of vasorelaxation to testosterone in the rat aorta. *Eur J Pharmacol.* 2003 Mar 28;465(1-2):125-32.

[39] Won E, Won J, Kwon S, Lee Y, Nam T, Ahn D. Testosterone causes simultaneous decrease of [Ca2+]I and tension in rabbit coronary arteries: by opening voltage dependent potassium channels. *Yonsei Med J.* 2003 Dec 30;44(6):1027-33.

[40] Jones RD, English KM, Jones TH, Channer KS. Testosterone-induced coronary vasodilatation occurs via a non-genomic mechanism: evidence of a direct calcium antagonism action. *Clin Sci (Lond).* 2004 Aug;107(2):149-58

[41] Scragg JL, Jones RD, Channer KS, Jones TH, Peers C. Testosterone is a potent inhibitor of L-type Ca(2+) channels. *Biochem Biophys Res Commun.* 2004 May 28;318(2):503-6

[42] Perusquia M, Navarrete E, Jasso-Kamel J, Montaño LM. Androgens induce relaxation of contractile activity in pregnant human myometrium at term: a nongenomic action on L-type calcium channels. *Biol Reprod.* 2005 Aug;73(2):214-21.

[43] Hutchison SJ, Browne AE, Ko E, Chou TM, Zellner C, Komesaroff PA, Chatterjee K, Sudhir K. Dehydroepiandrosterone sulfate induces acute vasodilation of porcine coronary arteries in vitro and in vivo. *J Cardiovasc Pharmacol.* 2005 Sep;46(3):325-32.

[44] Yildiz O, Seyrek M, Gul H, Un I, Yildirim V, Ozal E, Uzun M, Bolu E. Testosterone relaxes human internal mammary artery in vitro. *J Cardiovasc Pharmacol.* 2005 Jun;45(6):580-5.

[45] Hall J, Jones RD, Jones TH, Channer KS, Peers C. Selective inhibition of L-type Ca2+ channels in A7r5 cells by physiological levels of testosterone. *Endocrinology.* 2006 Jun;147(6):2675-80.

[46] Malkin CJ, Jones RD, Jones TH, Channer KS. Effect of testosterone on ex vivo vascular reactivity in man. *Clin Sci (Lond).* 2006 Oct;111(4):265-74.

[47] Scragg JL, Dallas ML, Peers C. Molecular requirements for L-type Ca2+ channel blockade by testosterone. *Cell Calcium.* 2007 Jul;42(1):11-5.

[48] Perusquia M, Navarrete E, González L, Villalón CM. The modulatory role of androgens and progestins in the induction of vasorelaxation in human umbilical artery. *Life Sci.* 2007 Sep 1;81(12):993-1002.

[49] Seyrek M, Yildiz O, Ulusoy HB, Yildirim V. Testosterone relaxes isolated human radial artery by potassium channel opening action. *J Pharmacol Sci.* 2007 Mar;103(3):309-16.

[50] Navarro-Dorado J, Orensanz LM, Recio P, Bustamante S, Benedito S, Martínez AC, García-Sacristán A, Prieto D, Hernández M. Mechanisms involved in testosterone-induced vasodilatation in pig prostatic small arteries. *Life Sci.* 2008 Oct 10;83(15-16):569-73.

[51] Montano LM, Calixto E, Figueroa A, Flores-Soto E, Carbajal V, Perusquia M. Relaxation of androgens on rat thoracic aorta: testosterone concentration dependent agonist/antagonist L-type Ca2+ channel activity, and 5beta-dihydrotestosterone restricted to L-type Ca2+ channel blockade. *Endocrinology.* 2008 May;149(5):2517-26

[52] Cairrao E, Alvarez E, Santos-Silva AJ, Verde I. Potassium channels are involved in testosterone-induced vasorelaxation of human umbilical artery. *Naunyn Schmiedebergs Arch Pharmacol.* 2008 Jan;376(5):375-83.

[53] Han DH, Chae MR, Jung JH, So I, Park JK, Lee SW. Effect of testosterone on potassium channel opening in human corporal smooth muscle cells. *J Sex Med.* 2008 Apr;5(4):822-32. Epub 2008 Jan 17.

[54] Yildiz O, Seyrek M, Irkilata HC, Yildirim I, Tahmaz L, Dayanc M. Testosterone might cause relaxation of human corpus cavernosum by potassium channel opening action. *Urology.* 2009 Jul;74(1):229-32.

[55] Marrachelli VG, Miranda FJ, Centeno JM, Burguete MC, Castello-Ruiz M, Jover-Mengual T, Pérez AM, Salom JB, Torregrosa G, Alborch E. Mechanisms involved in the relaxant action of testosterone in the renal artery from male normoglycemic and diabetic rabbits. *Pharmacol Res.* 2010 Feb;61(2):149-56. Epub 2009 Sep 13.

[56] Alvarez E, Cairrao E, Morgado M, Morais C, Verde I. Testosterone and cholesterol vasodilation of rat aorta involves L-type calcium channel inhibition. *Adv Pharmacol Sci.* 2010;2010:534184.

[57] Seyrek M, Irkilata HC, Vural IM, Yildirim I, Basal S, Yildiz O, Dayanc M. Testosterone relaxes human internal spermatic vein through potassium channel opening action. *Urology.* 2011 (In press, DOI:10.1016/j.urology.2011.03.003).

[58] Rosano GM, Leonardo F, Pagnotta P, Pelliccia F, Panina G, Cerquetani E, della Monica PL, Bonfigli B, Volpe M, Chierchia SL. Acute anti-ischemic effect of testosterone in men with coronary artery disease. *Circulation.* 1999 Apr 6;99(13):1666-70. Erratum in: Circulation 2000 Feb 8;101(5):584.

[59] Webb CM, Adamson DL, de Zeigler D, Collins P. Effect of acute testosterone on myocardial ischemia in men with coronary artery disease. *Am J Cardiol.* 1999 Feb 1;83(3):437-9.

[60] English KM, Steeds RP, Jones TH, Diver MJ, Channer KS. Low-dose transdermal testosterone therapy improves angina threshold in men with chronic stable angina: A randomized, double-blind, placebo-controlled study. *Circulation.* 2000 Oct 17;102(16):1906-11.

[61] Ong PJ, Patrizi G, Chong WC, Webb CM, Hayward CS, Collins P. Testosterone enhances flow-mediated brachial artery reactivity in men with coronary artery disease. *Am J Cardiol.* 2000 Jan 15;85(2):269-72.

[62] Kang SM, Jang Y, Kim JY, Chung N, Cho SY, Chae JS, Lee JH. Effect of oral administration of testosterone on brachial arterial vasoreactivity in men with coronary artery disease. *Am J Cardiol.* 2002 Apr 1;89(7):862-4.

[63] Jones RD, Rowell KO, Pugh PJ, Adam IR, Vaughan R, Rocco G Testosterone-induced vasodilatation of isolated human mesenteric and pulmonary resistance arteries is independent of the vascular endothelium. *Endocr Abstracts* 2003; 7:P66

[64] Fujimoto R, Morimoto I, Morita E, Sugimoto H, Ito Y, Eto S. Androgen receptors, 5 alpha-reductase activity and androgen-dependent proliferation of vascular smooth muscle cells. *J Steroid Biochem Mol Biol.* 1994;50:169-174.

[65] Benten WP, Lieberherr M, Stamm O, Wrehlke C, Guo Z, Wunderlich F. Testosterone signaling through internalizable surface receptors in androgen receptor–free macrophages. *Mol Biol Cell.* 1999;10:3113-23

[66] Perusquia M, Hernández R, Morales MA, Campos MG, Villalón CM. Role of endothelium in the vasodilating effect of progestins and androgens on the rat thoracic aorta. *Gen Pharmacol.* 1996 Jan;27(1):181-5.

[67] Gul H, Yildiz O, Seyrek M, Un I. Protein Kinase C Inhibition May Contribute To Testosterone Induced Relaxation In Human Internal Mammary Artery. *9th Balkan Military Medical Committee, Abstract book,* 2004; page: 422, P-291.

[68] Sader MA, Celermajer DS. Endothelial function, vascular reactivity and gender differences in the cardiovascular system. *Cardiovasc Res.* 2002 Feb 15;53(3):597-604. Review.

[69] Costarella CE, Stallone JN, Rutecki GW, Whittier FC. Testosterone causes direct relaxation of rat thoracic aorta. *J Pharmacol Exp Ther.* 1996 Apr;277(1):34-9.

[70] Hishikawa K, Nakaki T, Marumo T, Suzuki H, Kato R, Saruta T. Up-regulation of nitric oxide synthase by estradiol in human aortic endothelial cells. *FEBS Lett.* 1995 Mar 6;360(3):291-3.

[71] Goetz RM, Thatte HS, Prabhakar P, Cho MR, Michel T, Golan DE. Estradiol induces the calcium-dependent translocation of endothelial nitric oxide synthase. *Proc Natl Acad Sci U S A.* 1999 Mar 16;96(6):2788-93.

[72] English KM, Steeds R, Jones TH, Channer KS. Testosterone and coronary heart disease: is there a link? *QJM.* 1997 Dec;90(12):787-91.

[73] Rowell KO, Hall J, Pugh PJ, Jones TH, Channer KS, Jones RD. Testosterone acts as an efficacious vasodilator in isolated human pulmonary arteries and veins:evidence for a biphasic effect at physiological and supra-physiological concentrations. *J Endocrinol Invest.* 2009 Oct;32(9):718-23.

[74] Perusquia M, Stallone JN. Do androgens play a beneficial role in the regulation of vascular tone? Nongenomic vascular effects of testosterone metabolites. *Am J Physiol Heart Circ Physiol.* 2010 May;298(5):H1301-7. Review.

[75] White RE, Owen MP, Stallone JN. Testosterone-induced vasorelaxation of rat mesenteric microvasculature is K_ channel- and nitric oxidedependent but estrogen-independent (Abstract). *FASEB J* 21: 972.10, 2007.

[76] Sochorová R, Mosnárová A, Huzuláková I. The possible influence of testosterone on calcium ion transport (investigated) in guinea pig uterus. *Acta Physiol Hung.* 1991;77(1):19-24.

[77] Er F, Michels G, Brandt MC, Khan I, Haase H, Eicks M, Lindner M, Hoppe UC. Impact of testosterone on cardiac L-type calcium channels and Ca2+ sparks: acute actions antagonize chronic effects. *Cell Calcium.* 2007 May;41(5):467-77.

[78] Tosun M, Paul RJ, Rapoport RM. Intracellular Ca2+ elevation and contraction due to prostaglandin F2alpha in rat aorta. *Eur J Pharmacol.* 1997 Dec 11;340(2-3):203-8.

[79] Raymond V, Leung PC, Labrie F. Stimulation by prostaglandin F2 alpha of phosphatidic acid-phosphatidylinositol turnover in rat luteal cells. *Biochem Biophys Res Commun.* 1983 Oct 14;116(1):39-46.

[80] Berridge MJ. Inositol trisphosphate and diacylglycerol: two interacting second messengers. *Annu Rev Biochem.* 1987;56:159-93. Review

[81] Harder DR, Belardinelli L, Sperelakis N, Rubio R, Berne RM. Differential effects of adenosine and nitroglycerin on the action potentials of large and small coronary arteries. *Circ Res.* 1979 Feb;44(2):176-82.

[82] Sato K, Kanatsuka H, Sekiguchi N, Akai K, Wang Y, Sugimura A, Kumagai T, Komaru T, Shirato K. Effect of an ATP sensitive potassium channel opener, levcromakalim, on coronary arterial microvessels in the beating canine heart. *Cardiovasc Res.* 1994 Dec;28(12):1780-6.

[83] Shimizu S, Yokoshiki H, Sperelakis N, Paul RJ. Role of voltage-dependent and Ca(2+)-activated K(+) channels on the regulation of isometric force in porcine coronary artery. *J Vasc Res.* 2000 Jan-Feb;37(1):16-25.

[84] Yokoshiki H, Katsube Y, Sunagawa M, Sperelakis N. Levosimendan, a novel Ca^{2+} sensitizer, activates the glibenclamide-sensitive K^{+} channel in rat arterial myocytes. *Eur J Pharmacol.* 1997 Aug 27;333(2-3):249-59.

[85] Kunz L, Rämsch R, Krieger A, Young KA, Dissen GA, Stouffer RL, Ojeda SR, Mayerhofer A. Voltage-dependent K+ channel acts as sex steroid sensor in endocrine cells of the human ovary. *J Cell Physiol.* 2006 Jan;206(1):167-74.

[86] Yildiz O, Seyrek M, Un I, Gul H, Candemir G, Yildirim V. The relationship between risk factors and testosterone-induced relaxations in human internal mammary artery. *J Cardiovasc Pharmacol.* 2005 Jan;45(1):4-7.

[87] Yildiz O, Seyrek M. Vasodilating mechanisms of testosterone. *Exp Clin Endocrinol Diabetes.* 2007 Jan;115(1):1-6. Review.

[88] Irkilata HC, Yildiz O, Yildirim I, Seyrek M, Basal S, Dayanc M, Ulku C. The vasodilator effect of testosterone on the human internal spermatic vein and its relation to varicocele grade. *J Urol.* 2008 Aug;180(2):772-6. Epub 2008 Jun 13.

[89] Webb CM, McNeill JG, Hayward CS, de Zeigler D, Collins P. Effects of testosterone on coronary vasomotor regulation in men with coronary heart disease. *Circulation.* 1999 Oct 19;100(16):1690-6.

[90] Webb CM, Elkington AG, Kraidly MM, Keenan N, Pennell DJ, Collins P. Effects of oral testosterone treatment on myocardial perfusion and vascular function in men with low plasma testosterone and coronary heart disease. *Am J Cardiol.* 2008 Mar 1;101(5):618-24.

[91] Cornoldi A, Caminiti G, Marazzi G, Vitale C, Patrizi R, Volterrani M, Miceli M, Fini M, Spera G, Rosano G. Effects of chronic testosterone administration on myocardial ischemia, lipid metabolism and insulin resistance in elderly male diabetic patients with coronary artery disease. *Int J Cardiol.* 2010 Jun 25;142(1):50-5.

[92] Hougaku H, Fleg JL, Najjar SS, Lakatta EG, Harman SM, Blackman MR, Metter EJ. Relationship between androgenic hormones and arterial stiffness, based on longitudinal hormone measurements. *Am J Physiol Endocrinol Metab.* 2006 Feb;290(2):E234-42.

[93] Dockery F, Bulpitt CJ, Donaldson M, Fernandez S, Rajkumar C. The relationship between androgens and arterial stiffness in older men. *J Am Geriatr Soc.* 2003 Nov;51(11):1627-32.

[94] Webb CM, Collins P. Testosterone and coronary artery disease in men. *Maturitas.* 2010 Sep;67(1):15-9. Epub 2010 May 5. Review.

[95] Wiinberg N, Høegholm A, Christensen HR, Bang LE, Mikkelsen KL, Nielsen PE, Svendsen TL, Kampmann JP, Madsen NH, Bentzon MW. 24-h ambulatory blood pressure in 352 normal Danish subjects, related to age and gender. *Am J Hypertens.* 1995 Oct;8(10 Pt 1):978-86.

[96] Fogari R, Preti P, Zoppi A, Fogari E, Rinaldi A, Corradi L, Mugellini A. Serum testosterone levels and arterial blood pressure in the elderly. *Hypertens Res.* 2005 Aug;28(8):625-30.

[97] Hughes GS, Mathur RS, Margolius HS. Sex steroid hormones are altered in essential hypertension. *J Hypertens.* 1989 Mar;7(3):181-7.

[98] Phillips GB, Jing TY, Resnick LM, Barbagallo M, Laragh JH, Sealey JE. Sex hormones and hemostatic risk factors for coronary heart disease in men with hypertension. *J Hypertens.* 1993 Jul;11(7):699-702.

[99] Svartberg J, von Mühlen D, Schirmer H, Barrett-Connor E, Sundfjord J, Jorde R. Association of endogenous testosterone with blood pressure and left ventricular mass in men. *The Tromsø Study. Eur J Endocrinol.* 2004 Jan;150(1):65-71.

[100] Fang H, Tong W, Branham WS, Moland CL, Dial SL, Hong H, Xie Q, Perkins R, Owens W, Sheehan DM. Study of 202 natural, synthetic, and environmental chemicals for binding to the androgen receptor. *Chem Res Toxicol.* 2003 Oct;16(10):1338-58.

[101] Marin P, Holmäng S, Jönsson L, Sjöström L, Kvist H, Holm G, Lindstedt G, Björntorp P. The effects of testosterone treatment on body composition and metabolism in middle-aged obese men. *Int J Obes Relat Metab Disord.* 1992 Dec;16(12):991-7.

[102] Tenover JS. Effects of testosterone supplementation in the aging male. *J Clin Endocrinol Metab.* 1992 Oct;75(4):1092-8.

[103] Yaron M, Greenman Y, Rosenfeld JB, Izkhakov E, Limor R, Osher E, Shenkerman G, Tordjman K, Stern N. Effect of testosterone replacement therapy on arterial stiffness in older hypogonadal men. *Eur J Endocrinol.* 2009 May;160(5):839-46.

[104] Reckelhoff JF, Zhang H, Granger JP. Testosterone exacerbates hypertension and reduces pressure-natriuresis in male spontaneously hypertensive rats. *Hypertension.* 1998 Jan;31(1 Pt 2):435-9.

[105] Yanes LL, Reckelhoff JF. A new piece in the hypertension puzzle: central blood pressure regulation by sex steroids. *Am J Physiol Heart Circ Physiol.* 2009 Nov;297(5):H1583-4.

[106] Zhang XH, Melman A, Disanto ME. Update on corpus cavernosum smooth muscle contractile pathways in erectile function: A role for testosterone? *J Sex Med.* 2011 Feb 16. doi: 10.1111/j.1743-6109.2011.02218.x. [Epub ahead of print]

[107] Isidori AM, Giannetta E, Gianfrilli D, Greco EA, Bonifacio V, Aversa A, Isidori A, Fabbri A, Lenzi A. Effects of testosterone on sexual function in men: results of a meta-analysis. *Clin Endocrinol* (Oxf). 2005 Oct;63(4):381-94. Review.

[108] Morelli A, Filippi S, Zhang XH, Luconi M, Vignozzi L, Mancina R, Maggi M. Peripheral regulatory mechanisms in erection. *Int J Androl.* 2005 Dec;28 Suppl 2:23-7. Review.

[109] Zhang XH, Morelli A, Luconi M, Vignozzi L, Filippi S, Marini M, Vannelli GB, Mancina R, Forti G, Maggi M. Testosterone regulates PDE5 expression and in vivo responsiveness to tadalafil in rat corpus cavernosum. *Eur Urol.* 2005 Mar;47(3):409-16; discussion 416.

[110] Traish AM, Guay AT. Are androgens critical for penile erections in humans? Examining the clinical and preclinical evidence. *J Sex Med.* 2006 May;3(3):382-404; discussion 404-7. Review.

[111] Traish AM, Park K, Dhir V, Kim NN, Moreland RB, Goldstein I. Effects of castration and androgen replacement on erectile function in a rabbit model. *Endocrinology.* 1999 Apr;140(4):1861-8.

[112] Aversa A, Bruzziches R, Francomano D, Natali M, Gareri P, Spera G. Endothelial dysfunction and erectile dysfunction in the aging man. *Int J Urol.* 2010 Jan;17(1):38-47. Review

[113] McClamrock HD, Adashi EY. Gestational hyperandrogenism. *Fertil Steril.* 1992 Feb;57(2):257-74. Review.

[114] Benagiano G, Mancuso S, Mancuso FP, Wiqvist N, Diczfalusy E. Studies on the metabolism of C-19 steroids in the human foeto-placental unit. 3. Dehydrogenation and reduction prducts formed by previable foetuses with androstenedione and testosterone. *Acta Endocrinol* (Copenh). 1968 Feb;57(2):187-207.

[115] Perusquia M, Jasso-Kamel J. Influence of 5alpha- and 5beta-reduced progestins on the contractility of isolated human myometrium at term. *Life Sci.* 2001 May 18;68(26):2933-44.

[116] Ibrahim II, Abdalla MI, Girgis SM, Osman MI, Bayad MA, El-Karaksy A, Hafez ES. FSH, LH, E2, progesterone, and testosterone in peripheral blood, spermatic vein, and semen of subfertile men with varicocele. *Arch Androl.* 1983 May;10(2):173-7.

[117] Pirke KM, Doerr P, Sintermann R, Vogt HJ. Age dependence of testosterone precursors in plasma of normal adult males. *Acta Endocrinol (Copenh).* 1977 Oct;86(2):415-29.

[118] Scholler R, Nahoul K, Grenier J, Charles JF, Netter A. Proceedings: Concentrations of 7 steroids in the spermatic vein in man. Comparison with peripheric concentrations. *Ann Endocrinol (Paris).* 1975 Nov-Dec;36(6):353-4.

[119] Marin P, Lönn L, Andersson B, Oden B, Olbe L, Bengtsson BA, Björntorp P. Assimilation of triglycerides in subcutaneous and intraabdominal adipose tissues in vivo in men: effects of testosterone. *J Clin Endocrinol Metab.* 1996 Mar;81(3):1018-22.

[120] Labrie F, Bélanger A, Cusan L, Gomez JL, Candas B. Marked decline in serum concentrations of adrenal C19 sex steroid precursors and conjugated androgen metabolites during aging. *J Clin Endocrinol Metab.* 1997 Aug;82(8):2396-402.

[121] Liu PY, Death AK, Handelsman DJ. Androgens and cardiovascular disease. Endocr Rev. 2003 Jun;24(3):313-40. Review.

[122] Perusquía M, Villalón CM. The vasodepressor effect of androgens in pithed rats: potential role of calcium channels. *Steroids.* 2002 Dec;67(13-14):1021-8.

Index

D

E

F

G

H

I

J

K

L

M

N

O

P

Q

R

S

T

U

V

W